THE
ESSENTIAL GUIDE
TO VITAMINS
AND MINERALS

THE ESSENTIAL GUIDE TO VITAMINS AND MINERALS

Elizabeth Somer, M.A., R.D.

AND

Health Media of America

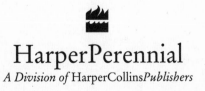

HarperPerennial
A Division of HarperCollinsPublishers

The Essential Guide to Vitamins and Minerals is intended as a reference volume only, not as a medical manual or a guide to self-treatment. If you suspect you have a medical problem, you should seek competent medical help. Keep in mind that nutritional needs vary from person to person, depending on age, sex, health status, and total diet. Information here is intended to help you make informed decisions about your diet, not to substitute for any treatment that may have been prescribed by your physician. The authors and publishers disclaim any liability for any adverse efects resulting from the use of any information discussed in this book.

*To Victoria Dolby for her invaluable help
in preparing the research for this book.*

Contents

SECTION 2
VITAMINS AND MINERALS IN THE PREVENTION AND
TREATMENT OF DISEASE

SECTION 3
THE VITAMIN/MINERAL-RICH DIET

CHAPTER 1

Nutrition as a Way of Life

People want to feel and look their best no matter what their ages. Most people want the energy, enthusiasm, and good health to enjoy life and they want freedom from crippling disorders that interfere with that enjoyment. Although a person's level of health throughout life will vary based on hereditary uniqueness, achieving optimal health depends in large part on what and how much a person eats.

The phrase "you are what you eat" is now supported by scientific research. A balanced diet of wholesome, nutritious, low-fat foods reduces a person's risk for developing many of the common degenerative diseases, such as heart disease, stroke, high blood pressure, cancer, diabetes, osteoporosis, and obesity. A diet that supplies optimal amounts of vitamins and minerals helps a person not only avoid disease, but also feel his or her best, with the emotional and physical health and energy necessary to enjoy life to its fullest.

The opposite is also true. A diet unbalanced in favor of high-fat, high-sugar, low-fiber, or salty foods is associated with low vitamin and mineral intake and a higher risk for developing disease, or at best not feeling "up to par." Since people do not possess a natural instinct for choosing nutritious, wholesome foods, it is important to learn which nutrients the body needs and what to eat to meet these nutrient needs. "You are what you eat" is a promise of better health if a person takes the time to choose nutritious foods and to practice good eating habits.

THE CHANGING AMERICAN DIET

The typical American diet today is much different than the diet chosen at the beginning of the century. Many traditional foods, such as milk, broccoli, bread, and meat, still grace American dining tables, but they are now outnumbered by thousands of new processed, refined, or convenience foods, such as French fries, soda pop, frozen dinners, and ready-to-eat cereals. In some ways the changes in the way individuals in America eat are an improvement; in other ways good eating habits in this country are on the decline.

Advertising has proven "you are what you are told to eat." Millions of dollars are spent each year by large food and restaurant corporations to convince people they should eat one processed food or another. Food selection has changed dramatically as a result. The marketing of food, however, is motivated by sales, not nutrition, and can cause a person to make food choices based on generalities, misconceptions, half-truths, and superstitions.

For example, a person concerned about nutrition might choose a commercial granola cereal because it is "natural," contains no "additives," or does not include white sugar. The cereal, however, might provide more than 30 percent of its calories from a highly saturated fat called coconut oil. Another person might choose a bag of "fat-free" cookies, not realizing the product is very high in sugar and calories. One person might swallow a half dozen vitamin and mineral supplements instead of taking the time to make good food choices while another person grabs a "breakfast bar," containing more sugar than is found in a candy bar, in an effort to lose weight. In most cases, these unhealthful food choices are based on misconceptions and marketing strategies.

Food selections have never been greater. Approximately 500 new foods enter the marketplace each year, most of them sweetened or highly processed snacks and desserts. However, more than one-half of all foods are processed or refined and their nutrient quality never equals their natural, unprocessed counterparts. Most advertisements are for convenience foods high in fat, salt, sugar, air, or water. Seldom are fresh fruits and vegetables, whole grain breads, nonfat milk products, or extra-lean beef advertised.

Changes in the family structure also have influenced eating patterns. Dual-career and single-parent families have increased the demand for time-saving, highly processed convenience foods. In addition, people today as compared to people in 1910 are more likely to skip meals, snack, diet, and eat away from home.

Today, people consume fewer calories than did their ancestors. The reduced food intake means these diets cannot always guarantee daily recommended amounts of vitamins and minerals, especially for those people who diet, have irregular eating habits, skip meals, or choose poorly from the wealth of food selections available. Consequently, the nutritional changes in the American diet since 1910 include a substantial increase in fat and sugar consumption, and a decrease in complex carbohydrate (starch) consumption. And, as fat and sugar intake increase, vitamin and mineral intake decrease. The influences of these dietary changes are reflected in the disease statistics in the United States since 1910. The incidence of cardiovascular disease, including heart disease, high blood pressure, and stroke; cancer; diabetes; and obesity has increased.

Major national surveys repeatedly show that diets consumed by many Americans are not well balanced. Inadequate intake of vitamins and minerals are frequently reported, including vitamin A, vitamin C, vitamin B1, vitamin B2, folic acid, vitamin B6, calcium, chromium, copper, iron, magnesium, manganese, and zinc. In addition, only one person in every 10 consumes the recommended foods outlined in USDA's Food Guide Pyramid.

Although more than 80 percent of adult consumers think "it is alright to eat what you want when you want it," good eating habits are not instinctive. The body and mind do not automatically choose nutritious foods, especially in light of modern distractions and highly sophisticated marketing and advertising techniques. Even the well-planned diet can be lacking in vitamins and minerals when processed foods are overused or foods are not stored or prepared properly. If an individual chooses a diet that contains less than 2,000 calories, he or she cannot be guaranteed an optimal supply of all vitamins and minerals.

The best way to guarantee optimal intake of all vitamins and minerals is to understand which of the nutrients in the diet are most likely to be low and to learn how to design and consume a nutritious diet based on individual needs. At no other time in history has nutritious and safe food been more accessible. The challenge is learning how to wisely select the most healthful food while planning a diet that tastes good, looks good, and fits into your lifestyle.

HOW TO USE THIS BOOK

Interest in nutrition has substantially increased with the transition from treatment to prevention in health care. Self-responsibility, including healthful lifestyle and dietary habits, is now recognized as the most important factor in the prevention and treatment of many diseases. However, even when you know nutrition is important, it is sometimes difficult to find accurate, reliable information on which you can depend.

The Essential Guide to Vitamins and Minerals is unique. It dispels the myths and accurately reports the facts and current findings on vitamins and minerals. It is a comprehensive guide to nutrition, including basic information as well as the latest findings in nutrition research. It also includes practical suggestions on how to apply this information to individualized menu planning, weight control and maintenance, and the achievement of optimal health. No other book combines the fundamentals of nutrition with current research in a documented format. In a time when nutrition information is doubling every 18 months and misinformation is rampant, *The Essential Guide to Vitamins and Minerals* provides you with accurate and timely information substantiated by credible research.

This book is not meant to replace the advice and supervision of a physician during illness or medication use. Your doctor will consider other aspects of your condition, such as your medical history and special circumstances, not included in the pages of this book and from that additional information can form a more precise diagnosis before recommending treatment.

This book provides the most current and reliable information on vitamins and minerals, but it does not provide the absolute truths about all aspects of nutrition. The science of nutrition is new and is changing rapidly. Many important concepts have been identified and these have been discussed in this book, but even more information remains to be discovered and revised. For this reason, the use of the word "might" has been used judiciously throughout the book in regards to the suspected role a nutrient might play in the prevention, treatment, or promotion of a disease or a condition. The reader is reminded to consider any statement that uses the word "might" as a possibility, not a concrete fact.

WHERE YOU BEGIN

You can do much to obtain and maintain optimal health and to prevent the development of many disorders and nutritional deficiencies. This book serves as an aid in assessing and monitoring personal nutritional status as it relates to health and the treatment of disease. Your full participation in this process can be a rewarding experience of self-discovery in maximizing your health potential.

SECTION 1

VITAMIN AND MINERAL BASICS

CHAPTER 2

Vitamins, Minerals, and the Body

The body requires more than 45 nutrients from the diet to maintain health. Those 45-plus nutrients can be obtained from a variety of foods and diet patterns within a wide range of calorie intakes. Although in theory it is a simple task to meet the body's daily nutritional needs, in practice many people make the wrong food choices, consume too many calories or too few vitamins or minerals, or choose foods that promote rather than prevent the development of degenerative diseases.

For example, Gladys Block, Ph.D. at the University of California at Berkeley recently reviewed the data from three major national nutrition surveys and found that one in every two women consumes inadequate amounts of just about every vitamin and mineral studied, from vitamin A to zinc. On any four consecutive days, 86 percent of women fail to include even one dark green leafy vegetable in their diets. This explains why our diets fall far short of optimal for beta carotene, iron, and folic acid, increasing our risks for cancer, anemia, and birth defects. Almost half of all women avoid fruit, which is why the intake of the vitamin C is embarrassingly low and possibly a contributor to an escalating incidence of heart disease and cancer.

In addition, undetected marginal deficiencies of vitamins and minerals can interfere with the quality and length of life. The epidemic of cancer, cardiovascular disease, adult-onset diabetes, osteoporosis, iron deficiency anemia, and obesity in the United States will attest to the difficulty some people have in designing an optimal diet for life (Table 1).

7

Table 1
THE ESSENTIAL NUTRIENTS

CARBOHYDRATE
Glucose

AMINO ACIDS

Arginine	Methionine
Histidine	Phenylalanine
Isoleucine	Threonine
Leucine	Tryptophan
Lysine	Valine

FATS

Linoleic Acid	Omega 3 Fatty Acids

VITAMINS

Vitamin A	Vitamin B6
Vitamin D	Folic Acid
Vitamin E	Vitamin B12
Vitamin K	Biotin
Vitamin B1	Pantothenic Acid
Vitamin B2	Vitamin C
Niacin	

MINERALS

Calcium	Molybdenum
Chloride	Nickel
Chromium	Phosphorus
Cobalt	Potassium
Copper	Selenium
Fluoride	Silicon
Iodine	Sodium
Iron	Sulfur
Magnesium	Vanadium
Manganese	Zinc

WATER

The first step in providing the best nutrition for the body is to understand the basics about nutrients, how information about individual nutrients can be organized into simple guidelines for dietary intake, and the importance of designing a diet that provides optimal, not minimal, amounts of all vitamins and minerals.

THE NUTRIENT CATEGORIES

A nutrient is a substance obtained from food and used by the body for growth, maintenance, or repair of tissues. Nutrients are divided into six categories: protein, carbohydrate, fat, vitamins, minerals, and water. Water is the most abundant nutrient in the body, followed in descending order by protein, fat, and carbohydrate. Vitamins and minerals constitute the smallest percentage of body weight, but are just as important as the other four nutrient categories.

Three categories of nutrients—protein, carbohydrate, and fat—provide calories. They are called the energy nutrients. The energy they provide is used by the body to fuel the billions of chemical reactions that sustain life each day, heat the body and maintain body temperature, move muscles, build structures such as bones, or is stored as fat for later use. (See Appendix, page 367, for more information on calories.) The primary role of protein is to build tissues and other essential compounds, such as hormones. Vitamins and minerals are important in the regulation of all body processes and some minerals, such as calcium and magnesium, also act as structural components in bone and other tissues, but they do not provide calories or energy.

Alcohol also supplies calories, but is not a nutrient because it does not contribute to the maintenance, repair, and growth of body tissues. In contrast, it is damaging to tissues when consumed in even moderate amounts or over long periods of time. Calories from alcohol can be converted to fat when total calorie consumption exceeds the daily requirement.

Most foods provide a combination of the six categories of nutrients. For example, chicken is a protein-rich food that contains a generous supply of niacin, iron, and other trace minerals and B vitamins. Whole wheat bread is called a carbohydrate-rich food, but also supplies protein, vitamins, minerals, and small amounts of fat and water. Milk is more than a source of calcium; it also contains vitamin B2, protein, carbohydrate, vitamin D, water, magnesium, and other nutrients. The exceptions to this rule are sugar, which is pure carbohydrate, and oils or other fats, which are pure fat.

Essential nutrients are substances the body is unable to make in adequate amounts to sustain life and therefore must be obtained from the diet. Up to 8 or 10 amino acids (the building blocks of protein), most of the 13 vitamins, 15 to 20 minerals, and 2 categories of fats, linoleic acid and possibly the omega 3 fatty acids, are essential nutrients. Carbohydrates can be made from amino acids, but this is an inefficient use of protein; therefore, dietary sources of carbohydrate, such as starchy foods, are also important in the daily diet. Most fats, including cholesterol, are manufactured from other substances in the diet and body and are nonessential nutrients. Vitamin D must be obtained from dietary sources and is considered an essential nutrient if a person is not exposed to sunlight. Niacin becomes an essential nutrient when the diet supplies insufficient amounts of the amino acid tryptophan, which the body can convert to niacin. Essential does not only mean necessary, as nonessential nutrients are also necessary, but refers to the body's dependency on the diet for an optimal source of the nutrient.

Nutrients always work as teams; no vitamin or mineral works alone in the body. For example, the B vitamins are essential for extracting energy from the calorie-containing nutrients. Calcium, phosphorus, and magnesium are essential components of bones. Nerve impulses require adequate amounts of sodium, potassium, and chloride, as well as calcium and vitamin B12. The digestion of food requires a healthy digestive tract dependent on a constant supply of all vitamins and minerals. Healthy skin requires a frequent supply of most nutrients, including vitamin B2, niacin, folic acid, iron, vitamin E, and the essential fat linoleic acid. Red blood cell formation and the maintenance of a constant oxygen supply to the brain and body tissues are dependent on a constant supply of iron, vitamin C, copper, vitamin B6, vitamin B12, folic acid, and protein.

A person eats only two to six times a day, but the tissues require a constant supply of nutrients. The body is efficient in regulating the storage and release of nutrients entering from the digestive tract so that constant blood levels of vitamins, minerals, and other substances are maintained if the diet is adequate. The liver is a primary organ in the control and storage of many nutrients. For example, vitamin A entering from the digestive tract is transported in the blood to the liver where small amounts are released gradually to maintain blood levels while the rest is stored for later use. Calcium is stored in bones and constantly released in small amounts to maintain blood calcium levels. Excess calories are stored in fat tissue and released when extra energy is needed.

Optimal and regular intake of all vitamins and minerals is necessary to maintain storage levels and readily available supplies of nutrients for all body functions. The Recommended Dietary Allowances (RDAs) are the most commonly used guidelines for determining how much of each vitamin and mineral people need to maintain health.

THE RECOMMENDED DIETARY ALLOWANCES

The Recommended Dietary Allowances (RDAs) are suggested levels of intake for several essential nutrients. They are established by the Food and Nutrition Board, National Research Council of the National Academy of Sciences—a group composed of scientists and other nutrition experts. The RDAs have become the primary nutrient standards used in the United States and throughout the world. Since 1943 they have evolved and are updated from current research approximately every 5 years. The RDAs are based on a person's age, weight, height, and gender. The RDAs provide dietary intake guidelines for:

Calories	Vitamin C	Vitamin K
Protein	Calcium	Magnesium
Vitamin A	Vitamin D	Niacin
Vitamin B1	Vitamin E	Phosphorus
Vitamin B2	Folic acid	Selenium
Vitamin B6	Iodine	Zinc
Vitamin B12	Iron	

Additional tables of Safe and Adequate Ranges provide daily dietary intake ranges for biotin, pantothenic acid, copper, manganese, fluoride, chromium, molybdenum, sodium, potassium, and chloride.

The RDAs replaced the outdated "Minimum Daily Requirements" or MDRs. The RDA for each nutrient is designed to meet or exceed most people's requirement for that nutrient and, in most cases, the RDA contains a wide margin of safety. What does this margin of safety mean? It means that the "R" in RDA stands for recommendation, not requirement, and that the RDAs are not minimum requirements, but meet the nutrient requirements and contain an extra allowance for most people.

The RDAs are the "best game in town" when it comes to deciding the nutritional adequacy of a person's diet. However, they are not without limitations. The RDAs are designed for the "reference" person, the average woman, man, or child with an average weight, body fat percentage, nutrient absorption and excretion rate, stress level, and heredity pattern. The RDA for many nutrients would require adjustment if one falls outside these descriptions.

The RDAs are only estimates of nutrient needs. In many cases the available research on a nutrient is scarce and a recommendation is based on the amount of a nutrient found in the "normal" diet. In addition, the following considerations influence the usefulness of the RDAs:

1. The RDAs are expressed as daily amounts, but actually are averages for each nutrient to be consumed over a week's time.
2. The RDAs are based on nutrient requirements for healthy persons and might not be adequate during illness or chronic use of medications, for the elderly, or when other factors alter nutrient requirements. They are recommendations for maintenance of nutrient status and might be inadequate if a person needs to restore depleted vitamin and mineral stores because of long-term illness or poor dietary habits.

3. Recommendations for some nutrients, especially the nutrients included in the Safe and Adequate Ranges are based on limited information and can be considered, at best, estimates of nutrient needs.

4. Interactions between nutrients or between nutrients and other substances in the diet were not considered in the development of the RDAs but could affect absorption, utilization, and excretion of vitamins and minerals. For example, excessive intake of calcium or protein might interfere with absorption and use of magnesium. Large doses of iron upset the absorption of zinc and copper.

5. The RDAs are based on the assumption that people will store and prepare foods with reasonable care to ensure retention of vitamins and minerals. Improper storage or preparation techniques could result in excessive loss of nutrients from food and potential vitamin or mineral deficiencies.

6. The RDAs are recommendations to prevent classical nutrient deficiency diseases and to maintain growth, maintenance, and repair of tissues. They do not consider the relationship between nutrients and the prevention of disease. For example, the RDA for vitamin A is based on maintenance of normal blood levels of the fat-soluble vitamin and the prevention of vitamin A deficiency symptoms. The dietary advice from the Institute of Medicine of the National Academy of Sciences (a different branch of the same umbrella organization that oversees the development of the RDAs) and the Cancer Institute of the National Institutes of Health includes a recommendation to increase dietary intake of vitamin A to reduce the risk of developing cancer. This recommendation and the research on which it is based are not considered in the RDA for vitamin A.

7. Several substances in foods, such as beta carotene and choline, are now recognized as possibly essential nutrients in the diet. However, no RDA has been set for these substances.

Until more precise recommendations are developed, or the RDAs are revised to include recommendations for optimal health and the prevention of degenerative diseases, it is wise for a person to consider the following when designing an individualized nutritious diet:

1. The RDAs are the best guidelines available for vitamin, mineral, protein, and energy intakes; however, they are not perfect. They are based on the most reliable information available, but still remain only estimates of nutrient needs. Although the RDAs are generous in their recommendations, it is wise to strive for an average dietary intake that meets 100 percent of the RDAs.

2. When some is good, more is not necessarily better. Excessive intake of one or more nutrients can be dangerous, can upset the delicate balance between nutrients and result in secondary deficiencies of other vitamins or minerals, and can result in temporary or permanent damage to the body. Vitamins in large doses can act more like drugs than nutrients, and megadoses should be taken only with the supervision of a physician.

MARGINAL DEFICIENCIES

Classical nutrient deficiency symptoms are described in detail in all nutrition textbooks and are memorized by all conscientious nutrition authorities. However, scurvy (the classic disease of vitamin C deficiency), beriberi (an extreme deficiency of vitamin B1), and xerophthalmia (the final stage of vitamin A deficiency) are unusual in the United States. These symptom-diseases are characteristic of long-term and severe vitamin or mineral deficiencies. Long before the gums recede in scurvy or dermatitis develops in beriberi, a series of harmful, yet subtle, changes have taken place in the body. These subclinical changes are characteristic of marginal nutrient deficiencies.

A marginal nutrient deficiency is a condition where the body's vitamin or mineral stores are gradually drained, resulting in loss of optimal health and impairment of body processes that depend on that nutrient. Marginal nutrient deficiencies can develop from long-term poor dietary intake; altered absorption, use, or excretion of a nutrient; or chronic use of medications or alcohol, which interfere with the absorption or use of a nutrient.

Nutrient deficiencies develop in stages. During the initial stage, marginal deficiencies develop over time as body stores are gradually emptied. The second stage of deficiency is characterized by impairment of body processes dependent on the nutrient. No signs of a deficiency are visually detected during these two stages of nutrient loss. During the third stage of a nutrient deficiency the loss becomes so great that personality and emotions are affected. A person might feel depressed, irritable, or anxious. The loss of health is not severe and the person does not usually seek medical care. However, some quality of life is lost. The initial stages in nutrient deficiency are actually a gradual continuum with no clearly defined separation between stages. Classical deficiency symptoms develop if the nutrient deficiency continues to the fourth stage. The fifth and final stage is when death is likely if immediate action is not taken to restore the lacking nutrient (Table 2).

Table 2
SEQUENCE OF EVENTS IN THE DEVELOPMENT OF A VITAMIN DEFICIENCY

Deficiency Stage	Symptoms
1. Preliminary	1. Depletion of tissue stores (caused by diet, poor absorption, abnormal metabolism, etc.). Urinary excretion of the nutrient is decreased.
2. Biochemical	2. Enzyme activity is reduced because of nutrient lack. Urinary excretion of nutrient is negligible.
3. Physiological/Behavioral	3. Loss of appetite, reduced body weight, insomnia or excessive sleepiness, irritability, personality changes.
4. Clinical	4. Nonspecific symptoms worsen. Specific deficiency syndrome appears.
5. Anatomical	5. Clear specific syndromes with tissue damage. Death ensues unless treated.

A marginal nutrient deficiency occurs somewhere between optimal nutritional status and a classical nutrient deficiency disease. The symptoms of a marginal deficiency are vague and poorly defined and often are described as "feeling under the weather" or "not at one's best." General feelings of tiredness, irritability, insomnia, poor concentration, or depression are common symptoms of marginal nutrient deficiency. These emotional or behavioral changes also result from numerous other factors such as lack of sleep, stress, or the presence of disease, which makes it difficult to establish the primary cause of the mood or behavior change. Marginal nutrient deficiencies consequently often progress undetected, undermining the quality of life and health.

The subject of marginal deficiencies is controversial. Many nutrition experts presume a person is adequately nourished if he or she shows no clinical signs of classical deficiency disease, such as scurvy, beriberi, or anemia. These deficiency diseases are diagnosed by simple physical or blood examinations. Other nutrition experts support the presence and importance of marginal deficiencies.

Treating a disease in its early stages is more advantageous than waiting until the disease has progressed to final and severe stages. For example, the identification and treatment of cell changes on the cervix found during an annual Pap smear has an almost 100 percent cure rate as compared to the poor prognosis if cervical cancer is allowed to progress. If other diseases develop in a progressive fashion from early to advanced stages, it is only reasonable to suspect nutritional deficiencies proceed through similar stages.

More advanced tests for nutritional status have proven this theory correct. As researchers learned more about vitamins and minerals and their chemical pathways and storage in the body, they recognized classical deficiency diseases to be one of the final stages in long-term depletion of vitamin or mineral status. Current laboratory tests can assess the vitamin or mineral concentrations in blood, urine, and more specifically in the cells or tissues. Marginal nutrient status is detected at this level long before overt symptoms are recognized. For example, iron deficiency anemia is the fourth or clinical stage of iron deficiency. Iron levels in the tissues slowly have been drained for weeks, months, even years before overt signs of anemia develop. Poor concentration and changes in personality or mood are likely to develop during the stages of marginal iron deficiency, although no signs of iron loss, indicative of the clinical stage of deficiency, are detected in routine blood tests, such as the hemoglobin and hematocrit tests.

How Common Are Marginal Deficiencies?

Marginal nutrient deficiencies are found in all segments of the population, especially in pregnant women, alcoholics and drug abusers, smokers, children, and the elderly. School children who consume diets low in zinc develop a marginal zinc deficiency and as a result are shorter in stature than children who consume optimal amounts of zinc. Marginal nutrient deficiencies are common in hospitalized patients who consume inadequate diets during illness and stress, when nutrient needs are highest. Poor nutrition during times of illness can weaken the body's natural defense against disease and infection and can hamper the healing process. Vague discomfort and muscle weakness in the elderly has been attributed to marginal intake and status of vitamin C. The body is more susceptible to colds and infections when dietary intake of vitamins and minerals, especially iron, zinc, vitamin A, vitamin B12, vitamin B6, and folic acid, is marginal. Depression, anxiety, and nausea are reported long before the appearance of clinical signs of nutrient deficiency when people consume a diet marginal in vitamin B1.

Long-term marginal intake of nutrients might be associated with the development of the degenerative diseases. Low intake of chromium is associated with high blood sugar levels and adult-onset diabetes, which in some cases is corrected or improved when intake of chromium is increased. Suboptimal consumption of magnesium is linked to an increased risk for sudden death from heart attack, and the risk for experiencing a heart attack or irregular heartbeat associated with heart disease declines when adequate amounts of magnesium are consumed. Low dietary intake or blood levels at the low end of the normal range for vitamin A are associated with an increased risk for developing several forms of cancer. Low blood or tissue levels of calcium or long-term poor dietary intake of the mineral are associated with an increased risk for developing high blood pressure and osteoporosis.

In all cases, the diet contains some of the nutrient but not enough to either maintain adequate tissue stores or prevent disease. Many degenerative diseases, such as osteoporosis and heart disease, once thought to be the natural result of aging, are now recognized as preventable, in many cases, with a lifetime of healthy habits.

Many questions remain to be answered about marginal nutrient deficiencies.

- What are the long-term effects of suboptimal nutrient intakes?
- Do marginal nutrient deficiencies produce subtle changes in mood and personality that current tests are unable to detect?
- How do marginal vitamin or mineral deficiencies affect the body's immune system and ability to ward off disease and infection?
- Are there additional signs of malnutrition as yet not identified?

It is hoped that future well-designed research studies might provide more information and answers to these questions. In the meantime, it is important to consume a diet optimal in all vitamins and minerals to avoid the potential effects of even marginal intake of nutrients.

CHAPTER 3

The Vitamins

Vitamins are essential, noncaloric substances—needed in very small amounts from the diet—that promote growth, health, and life. They are produced by living material, such as plants and animals, as compared to minerals that originate from the soil. The 13 recognized vitamins cannot be made by the body in sufficient amounts to maintain life, so they must be obtained from the diet.

Vitamins participate in a variety of life-building processes, including the formation and maintenance of blood cells, hormones, nervous system chemicals, genetic material, and all the cells and tissues of the body. Characteristic deficiency symptoms develop if the diet does not supply optimal amounts of a vitamin. For example, poor dietary intake of folic acid or vitamin B12 results in anemia, inadequate intake of vitamin A affects vision, and a vitamin B6 deficiency is characterized by mood disorders and nausea. If a substance does not produce a deficiency symptom when it is removed from the diet, it is not considered a vitamin. Each vitamin functions in many diverse roles and always with other essential nutrients. A deficiency interferes with many different body processes, including how the body uses other nutrients.

Unlike carbohydrates, protein, and fat, vitamins do not supply energy. Only calories provide energy, and vitamins do not contain calories. Several vitamins, however, do help convert the calories in carbohydrates, protein, and fat into usable energy for the body. They are like the ignition switch that sparks the fuel and keeps the engine running.

Vitamins are grouped into two categories: fat-soluble and water-soluble. The fat-soluble vitamins A, D, E, and K are found in the fat or oil of food and require some dietary fat to be absorbed. The water-soluble vitamin C and the B vitamins—B1, B2, niacin, B6, folic acid, B12, pantothenic acid, and biotin—are found in the watery portion of foods, are easily lost when foods are overcooked, and do not require fat for their absorption. Fat-soluble vitamins generally are stored in the body, while water-soluble vitamins mix easily in the blood, are excreted in the urine, and only small amounts are stored in the tissues.

The vitamin content of food varies depending on how and where the food is grown, when it is harvested, and how it is stored and processed. In general, the fresher the food, the colder the storage temperature (below 40° F for refrigeration), and the shorter the cooking and holding time, the higher the vitamin content.

VITAMIN A (RETINOL AND RETINAL)

Overview

Vitamin A was the first vitamin to be discovered. The substance was termed vitamin A in 1913 after studies found that the eyes of animals became inflamed and infected when the diet lacked sufficient amounts of foods now recognized as rich sources of vitamin A. In 1932 researchers discovered that a substance in plants, called beta carotene, could be converted in the body to vitamin A and was as useful as cod liver oil in preventing eye disorders.

Vitamin A is a family of compounds that includes retinol, retinal, and the carotenoids. Retinol and retinal are found in foods of animal origin, such as liver and eggs. These forms of vitamin A are ready to be used by the body directly from the food source and are called pre-formed vitamin A. The carotenoids, of which beta carotene is the most publicized, are a group of fat-soluble pigments found in orange, dark yellow, and dark green vegetables and fruits. Some carotenoids, including beta carotene, can be converted to vitamin A once ingested and are called a building block or provitamin form of vitamin A, although beta carotene has many functions independent of vitamin A. The vitamin A content of the diet is a combination of the pre-formed vitamin A and the provitamin beta carotene. (See the section on beta carotene below.)

The factors that affect fat absorption also influence the absorption of dietary vitamin A. A small amount of fat is needed in the diet to stimulate the secretion of digestive juices that aid in fat digestion. In contrast, absorption of vitamin A decreases if a person has an intestinal disorder that alters or reduces the absorption of dietary fat. One form of vitamin A found in some supplements, retinyl palmitate, can be absorbed even in the absence of dietary fat and is useful for people with long-term intestinal disorders.

Functions

CANCER. Ample intake of vitamin A and normal to high levels of vitamin A in the blood are associated with a reduced risk for developing certain forms cancer, such as breast, stomach, cervical, and lung cancer. Vitamin A might help prevent cancer by maintaining healthy epithelial tissues, by discouraging the formation of abnormal cells, or by strengthening the immune system.

EPITHELIAL TISSUE. Vitamin A helps develop and maintain moist, healthy epithelial tissue, the tissue that lines the body's external and internal surfaces. In this capacity, vitamin A is necessary in the maintenance of the cornea in the eye, all mucous membranes, the digestive tract, the urinary tract, the reproductive tract, the skin, and the lungs. Adequate vitamin A intake also maintains the lining of the stomach and might aid in the prevention and treatment of gastric ulcer.

EYES AND VISION. Vitamin A is essential for normal eyesight. The vitamin combines with a specialized protein in the retina of the eye that is necessary for night vision.

GROWTH AND BONE FORMATION. Vitamin A is important in normal body growth and the formation of bones and soft tissue. The formation of tooth enamel and the proper spacing of teeth are also dependent on adequate amounts of vitamin A in the body.

IMMUNITY. Vitamin A is called the "anti-infective vitamin" because it functions in the development and maintenance of the body's barriers to infection, such as the skin, lungs, and linings of the mouth and throat. This vitamin also enhances the activity of the immune system, the body's natural defense system against infection and disease. Vitamin A, when given before or shortly after exposure to a bacteria, reduces infection. Optimal intake and high blood levels of vitamin A also reduce the onset and duration of measles in children, and reduce the chances of complications from this infectious disease, such as pneumonia and debilitation that leads to hospitalization. Vitamin A's influence on immunity might be one of the ways this vitamin helps prevent the initiation or promotion of cancer.

LIVER DISORDERS. Adequate intake of vitamin A might help prevent liver damage caused by exposure to toxic chemicals.

REPRODUCTION. Vitamin A might assist normal pregnancy and lactation (breastfeeding). How vitamin A functions in the reproductive system is unclear, but it might encourage the activity of certain hormones or aid in the normal changes in cells characteristic of early growth in the developing baby.

Deficiency

Prolonged deficiency of vitamin A results in changes in the skin, eyes and eyesight, and teeth.

CANCER. A low intake of vitamin A has been linked to the development and promotion of certain types of cancer. For example, people who smoke cigarettes, cigars, or pipes, or chew tobacco show low levels of vitamin A and an increase in the amount of precancerous cells in the tissues of the mouth, throat, and lungs.

EYES AND VISION. Chronic, severe vitamin A deficiency results in ulceration and distortion of the cornea of the eye and blindness. This vitamin deficiency disease, called xerophthalmia, begins as dryness, thickening, and wrinkling of the conjunctiva, the membrane that covers the eye. If poor dietary intake of vitamin A continues, the condition worsens, hardened patches (Bitot's spots) appear on the eye, and a milky appearance to the eye develops that eventually results in infection of the iris, the formation of scar tissue, and blindness. Xerophthalmia is common in third world countries, especially in infants and children, but is seldom found in the United States.

A specialized protein in the eye cannot be formed without adequate supplies of vitamin A. As a result, night vision is diminished or lost. Night blindness is a primary symptom of vitamin A deficiency.

GROWTH. Poor intake of vitamin A results in growth retardation, loss of appetite, weight loss, and bone deformities. Because the tongue is lined with epithelial tissue, a vitamin A deficiency results in keratinosis (hardening) of the taste buds and loss of appetite.

SKIN. Long-term poor intake of vitamin A results in skin problems called "goose flesh" or "toad skin." The skin develops small hard bumps because the hair follicles are plugged with a hardened protein called keratin. The skin becomes dry, scaly, and rough. The condition is called xeroderma or follicular keratinosis. The most common locations are the shoulders, neck, back, forearms, thighs, and abdomen.

TOOTH FORMATION. Inadequate intake of vitamin A during the formative years can result in improper tooth formation, crooked teeth, and poor spacing between teeth.

Groups at high risk for developing vitamin A deficiency are alcohol abusers; people with celiac disease and other intestinal malabsorption disorders; adolescents; people with liver disease; people who use tobacco; and people who consume few or irregular amounts of dark green, dark yellow, or orange fruits and vegetables. Low-income groups, cancer patients, and people at risk for developing cancer might have low blood levels of the vitamin, which indicates inadequate dietary intake or poor absorption of the vitamin.

Daily Recommended Intake

The need for vitamin A increases with increasing body size and weight. The Recommended Dietary Allowances (RDAs) for vitamin A are expressed in either RE (retinol equivalents) or mcg (micrograms). One RE is equivalent to 1mcg of retinol (and 6 mcg of beta carotene). The 1989 RDAs for vitamin A are:

	Retinol Equivalents/ Micrograms(RE/mcg)
INFANTS	
0 to 1.0 year	375
CHILDREN	
1 to 3 years	400
4 to 6 years	500
7 to 10 years	700
Males 11+ years	1,000
Females 11+ years	800
Pregnant	800
Lactating, 1st 6 mo.	+500
Lactating, 2nd 6 mo.	+400

The RDAs for infants are based on the normal vitamin A content in breastmilk. The RDA for women is approximately 80 percent of the RDA for men based on the assumption that women generally weigh less and therefore probably need a smaller intake of the vitamin. Exact daily requirements have not been determined for any age or sex group. Some researchers suggest that doses larger than the RDAs, between 2,000RE and 5,000RE for adults, might be necessary to decrease the risk for developing cancer. However, more evidence is necessary before higher recommendations can be made.

Sources in the Diet

The dietary sources of preformed vitamin A are liver, kidney, egg yolk, butter, fortified margarine, cheese made with whole milk or cream, fortified nonfat milk, whole milk, and cream. However, with the exception of nonfat milk, these dietary sources also are high in saturated fat and cholesterol. Cod liver oil is a low-cholesterol, low-saturated fat, but high polyunsaturated fat, source of vitamin A (Table 3).

Table 3
THE VITAMIN A CONTENT OF SELECTED FOODS

Food	Amount	Vitamin A (RE)
Liver, beef	3 ounces	9,011
Liver, lamb	3 ounces	6,366
Mackerel	1 can	470
Kidney, beef	3 ounces	312
Milk, nonfat	1 cup	149
Egg yolk	1	197
Oyster	1	686
Cheese, cheddar	1 ounce	86
Milk, whole	1 cup	76
Butter	1 tsp	35

Dietary sources of vitamin A are preferable to supplements, since it is difficult to obtain toxic levels of this fat-soluble vitamin from food alone.

Toxicity

The preformed vitamin A is not excreted and can accumulate in the body to toxic levels if large amounts are consumed over long periods of time. In some adults, prolonged daily intake of 10,000RE to

20,000RE can cause vomiting, nausea, loss of appetite and weight, joint pain, abdominal discomfort, irritability, bone deformities, itching, hair loss, liver enlargement, or dry and cracked lips. Headaches are reported in adults who daily consume between 12,000RE and 68,200RE or more of vitamin A. Children develop toxicity symptoms more readily than adults and can experience the above symptoms as well as slowed growth when much smaller doses, such as 5,000RE, are consumed.

Birth defects have occurred in animals and humans who received overdoses of vitamin A. During the first trimester in humans, dietary intake of vitamin A must be closely regulated to ensure that the developing baby is exposed to neither too little nor too much vitamin A, since both conditions can cause birth defects.

Other than in the case of birth defects, symptoms disappear quickly when vitamin A toxicity is detected and the vitamin therapy is discontinued. Individual tolerance to vitamin A varies widely among people. Vitamin A toxicity from dietary sources is rare and is associated primarily with arctic explorers who consumed excessive amounts of polar bear liver.

Nutrient-Nutrient Interactions

- Beta carotene can be converted in the body to vitamin A.
- Vitamin A's function is enhanced by the amount of vitamin E in the body.
- Adequate intake of zinc is necessary for the proper use and transportation of vitamin A within the body. Deficiency symptoms of vitamin A can occur when intake is adequate, but the diet is low in zinc.
- Vitamin A is important for calcium metabolism in the formation of healthy bones and teeth.

BETA CAROTENE

Overview

Beta carotene is just one of the more than 560 carotenoids found in dark green, yellow, and dark orange fruits and vegetables. Other carotenoids include lycopene, alpha carotene, and canthaxanthin. Beta carotene, however, is the carotenoid most readily converted by the body to vitamin A. Although in the early part of this century researchers realized that a substance in many plants known as beta carotene could be converted in the body to vitamin A, it was not until the 1980s that research supported the contention that beta carotene had functions independent of its vitamin A activity.

Functions

Although beta carotene and vitamin A are interrelated in many ways, in the past decade, numerous studies have shown that beta carotene has health-enhancing and disease-preventing capabilities, including strengthening of immune functions, antioxidant capabilities, the prevention of cancer, and cell communication.

ANTIOXIDANT. As an antioxidant, beta carotene disarms highly reactive substances called free radicals that, left unguarded, trigger the development of numerous diseases, from heart disease and cancer to arthritis and cataracts. Ample intake of beta carotene protects cells by discouraging abnormal cell formation and limiting free-radical damage to fatty parts of cell membranes. In fact, up to 1,000 free radicals can be destroyed by just one molecule of beta carotene. Beta carotene's effective antioxidant capabilities might underlie its role in the prevention of numerous diseases from heart disease to cancer. (See pages 150–153 for more information on antioxidants and free radicals.)

CANCER. Numerous studies report that a low blood beta carotene level is a red flag for increased cancer risk. In contrast, eating more beta carotene-rich foods reduces a person's cancer risk. Even smokers are less prone to lung cancer when they consume ample amounts of carotene-rich fruits and vegetables. Beta carotene also might protect the skin from damage and cancer caused by overexposure to sunlight and its harmful ultraviolet (UV) light.

Another phenomena called "tissue specific" deficiency links beta carotene to cancer. Researchers at Albert Einstein College of Medicine in the Bronx report that women with low beta carotene levels in their cervical tissues, even when blood levels are normal, are at risk for developing cervical cancer. Increasing dietary intake of beta carotene might prevent this deficiency and avoid cancer.

A recent Finnish study raised controversy over the role of beta carotene in cancer prevention. This study reported that taking a moderate-dose supplement of beta carotene after 36 years of heavy smoking slightly raised the incidence of lung cancer. Even then, the subjects in this study with the lowest initial beta carotene levels were at the greatest risk of developing lung cancer during the study. While it always is best to remain cautious regarding any aspect of nutrition, the weight of the research shows that beta carotene is effective in lowering the risk of many types of cancer, including lung cancer.

CELL COMMUNICATION. A recent review by George Wolf, Ph.D., from the Department of Nutritional Sciences at the University of California, Berkeley states that beta carotene stimulates cell communication through "gap junctions" or protein pores in cell membranes. The better the cells can "talk" through these gap junctions, the stronger are their defenses against cancer. Beta carotene increases the synthesis of gap junction proteins. This helps prevent the communication shutdown that allows uncontrolled growth of abnormal and cancerous cells. Theoretically, increased beta carotene levels should reduce the likelihood of cancer cell growth.

IMMUNITY. Beta carotene stimulates the immune system by increasing the numbers of immune cells such as the T and B lymphocytes (white blood cells forming the core of immune response) and natural killer cells (white blood cells that recognize and kill tumor cells and other foreign bodies). Immune enhancement has been documented in animal and laboratory studies, but future research of beta carotene and humans is needed to confirm the immune system benefits of this nutrient. (See pages 153–157 for more information on beta carotene and cancer.)

Deficiency

Although there is no established level to identify beta carotene deficiency, diets low in carotene-rich fruits and vegetables are associated with an increased risk of heart disease and cancers of the lung, cervix, colon, stomach, and oral cavity. Inadequate beta carotene intake also might decrease the effectiveness of the free radical scavenging and immune systems, thus undermining the body's basic defense systems against infection and disease. In contrast, people who eat carotene-rich diets are at low risk for several types of cancer and show improved immunity to disease and infection.

Daily Recommended Intake

There is no established RDA for beta carotene. The Alliance for Aging Research, a nonprofit group comprised of well-respected researchers in the nutrition field, is the first national group to establish recommendations for beta carotene intake. The Alliance recommends a daily intake of 10 to 30mg for health promotion and disease prevention.

Sources in the Diet

Good dietary sources of beta carotene are dark green, dark yellow, and orange vegetables, such as spinach, collard greens, broccoli, carrots, and sweet potatoes, and yellow fruits, such as apricots and peaches. These foods supply significant amounts of beta carotene and are low in fat and calories. The deeper the green, yellow, or orange color, the higher the content of beta carotene. At least one serving of a dark green or orange vegetable and four additional servings of other vegetables and fruits should be included in the diet daily (Table 4).

Table 4
THE BETA CAROTENE CONTENT OF SELECTED FOODS[1]

Food	Amount	Beta Carotene (mg)
Carrot, raw	1 medium	12.15
Sweet potato, baked	1 small	14.29
Spinach, cooked	½ cup	5.25
Apricots, dried	8 large halves	1.21
Beet greens, cooked	½ cup	.67
Squash, winter	½ cup	.32
Cantaloupe, cubed	1 cup	3.10
Broccoli, steamed	½ cup	.66
Peach	1 medium	28.00
Lettuce, romaine	1 cup	.88
Peas, cooked	½ cup	.41
Orange	1 medium	.16
Apple	1 medium	.04
Celery, raw	1 stalk	.03

[1] 1 RE is equal to .006mg or 6mcg of beta carotene.

Toxicity

Unlike preformed vitamin A, beta carotene is relatively non-toxic, even when consumed in large amounts over long periods of time. Blood levels of beta carotene fluctuate with dietary intake. Consequently, as intake increases, so does blood levels, with higher blood levels associated with a reduced risk for developing several diseases including cancer. The only adverse side effect to consuming large amounts of dark green, yellow, or orange fruits and vegetables is a yellowing of the skin as carotenes are deposited into the fatty cell membranes of skin cells. Even this condition disappears when fruit and vegetable intake is reduced.

Preliminary research shows that other carotenoids in dark green vegetables, such as canthaxanthin and lycopene, also might reduce a person's risk for developing cancer. These findings suggest that there are other substances in carotene-rich foods not found in supplements that are beneficial to health.

Nutrient-Nutrient Interactions

- Beta carotene can be used by the body as a provitamin to form vitamin A.
- Beta carotene's function is enhanced by the amount of vitamin E and selenium in the body.

VITAMIN D (CALCIFEROL, CHOLECALCIFEROL, ERGOCALCIFEROL)

Overview

Vitamin D was recognized as an essential substance in cod liver oil almost a decade after the discovery of vitamin A. Vitamin D is a family of compounds labeled vitamins D1, D2, and D3.

Vitamin D is unique from other essential nutrients because it can be produced in the body after exposure to sunlight or it can be obtained from the diet. The production of vitamin D in the body is blocked by several factors such as skin pigment (the darker the skin, the less readily vitamin D is formed) or substances that screen the sun's ultraviolet rays (smog, fog, smoke, clothing, screens and windows, or hats). In addition, as a person ages, his or her ability to manufacture vitamin D decreases and longer exposure to sunlight or a greater dependency on dietary sources is required to meet daily needs. A healthy, young, fair-skinned person can theoretically produce up to 10,000IU of vitamin D in one day. Adequate annual stores of vitamin D probably are obtained with 10 minutes of sunbathing daily during the summer months.

The second source of vitamin D is the diet. As with other fat-soluble vitamins, vitamin D requires at least a small amount of fat in the diet for absorption and any intestinal disorder that alters absorption of fat could affect dietary vitamin D absorption. Vitamin D from both the diet and internal production is not readily excreted and is stored in the liver, skin, brain, bones, and other tissues.

Functions

BONES AND TEETH. The primary function of vitamin D is to regulate the absorption and use of calcium and phosphorus and to aid in the formation of normal bones and teeth. Vitamin D also stimulates the specialized cells in the small intestine to absorb calcium and phosphorus, prevents excessive urinary loss of calcium and phosphorus, maintains normal blood levels of calcium and phosphorus to support normal mineralization of bones and teeth, and aids in the deposition of calcium into bones and teeth.

CANCER. Vitamin D might aid in the prevention or treatment of cancer. The vitamin might alter the growth of several different types of cancer, including cancers of the colon, breast, and prostate, and non-Hodgkin's lymphoma.

HEARING. Vitamin D aids in the maintenance of all bones, including the small bones of the ear.

IMMUNITY. Vitamin D might assist the regulation of normal immune function and, therefore, would function to defend the body against infection and disease.

INSULIN SECRETION. Vitamin D might function in the normal production or secretion of the hormone insulin from the pancreas. In this capacity, the vitamin might aid in the regulation of normal blood sugar.

NERVES AND MUSCLES. Vitamin D aids in the maintenance of a healthy nerve and muscle system by regulating the level of calcium in the blood. Calcium is necessary for normal nerve transmission and muscle contraction (including the heartbeat), and the nerves and muscles depend on a constant supply of this mineral from the blood.

SKIN. Vitamin D might prevent, or at least reduce the severity of some inflammatory skin conditions such as psoriasis, a chronic skin disorder characterized by scaly, reddish skin patches.

OTHER FUNCTIONS. Vitamin D has grown beyond just bone metabolism. Vitamin D receptors are located on other target tissues, in addition to the intestine, bone, and kidney. In fact, a large number of tissues are receptive to vitamin D, including the islet cells of the pancreas that produce the hormone insulin, the bone marrow cells responsible for the production of specialized immune cells called monocytes, the parathyroid gland, the ovaries, certain brain cells, developing heart muscle, and breast cells. These new roles are only partially understood. For example, vitamin D suppresses both the parathyroid glands and a hormone from this gland, thus showing significant therapeutic benefits in the treatment of an over-active parathyroid gland or hyperparathyroidism.

Deficiency

Prolonged deficiency of vitamin D results in changes in the bones of children and adults, and possible hearing loss with aging.

HEARING LOSS. Slow, progressive hearing loss might be caused by an inadequate intake of vitamin D. A lack of vitamin D causes a small, snail-shaped bone in the inner ear, called the cochlea, to become porous. The cochlea is then unable to transmit messages to the nerves that lead to the brain and hearing loss can result. In some cases, the loss will respond to vitamin D supplementation. Supplementation is not effective when hearing loss is a result of causes other than vitamin deficiency (Figure 1).

Figure 1

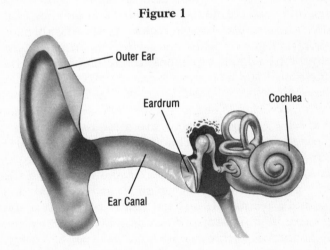

Vitamin D might improve hearing by strengthening the inner bones of the ear, including the cochlea.

OSTEOPOROSIS. Low levels of vitamin D increase the risk of osteoporosis by reducing bone mass and density. Supplementation with vitamin D and calcium significantly reduces the rate of bone loss and the incidence of bone fractures associated with osteoporosis. In addition, a gene regulating vitamin D receptors on cell membranes might influence bone density and result in a genetic predisposition to osteoporosis. It is likely that in the future a diagnostic test for vitamin D metabolism will help in the evaluation of osteoporosis risk.

RICKETS AND OSTEOMALACIA. Rickets is a childhood nutrient-deficiency disease caused by a lack of vitamin D in the diet or inadequate exposure to sunlight. As a result of this disease, the bones are malformed and weak from poor calcium and phosphorus deposition. The weight-bearing bones buckle under the strain of supporting the body, the chest bone bows to resemble a pigeon breast, the head is malformed, and the wrists and ankles are enlarged. Less severe symptoms occur when the deficiency is mild.

Often rickets is not detected in infants until they begin to walk. Prior to this time, the infant is restless, may sweat profusely, and repeatedly turns his or her head from side to side. Delayed development of teeth could be a sign of mild vitamin D deficiency. Death can result when internal organs are impaired by the weakened surrounding bone structure.

Rickets was more common in the past, prior to vitamin D fortification of milk. It is still seen in some parts of the world, especially in northern climates where sunlight is limited and the intake of vitamin D fortified foods is inadequate. Prolonged breastfeeding of infants without supplementation with vitamin D or inadequate consumption of vitamin D-fortified milk by children can result in rickets. Black children in the United States are more prone to rickets than are white children because dark skin pigment limits the amount of vitamin D produced during exposure to sunlight. Children on long-term anticonvulsant therapy for epilepsy or who have a fat-malabsorption disorder such as celiac disease are at risk for vitamin D deficiency and rickets.

Osteomalacia is the adult form of rickets and results from long-term poor dietary intake of vitamin D or exposure to sunlight. (See pages 263–264 for more information on vitamin D and osteomalacia.)

Rickets and osteomalacia respond well to vitamin D supplementation and there is improvement in symptoms within two months of initiating vitamin D therapy. Most bone loss can be corrected, but some damage might be irreversible. However, supplementation will prevent further deformities.

Daily Recommended Intake

There is no established requirement for vitamin D. The main function of the RDAs is to emphasize that the vitamin is needed throughout life. However, if an individual is healthy and the skin is frequently exposed to unfiltered sunlight, no dietary intake is necessary. Dietary sources are necessary if a person lives in a smoggy, foggy, or overcast environment; wears heavy clothing; is indoors or exposed to sunlight only through windows or screens; or is housebound. The body's ability to synthesize vitamin D from ultraviolet light diminishes with age. Therefore, seniors require greater or more frequent exposure to sunlight or possibly greater than current RDA levels of this vitamin, i.e., 400IU rather than the current 200IU. People with darker skin pigments are most dependent on dietary sources of vitamin D as their skin can screen out as much as 95 percent of the vitamin D- producing ultraviolet rays. The 1989 RDAs for vitamin D are:

	Micrograms (mcg)	International Units (IU)
INFANTS		
0 to 0.5 year	7.5	300
INFANTS, CHILDREN, AND YOUNG ADULTS		
0.5 year to 24 years	10	400
Adults (25+)	5	200
Pregnant and Lactating	10	400

Sources in the Diet

The most reliable dietary source of vitamin D in the U.S. is vitamin D-fortified milk. One quart of whole, low-fat, or nonfat milk supplies 400IU of vitamin D, or the RDA for infants, children, adults up to 24 years old, and pregnant and lactating women. Some dried or evaporated milks contain vitamin D. Unfortunately, a recent analysis of vitamin D levels in fortified milk across the United States and Canada found wide variation in concentrations. Eighty percent of samples contained more or less vitamin D than labels indicated. Fourteen percent had no detectable vitamin D at all. More effort must be paid to monitoring the process of vitamin D fortification to ensure that proper amounts of this vitamin are included in the food supply.

Other dairy products, such as cheese, yogurt, cottage cheese, cream cheese, raw milk, and goat's milk, do not contain vitamin D, as fortified milk seldom is used in the production of these products. Liver, egg yolk, butter, and cream contain varying amounts of the vitamin and are not reliable sources. Some ready-to-eat processed breakfast cereals are fortified with vitamin D. Vitamin D supplementation is recommended for breastfed infants. Cod liver oil and other fish oils are excellent sources of vitamin D. Salmon, herring, mackerel, and sardines contribute substantial amounts of vitamin D if consumed frequently.

Foods from plant sources are poor sources of the vitamin and people on strict vegetarian diets have few dietary choices in meeting their requirement of vitamin D other than processed, fortified foods or supplements (Table 5).

Table 5
THE VITAMIN D CONTENT OF SELECTED FOODS

Food	Amount	Vitamin D (IU)
Sardines, canned	3 ½ ounces	1,150–1,570
Mackerel, fresh	3 ½ ounces	1,100
Herring, fresh	3 ½ ounces	315
Salmon, fresh	3 ½ ounces	154–550
Shrimp	3 ½ ounces	150
Milk, fortified	1 cup	100
Egg yolk	1 average	25
Liver, beef	3 ½ ounces	9–42
Cheese	1 ounce	4
Butter	1 pat	1.8

Toxicity

Vitamin D can be toxic if taken in doses more than four times the RDA. The symptoms of vitamin D overdose include diarrhea, dermatitis, headache, nausea, weakness, loss of appetite, calcium deposits in soft tissues (kidney, arteries, heart, ear, and lungs), irreversible kidney or heart damage, retarded growth, and mental retardation. Large doses of vitamin D also are linked to increased risk for premature heart attack, atherosclerosis, and possibly kidney stones in people who are predisposed to kidney problems. Vitamin D overdose develops over time and there is wide variation among individuals in their tolerance to toxicity.

Children and infants are more susceptible than adults to vitamin D toxicity. A parent should monitor vitamin D intake as toxic levels could accumulate in the child's small body from regular combined ingestion of fortified milk or formula, children's vitamin supplements, and fortified cereals. Pregnant women also should avoid large doses of vitamin D. Toxicity can be reversed by the removal of excess vitamin D from the daily diet; however, the deposition of calcium into soft tissues could cause irreversible organ damage.

Prolonged exposure to sunlight does not cause vitamin D toxicity. The body has an efficient feedback system and reduces the production of vitamin D with increased exposure to sunlight.

Nutrient-Nutrient Interactions

- Vitamin D is important for the absorption of calcium and phosphorus and for the normal depositing of these minerals into bone.
- Cadmium can block the production of vitamin D.
- Fat must provide at least 10 percent of the total dietary calories for adequate absorption of vitamin D.
- Pantothenic acid is necessary for the synthesis of vitamin D.
- Vitamin D might improve zinc status in kidney disease patients on dialysis.

VITAMIN E (TOCOPHEROL)

Overview

Vitamin E was discovered in the 1920s and is a family of fat-soluble compounds, including the tocopherols. Alpha tocopherol is the most common and most potent form of the vitamin and requires a small amount of dietary fat for absorption.

Functions

ANTIOXIDANT. The main function of vitamin E is as an antioxidant. In this capacity, vitamin E stabilizes cell membranes and protects the cells and tissues from damage, protects the tissues of the lungs and mouth from damage by air pollutants, and might aid in the prevention of tumor growth. Vitamin E protects tissues of the eyes, skin, liver, nerves, breast, and calf muscles; helps regulate the use and storage of vitamin A; and protects red blood cells from damage, thus preventing a special form of anemia called hemolytic anemia. Vitamin E also might affect the production of hormone-like substances in the body called prostaglandins that regulate a variety of body processes including blood pressure, reproduction, and muscle contraction.

AGING. Vitamin E might aid in the prevention of premature aging because of its role as an antioxidant. Free radicals destroy connective tissues that provide firmness to tissues such as the skin, might contribute to the development of atherosclerosis, and accumulate during the aging process. The combination of vitamin E and vitamin C reduces free-radical levels by up to 26 percent in older adults. Whether or not this reduction slows the aging process is unclear.

Preliminary reports show that vitamin E might aid in the maintenance of normal, active brain function. Accumulation of free radicals in brain tissue has been associated with age-related memory loss, and antioxidants might prevent this sign of premature aging.

CANCER. Vitamin E might prevent several forms of cancer, including cancers of the lung, colon, rectum, and cervix. Additional research indicates risk reduction for oral, pancreas, and liver cancer. However, most studies show the effective level of vitamin E to protect against cancer far exceeds that provided by the typical diet. Vitamin E in topical form reduces sun-induced skin damage and might slow the development of skin cancer (Graph 1).

Graph 1
THE EFFECT OF VITAMIN E AND SELENIUM
ON THE PROTECTION OF CELL MEMBRANES

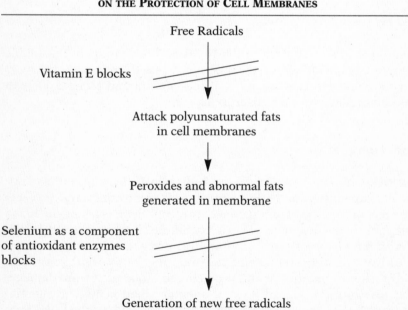

Free Radicals

Vitamin E blocks

Attack polyunsaturated fats
in cell membranes

Peroxides and abnormal fats
generated in membrane

Selenium as a component
of antioxidant enzymes
blocks

Generation of new free radicals

(See pages 150–153 and 188 for more information on vitamin E, antioxidants, and cancer.)

DIABETES. Vitamin E might reduce blood sugar levels in some diabetics. In one study, blood sugar levels decreased 20 percent when patients increased vitamin E intake to 2,000IU a day. Limited evidence also shows vitamin E might help modulate insulin activity.

EXERCISE. Free-radical levels in the blood and tissues might increase during exercise and contribute to tissue damage, fatigue, and extended recovery times for athletes. Animal studies show an increased need for vitamin E during endurance exercise and rats deficient in vitamin E are more vulnerable to free-radical damage. In humans, supplementation with 400IU of vitamin E daily reduced exercise-induced free-radical damage and helped maintain a high level of physical performance.

EYES. Vitamin E is essential for normal development of the retina of the eye and protects the blood vessels of the eyes from free-radical damage. Oxygen in the air diffuses directly into the eye through the cornea and the retina is at particular risk of damage from these oxygen fragments unless vitamin E is present to counter this attack. Vitamin E also protects vitamin A in the eye from damage.

HEART DISEASE. Vitamin E performs numerous functions in the prevention and treatment of heart disease. A recent study from Harvard School of Public Health found that people who supplemented their diets with 100IU of vitamin E daily reduced their risk of developing heart disease by up to 40 percent. The vitamin might help prevent or treat heart disease by

1. inhibiting the clumping of blood cell fragments called platelets that are associated with the development and progression of atherosclerosis,
2. increasing levels of a hormone-like substance called PGE2 that helps reduce platelet clumping,
3. decreasing the formation of lesions in the lining of blood vessels that are associated with atherosclerosis,
4. protecting LDL-cholesterol from free-radical damage called "oxidation," (oxidized LDL-cholesterol are more likely than un-oxidized LDL-cholesterol to lead to the formation of artery-clogging plaque, which causes heart disease),
5. improving blood cholesterol levels, and
6. reducing the tissue damage associated with ischemia (reduced blood and oxygen flow to the heart) and open-heart surgery thus limiting tissue damage associated with heart disease and surgery and helping speed recovery, and
7. reducing the pain and tension in the legs associated with intermittent claudication in heart-disease patients.

LUPUS ERYTHEMATOSUS. Recent evidence shows that vitamin E might be effective in the treatment of lupus erythematosus. The skin disorder associated with lupus usually appears on the face and might be a result of alteration of cell membranes in skin tissue. Doses between 800IU and 2,000IU of vitamin E relieve symptoms in some individuals with no apparent side effects. Sensitivity to sunlight in some patients with lupus is also reduced or eliminated with use of vitamin E.

PREMENSTRUAL SYNDROME (PMS). A few studies show that vitamin E supplementation (in doses between 150IU and 600IU) might alleviate some symptoms of PMS, such as breast tenderness. Researchers speculate that vitamin E might affect neurotransmitters and regulate the hormone-like substances called prostaglandins that are implicated in the development of PMS. However, this research is controversial and more evidence from well-designed scientific studies is needed before recommendations can be made.

RHEUMATOID ARTHRITIS. Limited evidence exists that vitamin E in conjunction with selenium might help alleviate some of the pain and morning stiffness of rheumatoid arthritis.

There is no scientific evidence that vitamin E is effective in the following disorders:

Muscular dystrophy
Rheumatic fever
Sterility and impotence
Pre-eclampsia in pregnancy

Deficiency

A deficiency of vitamin E is difficult to diagnose, as low intakes of the vitamin develop in a variety of ways in different animals. Symptoms of vitamin E deficiency in animals include nervous system disorders, infant malformations, muscular dystrophy, anemia, degeneration of heart tissue, damage to liver tissue, and destruction of tissues in the testes. Anemia in infants and nerve damage in adults are the only known disorders that occur as a result of vitamin E deficiency. Premature infants have not accumulated ample amounts of the fat-soluble vitamin in their tissues and are susceptible to a type of anemia where the red blood cells break easily. Breastmilk contains enough vitamin E to prevent this "hemolytic" anemia in normal term infants. Infant anemia in formula-fed infants is rarely seen as most formulas now contain vitamin E.

People with rare fat malabsorption syndromes, such as celiac disease, cystic fibrosis, and sprue, are susceptible to nerve damage, muscle weakness, poor coordination, involuntary movement of the eyes, damage to the eyes, and anemia probably caused by vitamin E deficiency. Symptoms are improved or alleviated with vitamin E supplementation. Low tissue levels are also found in people who abuse alcohol.

NERVE FUNCTION. Chronic deficiency of vitamin E causes a syndrome of nerve dysfunction involving both the spinal cord and the retina of the eye in adults. Although poorly understood, the mechanism whereby vitamin E deficiency produces these symptoms probably relates to the vitamin's antioxidant role in protecting nerve membranes from free-radical damage.

Classic deficiency symptoms easily treated with minimal increases in vitamin E intake are still being identified. In addition, the growing wealth of evidence showing that greater than recommended levels of vitamin E reduce the risk for developing heart disease, cancer, and other disorders suggests that suboptimal intakes of vitamin E could have far-reaching effects on life-long health.

Daily Recommended Intake

The need for vitamin E increases with increasing body size and dietary intake of polyunsaturated fats, including fish oil. Vitamin E protects these fats from rancidity caused by oxygen fragments and other free radicals. Vigorous exercise also might increase the need for vitamin E.

The RDAs are only estimates based on the assumption that the average person consumes a diet that provides a 2:5 ratio of vitamin E (as a mix of different tocopherols) to polyunsaturated fat. More information is needed about the dietary factors that influence vitamin E requirements. The 1989 RDAs for vitamin E are:

	Milligrams (mg)	International Units of alpha-tocopherol (IU)
INFANTS		
0 to 1 year	3–4	4.5–6.0
CHILDREN		
1 to 10 years	6– 7	9.0–10.5
Males (11+)	10	15
Females (11+)	8	12
Pregnant	10	15
Lactating, 1st 6 mo.	12	18
Lactating, 2nd 6 mo.	11	16.5

The Alliance for Aging Research, a nonprofit group comprised of well-respected researchers across the United States, has issued recommendations for antioxidant vitamins that far exceed the RDAs. They recommend a daily vitamin E intake of 100IU to 400IU for adults.

Sources in the Diet

The primary dietary sources of vitamin E are vegetable oils, seeds, wheatgerm, and nuts. Varying amounts of different tocopherols are found in different vegetable oils. For example, 90 percent of the vitamin E in safflower oil is alpha tocopherol, the most potent or "biologically active" form of the vitamin. Corn oil is only 10 percent alpha tocopherol and soybean oil is primarily gamma tocopherol, a form of vitamin E with little potency. The diet is likely to be deficient in vitamin E if soybean oil, the major oil used in salad dressings, mayonnaise, and other commercial oils, constitutes the major source of polyunsaturated fat.

Other plant sources of the vitamin include avocados, peaches, whole grain breads and cereals, spinach, broccoli, asparagus, and dried prunes. Foods of animal origin are usually poor sources of vitamin E. Wide variations exist, however, and depend on the vitamin E content of the animal's diet (Table 6).

Table 6
THE VITAMIN E CONTENT OF SELECTED FOODS

Food	Amount	Vitamin E (IU)
Wheat germ oil	¼ cup	63.6
Safflower oil	¼ cup	19.5
Sunflower oil	¼ cup	18.3
French Dressing (Cottonseed oil)	¼ cup	13.0
Wheat germ	¼ cup	6.0
Spinach	½ cup	2.2–3.3
Peaches, canned	½ peach	2.1–2.4
Dried prunes	10 prunes	1.61–1.85
Asparagus	5 spears	1.1–1.6
Avocados	½ avocado	.95–2.0
Broccoli	3 stalks	.8–3.4
Whole wheat cereal, shredded	1 cup	.4–.6
Beef	3½ ounces	.33–1.0
Turkey	3½ ounces	0.09
Milk, whole	1 cup	0.02

Cooking and processing of foods reduce their vitamin E content. Vitamin E is lost when flours and oils are processed and bleached. So much vitamin E is lost from bleaching vegetable oils that the by-product is used for vitamin E supplements. The vitamin E content of a vegetable oil, such as soybean oil, is not always adequate to maintain an optimal ratio of vitamin E to polyunsaturated fat. Cold-pressed, unbleached vegetable oils, especially safflower oil, are the best sources of vitamin E.

It is virtually impossible to obtain 100IU or more daily of vitamin E from dietary intake alone. A person must consume 11½ ounces of almonds (1909 calories), 4½ cups of wheat germ, 18½ cups of spinach, or 44 tbsp. of Italian salad dressing (3,036 calories) to reach this amount. Consequently, amounts greater than 25IU must be obtained from supplements.

Toxicity

Unlike the other fat-soluble vitamins, vitamin E is relatively non-toxic, even when consumed in amounts far in excess of the RDAs. Large doses of the vitamin might interfere with vitamin K activity and result in prolonged bleeding time. This effect is most likely to occur in people who take anticoagulant medications for heart disease or in people with low amounts of vitamin K in the body because of liver disease.

Nutrient-Nutrient Interactions

- Vitamin E protects vitamin A, beta carotene, and vitamin C in foods from destruction by oxygen.
- Large doses of vitamin E can interfere with the coagulant functions of vitamin K.
- Selenium enhances the antioxidant capabilities of vitamin E.
- The antioxidant nutrients, including vitamin E, selenium, vitamin A, and vitamin C, work alone and in teams to protect tissues from hazardous oxygen fragments. For example, vitamin C might work with vitamin E to prevent premature aging, while vitamin E improves the use of vitamin A in the body.
- Vitamin E might be necessary for the conversion of vitamin B12 to its biologically active form.
- Vitamin E might reduce some of the symptoms of a zinc deficiency and a zinc deficiency might increase dietary requirements for vitamin E.
- Vitamin E provides protection from the toxic effects of silver, mercury, and lead.

VITAMIN K

Overview

There are two naturally-occurring forms of vitamin K and one synthetic form. All forms of the vitamin require the presence of a small amount of dietary fat in the small intestine for absorption.

Functions

BLOOD CLOTTING. The primary function of vitamin K is to regulate normal blood clotting. The vitamin is important for the production of prothrombin, a protein essential for blood coagulation.

BONES. Vitamin K-dependent proteins, such as osteocalcin, are found in bones and thought to be involved in calcium metabolism, bone turnover, and mineralization of tissue.

CANCER. Experiments on tumor cells removed from the body show that vitamin K might inhibit the growth of several forms of cancer, including cancer of the breast, ovary, colon, stomach, bladder, liver, and kidney. The effectiveness is enhanced when vitamin K is used in conjunction with the medication warfarin. However, the research on vitamin K is limited and more conclusive information is needed before recommendations can be made.

Deficiency

A classic deficiency of vitamin K is rare, except in newborn infants. The vitamin is synthesized by microorganisms in the mature intestinal tract, but the establishment of bacteria takes days to weeks to develop in the newborn. The mother is often given vitamin K supplements prior to delivery to increase the amount of vitamin K that crosses the placenta and is available in breastmilk. Additionally, vitamin K injections are often given to the baby at delivery.

A deficiency in the adult is likely only if the diet is low in dark green leafy vegetables or the growth of intestinal bacteria is inhibited by chronic use of antibiotic medications. Other medications that affect vitamin K absorption or use include coumarin, warfarin, heparin, and salicylates. In addition, any malabsorption syndrome that affects fat digestion would inhibit vitamin K absorption. Severe liver disease would hinder the utilization of the vitamin in the formation of prothrombin. These conditions require the attention of a physician and therapeutic doses of the vitamin to maintain normal blood clotting.

Poor dietary intake of vitamin K can produce a marginal deficiency, characterized by low blood levels of the vitamin, without affecting blood clotting ability. These marginal deficiencies are not corrected by moderate increases in vitamin K intake of 45mcg, suggesting that at least 100 percent of the RDA is needed to meet vitamin K requirements for these people.

Daily Recommended Intake

It is assumed that half of the daily intake comes from bacterial synthesis in the intestines; however, several studies cast doubt on the effectiveness of intestinal bacteria as a source of vitamin K. The RDAs are based on body weight and are approximately 1mcg/kg body weight per day.

The 1989 RDAs for vitamin K are:

	Vitamin K (mcg)
INFANTS	
0 to 0.5 year	5
0.5 to 1.0 year	10
CHILDREN	
1 to 3 years	15
4 to 6 years	20
7 to 10 years	30
YOUNG ADULTS AND ADULTS	
Males, 11 to 14 years	45
Males, 15 to 18 years	65
Males, 19 to 24 years	70
Males, 25+ years	80
Females, 11 to 14 years	45
Females, 15 to 18 years	55
Females, 19 to 24 years	60
Females, 25+ years	65
Pregnant	65
Lactating	65

Sources in the Diet

The vitamin K value of many foods is not available, those that are available are only approximate values. In fact, the vitamin K content of a specific food may vary by as much as 50 percent of the values listed in Table 7. Vitamin K is found in green or leafy vegetables, such as broccoli, turnip greens, romaine lettuce, and cabbage. Cheese, egg yolk, and liver contain small amounts of the vitamin (Table 7).

Table 7
THE VITAMIN K CONTENT OF SELECTED FOODS

Food	Amount	Vitamin K (mcg)
Turnip greens	²/₃ cup	650
Broccoli	²/₃ cup	200
Lettuce	2 cups	129
Cabbage	²/₃ cup	125
Spinach	²/₃ cup	89
Liver, beef	3¹/₂ ounces	92
Cheese	3¹/₂ ounces	35
Avocados	3¹/₂ ounces	20
Egg, yolk	1 medium	11
Peach	¹/₂ medium	8
Liver, pork	3¹/₂ ounces	7
Potato, baked	1 medium	6

Toxicity

Large doses of synthetic vitamin K can cause anemia in animals and a severe form of jaundice in infants that results in degeneration of the brain. The less potent forms of vitamin K found in alfalfa leaves have a wider range of safety. Vitamin K supplements are available only through prescription as the vitamin can be toxic.

Nutrient-Nutrient Interactions

- Large doses of vitamin E might interfere with the blood clotting functions of vitamin K.

VITAMIN B1 (THIAMIN)

Overview

Vitamin B1 was called "water-soluble B" until 1926 when it was found that the vitamin consisted of two substances. The first compound, vitamin B1, cured beriberi and was easily deactivated by heat. The second compound, niacin, cured another disease called pellagra and was not affected by heat.

Functions

Vitamin B1 is required for normal functioning of all body cells, especially nerves. It also is involved in releasing acetylcholine, the nerve chemical that regulates memory, from nerve cells. Increasing vitamin B1 intake might increase reaction time and hand-eye coordination. Vitamin B1 is involved in numerous body processes that break down carbohydrates, protein, and fat for energy and convert excess carbohydrate to fat for storage.

Deficiency

Symptoms of vitamin B1 deficiency occur primarily in the nervous, gastrointestinal, and cardiovascular systems. Early symptoms include fatigue, loss of appetite, weight loss, gastrointestinal upsets, nausea, and weakness. Caution must be exercised in self-diagnosing the problem at this stage, as these symptoms are vague and can be an indication of numerous other health or lifestyle problems unrelated to vitamin B1 intake. The following symptoms are signs of advanced clinical deficiency:

> Mental confusion or delirium
> Paralysis of the extremities
> Muscle fatigue
> Emaciation
> Enlargement of the heart
> Numbness

Personality changes also can develop and include memory loss, emotional instability, reduced attention span, irritability, confusion, and depression. Permanent damage to the nervous system can occur if a severe deficiency is not corrected in time.

Beriberi, the classic vitamin B1 deficiency disease, is classified into two main types: wet beriberi and dry beriberi. Wet beriberi is characterized by the accumulation of fluids in the tissues (edema), especially in the ankles, feet, and legs. This excess of fluid affects heart function and can be fatal. There is no accumulation of fluid in dry beriberi; instead there is severe muscle wasting, emaciation, and paralysis of the legs.

Although the causes of some symptoms of vitamin B1 deficiency are not fully understood, many deficiency symptoms are probably a result of either the accumulation of substances that cannot be completely broken apart for energy without vitamin B1 or interference of nerve functions dependent on the vitamin. The effects of this accumulation are felt in every cell in the body, especially those cells that depend primarily on carbohydrate for energy, such as the brain and nervous system, or tissues that have immediate contact with nerves, such as the muscles. Anything that increases the demand for the conversion of carbohydrate to energy (i.e., exercise, alcohol, and high intake of carbohydrate foods, especially sugary foods) will increase the likelihood of deficiency symptoms if the diet is low in vitamin B1.

Vitamin B1 deficiency occurs primarily in people who consume a diet comprised mainly of highly refined foods. For example, vitamin B1 deficiency can develop during fasting, chronic dieting, or when a person consumes a limited variety or amount of food. The tannins in tea also inhibit vitamin B1 absorption, so repeatedly drinking tea with meals might result in vitamin B1 deficiency.

People who abuse alcohol also are at high risk for developing vitamin B1 deficiency. Alcohol is associated with poor dietary intake, reduced absorption, increased requirements, and increased urinary loss of vitamin B1. Alcohol's effect on vitamin B1 status results in Wernicke-Korsakoff syndrome with loss of immediate memory, disorientation, jerky movements of the eyes, and a staggering gait. Many symptoms of this form of alcohol-induced nerve damage are reversible if the individual stops drinking alcohol and starts eating a nutrient-rich diet. However, if the problem is not treated, the brain can be permanently damaged leading to psychosis and death.

Enrichment of white rice and white bread with vitamin B1 has reduced the incidence of overt vitamin B1 deficiency, so beriberi is rare in the United States. However, subclinical or mild deficiencies might be more common. Vitamin B1 deficiency has been reported in up to 48 percent of elderly patients admitted to a hospital and research from autopsies indicates that deficiencies often progress unnoticed in many individuals.

The diet should be adequate in vitamin B1 if a person consumes at least 10 servings a day of nutrient-rich foods, such as fresh vegetables, whole grain breads and cereals, extra-lean meats or cooked dried beans and peas, and low-fat or nonfat milk products.

Daily Recommended Intake

Because vitamin B1 is water-soluble, excesses are excreted in the urine rather than stored, and a daily supply of the vitamin is necessary to maintain normal body processes. The daily need for vitamin B1 is based on the amount of calories consumed, especially calories from carbohydrates as the vitamin will be needed to convert those calories to energy. Other factors that affect vitamin B1 requirements are body weight, growth, and the small amount of vitamin B1 that is absorbed from bacterial synthesis in the intestines.

Deficiency symptoms have been noted when vitamin B1 intake drops below 0.2 to 0.3mg for every 1,000 calories. The RDAs are based on 0.5mg/1,000 calories. Daily intake of vitamin B1 on diets less than 2,000 calories should not drop below 1.0mg/day. Vitamin B1 needs increase during pregnancy and breastfeeding, and during physical or emotional stress.

The 1989 RDAs for vitamin B1 are:

	Vitamin B1 (mg)
INFANTS	
0 to 0.5 year	0.3
0.5 to 1 year	0.4
CHILDREN	
1 to 3 years	0.7
4 to 6 years	0.9
7 to 10 years	1.0
YOUNG ADULTS AND ADULTS	
Males, 11 to 14 years	1.3
Males, 15 to 50 years	1.5
Males, 51+ years	1.2
Females, 11 to 50 years	1.1
Females, 50+ years	1.0
Pregnant	1.5
Lactating	1.6

Sources in the Diet

Pork, organ meats, oysters, green peas, collard greens, oranges, dried beans and peas, and wheatgerm are the richest sources of vitamin B1. Other good sources of the vitamin include brewer's or nutritional yeast, fish, peanuts and peanut butter, whole grain breads and cereals, nuts, and cooked dried beans and peas. Moderate dietary sources include avocados, extra-lean meat, milk, spinach, cauliflower, and dried fruit (Table 8).

Table 8
THE VITAMIN B1 CONTENT OF SELECTED FOODS

Food	Amount	Vitamin B1 (mg)
Wheat germ	¹/₄ cup	.47
Ham	3 ounces	.40
Brewer's (nutritional) yeast	1 tbsp	.34
Oysters	³/₄ cup	.25
Liver, beef	3 ounces	.23
Peanuts	¹/₂ cup	.22
Green peas	¹/₂ cup	.22
Raisins	1 cup	.21
Collard greens	¹/₂ cup	.14
Orange	1	.13
Dried beans and peas (cooked)	¹/₂ cup	.13
Asparagus	1 cup	.12
Cauliflower	1 cup	.11
Milk, nonfat	1 cup	.09
Potato, small	1	.08
Bread, whole wheat	1 slice	.06
Brussels sprouts	¹/₂ cup	.06
Beef, extra-lean	3 ounces	.05
Chicken, meat only	3 ounces	.05

Vitamin B1 is lost when the cooking water is discarded or when baking soda is added to cooked vegetables to maintain their green color. Sulfur dioxide used in the drying of fruits destroys vitamin B1.

Toxicity

There are no known toxic levels of vitamin B1 when the vitamin is taken orally. As the vitamin is not stored well in the body, it is unlikely vitamin B1 could accumulate to toxic levels. Repeated intravenous injections of vitamin B1 might cause anaphylactic shock in some people. The safety levels for vitamin B1 appear to be at least 300mg/day, possibly higher. However, there is no known reason to consume this quantity and the consumption of a nutritious diet should supply a safe and ample intake of this B vitamin.

Nutrient-Nutrient Interactions

The B vitamins, especially vitamin B1, vitamin B2, niacin, biotin, pantothenic acid, and vitamin B6, are generally found in the same foods and they work together in converting dietary protein, carbohydrates, and fat to energy or storage fat. In humans, a deficiency of one B vitamin is usually associated with poor intake of several B vitamins.

VITAMIN B2 (RIBOFLAVIN)

Overview

Vitamin B2 is one of a number of compounds that have similar chemical structures. Vitamin B2 is easily absorbed from food, but only approximately 15 percent of the vitamin is absorbed when taken alone in supplemental form on an empty stomach. The vitamin is not well stored and excesses are excreted in the urine, giving the urine a fluorescent yellow color.

Functions

Vitamin B2, as with vitamin B1, is essential for the normal release of energy from carbohydrate, protein, and fat in food. Vitamin B2 is important for normal growth and development, the production of and regulation of certain hormones, and the formation of red blood cells. Vitamin B2, with other B vitamins, is involved in the metabolism of neurotransmitters, which might affect the development of depression. Vitamin B2 might be a necessary adjunct to iron supplementation in the treatment of anemia and it might aid in the prevention of prostate cancer.

Deficiency

Clinical symptoms of vitamin B2 deficiency are rare, except in alcohol abusers, and are usually accompanied by vitamin B1 or niacin deficiencies. Subclinical or mild deficiencies are more common.

Early symptoms include soreness and burning of the lips, mouth, and tongue; burning and itching of the eyes; loss of vision; sensitivity to light; and cracks in the corners of the mouth. As the deficiency progresses, the mucous membranes of the mouth become inflamed, the eyes redden, dermatitis with simultaneous dryness and greasy scaling develops, and/or depression or hysteria develop. A severe B2 deficiency in a pregnant mother might lead to retarded growth or malformations in the infant. Symptoms are difficult to detect as other nutrient deficiencies are most likely occurring simultaneously. Similar deficiency symptoms also occur as a result of niacin, iron, or vitamin B6 deficiencies. Supplementation usually reverses symptoms within a few days to weeks.

Daily Recommended Intake

The daily need for vitamin B2 increases as calorie intake increases, and the RDA is based on 0.6mg/1,000 calories. Vitamin B2 intake should not drop below 1.2mg/day regardless of calorie intake, as tissue reserves cannot be maintained on low intakes. Daily needs increase during pregnancy, lactation, and possibly during premenstrual syndrome (PMS), strenuous exercise, or use of birth control pills.

The 1989 RDAs for vitamin B2 are:

	Vitamin B2 (mg)
Infants	
0 to 0.5 year	0.4
0.5 to 1 year	0.5
Children	
1 to 3 years	0.8
4 to 6 years	1.1
7 to 10 years	1.2
Young Adults and Adults	
Males, 11 to 14 years	1.5
Males, 15 to 18 years	1.8
Males, 19 to 50 years	1.7
Males, 51+ years	1.4
Females, 11 to 50 years	1.3
Females, 51+ years	1.2
Pregnant	1.6
Lactating, 1st 6 mo.	1.8
Lactating, 2nd 6 mo.	1.7

Sources in the Diet

Small amounts of vitamin B2 are distributed in a variety of foods; however, the most concentrated sources of the vitamin include milk products, liver, and dark green vegetables. Children, adolescents, and adults who avoid milk products are likely to consume inadequate amounts of vitamin B2 as milk products supply up to half of the daily vitamin B2 most people consume in the United States (Table 9).

Table 9
THE VITAMIN B2 CONTENT OF SELECTED FOODS

Food	Amount	Vitamin B2 (mg)
Liver, beef	3 ounces	3.6
Milk, low-fat	1 cup	.52
Yogurt, low-fat	1 cup	.39
Oysters	¾ cup	.30
Avocado	½	.22
Collard greens	½ cup	.19
Chicken, meat only	3 ounces	.16
Salmon, canned	3 ounces	.16
Asparagus	½ cup	.13
Broccoli	½ cup	.12
Brussels sprouts	½ cup	.11
Spinach	½ cup	.11
Whole wheat bread	1 slice	.05

Vitamin B2 is stable to heat so little is lost in cooking, unless baking soda is added during the cooking of vegetables. The vitamin is easily destroyed in the presence of light. Foods stored in clear containers, such as milk in glass bottles, noodles and other grains in glass or clear plastic jars, sun drying of fruits and vegetables, or mushrooms and other vegetables left uncovered, will lose large portions of their vitamin B2 content in a short period of time.

Toxicity

No known toxicity levels are identified for vitamin B2. The vitamin is excreted in the urine in proportion to intake when intake is greater than 1.3mg/day. Riboflavin is an essential component of all body cells; however, in eye tissue this B vitamin also might be a double-edged sword. When oxidized by light, riboflavin metabolites are toxic. These toxic riboflavin fragments might be a contributing factor in the formation of lipofuscin, a fatty build-up that invades the retina and is a primary contributor in the development of macular degeneration. However, there is no evidence that dietary intake affects these levels.

Nutrient-Nutrient Interactions

- Vitamin B2 works with other B vitamins, such as vitamin B1, niacin, biotin, pantothenic acid, and vitamin B6 in the breakdown of the calorie nutrients (carbohydrate, protein, and fat) for energy. A deficiency of any of these nutrients will compromise the other vitamins' ability to function.
- Vitamin B2 might enhance the effectiveness of iron supplementation in the treatment of anemia.
- Vitamin B2 is necessary for the activation of vitamin B6.
- Vitamin B2 is needed to convert tryptophan to niacin. Although pellagra is the nutrient deficiency disease associated with niacin, it is actually a multiple deficiency of niacin, vitamin B6, tryptophan, and vitamin B2.

NIACIN (NICOTINIC ACID, NIACINAMIDE)

Overview

Niacin is the common name for two compounds: nicotinic acid and niacinamide (also called nicotinamide). The name niacin was chosen to avoid confusion with the toxic drug nicotine found in tobacco. Niacin is absorbed in the small intestine and, as it is a water-soluble vitamin, it is not stored in the body. Excess intakes of niacin are excreted in the urine.

Functions

CELL FUNCTION. Niacin functions in more than 50 body processes and is primarily important in the release of energy from carbohydrates. Niacin aids in the breakdown of protein and fats, in the synthesis of fats and certain hormones, in the formation of red blood cells, and in the detoxification of several drugs and chemicals. The diversity of niacin's roles makes it essential for the supply of energy to and the maintenance of all body cells.

BLOOD CHOLESTEROL. Large daily doses of niacin, as nicotinic acid, decrease blood cholesterol, LDL-cholesterol, and triglyceride levels; increase HDL-cholesterol levels; and reduce the risk for developing heart disease in people with elevated blood fat levels. Smaller doses of nicotinic acid can be used with similar effectiveness when this B vitamin is combined with vitamin A and vitamin E. The cholesterol-lowering effect of many medications is even more pronounced when nicotinic acid is included in the therapy. Nicotinic acid as a treatment for elevated blood cholesterol should be supervised by a physician as there are side effects. (See page 196 for more information on nicotinic acid and heart disease.)

DRUG TOXICITY. Adriamycin is a medication used in the treatment of cancer. One of the adverse side effects of adriamycin is possible damage to heart tissue. Niacin might reduce the toxic effects of this medication on heart tissue without reducing its effectiveness in the treatment of cancer.

EPILEPSY. Niacinamide might enhance the effectiveness of antiepileptic medications such as phenobarbital or primidone.

PSYCHIATRIC DISORDERS. Large doses of niacin have been used with varying success in the treatment of schizophrenia. The vitamin was first investigated because the psychiatric symptoms of pellagra resemble schizophrenia.

Some psychiatric disorders might be caused by a genetic defect in the absorption of substances necessary for normal brain function. Psychological symptoms, such as aggressive behavior, temper tantrums, restlessness, depression, hyperactivity, and sleep disturbances, are sometimes a result of impaired absorption of the amino acid tryptophan, but symptoms improve with increased daily intake of niacinamide. Treatment for psychological problems with niacin only should be used with the supervision of a physician.

Deficiency

In 1945 it was found that either an amino acid called tryptophan found in protein or niacin could cure pellagra, and later it was recognized that tryptophan could be converted to niacin in the body. In more recent years, pellagra has been suspected to be a more complex nutrient deficiency disorder that also involves vitamin B1, vitamin B2, and other nutrients.

Pellagra is the classic deficiency disease associated with niacin. All tissues are affected by inadequate intake of niacin, but those tissues where the cells are replaced more frequently, such as the skin and the digestive tract, show symptoms first. The nervous system is also a prime target for deficiency symptoms. The classic description of pellagra is the four "Ds": dermatitis, diarrhea, dementia, and death.

Early symptoms of niacin deficiency include weakness, loss of appetite, indigestion, skin eruptions, and lethargy. The four "Ds" of pellagra develop as the deficiency worsens. The dermatitis of pellagra is a scaly, dark pigmentation that develops on areas of the skin exposed to sunlight, heat, or mild irritation or trauma. The tongue is swollen, the person may experience tremors, and damage to the central nervous system can result in disorientation, irritability, headaches, insomnia, loss of memory, delirium, and emotional instability. These symptoms are often accompanied by other deficiency symptoms from poor intake of protein, vitamin B2, iron, vitamin B1, or vitamin B6.

Niacin deficiency is rare unless a person consumes a diet composed primarily of corn or cornmeal with little protein, or the diet is so poor that numerous vitamin, mineral, protein, and calorie deficits are present. The niacin and tryptophan content of corn is low and poorly absorbed. In Mexico, where corn is treated with lye before use, the alkali increases the absorption of the amino acid tryptophan in the corn. Once in the body, tryptophan is converted to niacin, which lowers the risk for deficiency. In fact, pellagra and niacin deficiency can be cured by increasing the dietary intake of tryptophan with no increased intake of niacin. Wheat and other grains contain a poorly absorbed form of niacin, but provide adequate amounts of tryptophan so their use is not associated with pellagra.

Daily Recommended Intake

The RDAs for niacin are based on calorie intake: 6.6mg of niacin/1,000 calories. No less than 13mg of niacin should be consumed each day to maintain tissue stores in adults.

The 1989 RDAs for niacin are:

	Niacin (mg)
INFANTS	
0 to 0.5 year	5
0.5 to 1 year	6
CHILDREN	
1 to 3 years	9
4 to 6 years	12
7 to 10 years	13
ADOLESCENTS AND YOUNG ADULTS	
Males, 11 to 14 years	17
Males, 15 to 18 years	20
Females, 11 to 18 years	15
ADULTS	
Males, 19 to 50 years	19
Males, 50+	15
Females, 19 to 50 years	15
Females, 50+	13
Pregnant	17
Lactating	20

Either adequate amounts of niacin or high-quality protein are needed to cure the symptoms of pellagra. More than half of the daily requirement for niacin is obtained by the conversion of tryptophan to niacin with the help of vitamin B6.

The total daily niacin intake is expressed as niacin equivalents and includes both the dietary intake of the vitamin and the amount of niacin formed as a result of tryptophan intake. Food composition tables provide information on the amount of niacin in a food but do not include the niacin from the tryptophan-to-niacin conversion. To estimate total niacin equivalents:

1. Estimate total grams of protein consumed in a day.
2. Multiply by 0.01 to determine total tryptophan intake (tryptophan constitutes 1 percent of total protein intake).
3. Convert grams to milligrams (1 gram = 1,000mg).
4. Divide by 60mg to determine niacin equivalents from tryptophan conversion (it takes 60mg of tryptophan to produce 1mg of niacin).
5. Add the niacin equivalents to the dietary intake of preformed niacin to determine total niacin available in the diet. Most diets

in the United States contain about 500 to 1,000mg or more of tryptophan and about 8 to 17mg of preformed niacin, for a total daily intake of 34mg of niacin equivalents (Table 10).

Table 10
THE NIACIN EQUIVALENT CONTENT OF SELECTED FOODS

Food	Amount	Niacin (mg)	Tryptophan (mg/100gr)	Niacin Equivalent (mg/serving)
Chicken	¹/₂	15.5	205	21.5
Salmon	3 ounces	6.8	200	9.6
Beef	2.9 ounces	4.4	198	7.1
Peanut butter	2 tbsp	4.8	305	6.2
Peas, green	1 cup	2.7	66	4.5
Potato	1 medium	2.7	33	3.6
Brewer's (nutritional) yeast	1 tbsp	3.0	429	3.6
Milk	1 cup	.2	50	2.2

Sources in the Diet

The best sources of niacin and tryptophan are protein-rich foods such as extra-lean meat, chicken, fish, cooked dried beans and peas, brewer's (nutritional) yeast, peanut butter, nonfat or low-fat milk and cheese, soybeans, and nuts. Milk contains little preformed niacin, but is a good selection because of its high tryptophan content. Fruit, except for orange juice, is a poor source of niacin.

The vitamin is relatively stable to heat and light and little is lost during cooking and preparation of food unless cooking water is discarded.

Toxicity

Daily doses of niacin up to 1,000mg appear to be safe. A single 1,000mg dose of nicotinic acid can cause dilation of the blood vessels and skin flushing, headaches, tingling, and burning within 15 minutes of ingestion. In the past, snake oils and medicinal elixirs often contained nicotinic acid. The characteristic flushing that occurred when the product was used was mistakenly attributed to the healing effects of the potion.

The flushing effect is caused by a sudden release of histamine and for this reason people with asthma or peptic ulcer disease are cautioned against taking large doses of nicotinic acid. Niacinamide does not produce these effects, regardless of the dose.

Niacin is likely to be toxic for some people who consume several gram doses of the vitamin. Large doses of niacin (more than 3 grams) also might increase the risk for liver damage and might increase uric acid levels. Therapeutic doses of niacin should be taken with physician (M.D.) monitoring.

Nutrient-Nutrient Interactions

- Niacin works closely with vitamin B1, vitamin B2, pantothenic acid, biotin, and vitamin B6 in energy metabolism and is found in similar foods. A deficiency of one of these nutrients usually means that other B vitamins are deficient, too.
- Protein, specifically the amino acid tryptophan, can partially or totally substitute for niacin in the prevention and treatment of pellagra.
- The addition of vitamin A and vitamin E to nicotinic acid therapy in the treatment of heart disease might reduce the dose necessary to obtain benefits.
- Vitamin B6 is needed to convert tryptophan to niacin in the body.
- Tryptophan competes with another amino acid, leucine, for absorption and use in the body. Chronic, excess intake of leucine can cause a secondary tryptophan and niacin deficiency.

VITAMIN B6 (PYRIDOXINE, PYRIDOXAMINE, PYRIDOXAL)

Overview

Vitamin B6 is a family of water-soluble compounds that includes pyridoxine, pyridoxamine, and pyridoxal. Excess intake is excreted in the urine.

Functions

Vitamin B6 is involved in the building and breakdown of carbohydrates, fats, and proteins; however, its primary role involves protein and its building blocks, the amino acids. Vitamin B6 aids in the conversion of one amino acid to another, the synthesis of new amino acids from carbohydrate, the conversion of amino acids to carbohydrate or fat for storage or energy, and the conversion of the amino acid tryptophan to niacin. Thus, vitamin B6 is involved in the manufacture of most protein-related compounds, such as hormones, hemoglobin in red blood cells, nerve chemicals such as serotonin that regulate nerve function, and many enzymes (the catalysts for all body processes).

In addition, vitamin B6 is necessary for the conversion of one type of essential fat to another and in the formation of fat-derived hormone-like substances called prostaglandins that regulate a variety of body processes including blood pressure, muscle contraction, and heart function. Vitamin B6 also aids in the formation and maintenance of the nervous system, and therefore is an essential nutrient in the regulation of mental processes and mood.

ASTHMA. Supplementation with vitamin B6 might be an effective aid in the treatment of asthma. Some people who consume additional vitamin B6 daily report a reduction in severity and frequency of wheezing and asthmatic attacks. Asthmatics might have an altered ability to use vitamin B6 and might require increased intake to maintain normal body functions. Vitamin B6 supplementation might reduce many of the side effects of theophylline therapy, a drug frequently used in asthmatic children.

BEHAVIOR. Adequate intake of vitamin B6 is critical for the development and function of the central nervous system. Even marginal intakes of the vitamin produce abnormal functioning of several enzymes responsible for the metabolism of a variety of nerve chemicals and nerve modulators, including serotonin, dopamine, and GABA, that regulate behavior. Too little vitamin B6 also results in the accumulation of toxic breakdown products from nerve chemicals that irritate the nerves and are linked to many nerve disorders from depression to seizures.

In addition, the mood swings and depression that are considered side effects of medications, such as estrogen, oral contraceptives, and anti-tuberculous drugs, might be caused by drug-induced suppression of vitamin B6 metabolism and the consequent underproduction of serotonin.

CARPAL TUNNEL SYNDROME. Carpal tunnel syndrome is a neurological disorder of the wrists and hands that often requires surgery. Supplementation with vitamin B6 might alleviate pain and stiffness and prevent the need for surgery.

DRUG TOXICITY. Vitamin B6 might reduce the harmful effects of some medications used in the treatment of cancer. The toxic effects of vincristine on the nervous system are reduced without affecting the medication's effectiveness in treating cancer when the intake of vitamin B6 is increased. Azauridine triacetate is another medication used in the treatment of cancer. Adverse side effects of this medication are alleviated when vitamin B6 intake is increased.

IMMUNITY. Adequate intake of vitamin B6 aids in the regulation and maintenance of a healthy immune system; however, large doses do not provide additional benefits. Older adults who consume a diet inadequate in vitamin B6 might be especially susceptible to infection and disease.

KIDNEY DISORDERS. Vitamin B6 might be beneficial in the treatment of certain kidney disorders, such as hyperoxaluria—an excess amount of oxalates in the urine that can lead to kidney stones—and kidney damage or failure. Vitamin B6 supplementation might lower the amount of oxalic acid in the urine and reduce the risk for kidney stone formation.

PREMENSTRUAL SYNDROME. Supplementation with vitamin B6 might relieve the symptoms of Premenstrual Syndrome (PMS) in some women. Reduction in depression, irritability, tension, breast tenderness, edema (fluid retention), headaches, and acne has been reported by some women who take vitamin B6 supplements (25 to 200mg/day). However, symptoms also improve in many cases when women take placebos, which are sugar tablets with no nutritional or medicinal value. More research is necessary before recommendations can be made about the effectiveness of vitamin B6 as a treatment for PMS.

Deficiency

Deficiency symptoms of vitamin B6 are widespread and vague because of the vitamin's variety of functions. Symptoms include depression, vomiting, increased susceptibility to disease and infection, dermatitis, anemia, inflammation of the nerves, oxalate kidney stones, nausea, and lethargy. Infants fed formulas lacking in vitamin B6 become irritable and, in severe cases, can develop convulsions. Deficiency symptoms can result from either inadequate intake of the vitamin or the use of antagonistic medications such as isoniazid, a medication used in the treatment of tuberculosis. A deficiency of vitamin B6 also might be associated with an increased risk for developing some forms of cancer.

Pregnant women show low blood levels of vitamin B6, possibly because of the developing infant's increased need for the vitamin. Vitamin B6 has been used as a treatment for the nausea and vomiting of pregnancy and for the depression experienced by some women on oral contraceptives. The below-normal blood levels of vitamin B6 found in these women result in lethargy, fatigue, and depression. Symptoms improve with increased intake of the vitamin.

Vitamin B6 deficiency can accompany alcohol abuse, as alcohol reduces liver function and interferes with normal vitamin B6 metabolism. Tobacco use interferes with vitamin B6 metabolism, often resulting in deficiency. However, vitamin B6 status normalizes within two years of not smoking.

Infants born with a defect in how their body uses vitamin B6 can develop mental retardation and uncontrollable convulsions. Treatment for the disorder requires physician supervision and large daily doses of vitamin B6 initiated in the early days of life.

A low intake of vitamin B6 might be associated with reduced bone width, malformation of bones, abnormal electroencephalographs (EEGs),or epileptic seizures.

DEPRESSION. The amount of serotonin manufactured by nerve cells is directly related to how much vitamin B6 and the amino acid tryptophan are available to the brain; the greater the B6 and tryptophan, the greater the synthesis of serotonin. Numerous studies, mostly on the elderly, report that when depressed people are given vitamin B6 supplements, their mood improves. In one study conducted at Harvard Medical School and USDA Human Nutrition Research Center at Tufts University, more than one out of every four depressed patients were deficient in vitamins B6 and B12. In fact, vitamin B6 deficiency is reported in as many as 79 percent of patients with depression, compared to only 29 percent of other patients. In many cases, giving these patients vitamin B6 supplements (in doses as low as 10mg a day) raises vitamin B6 levels in the blood and improves or even alleviates the depression, providing convincing evidence that the deficiency might be the cause, rather than the effect, of the depression. Depression associated with Premenstrual Syndrome (PMS), menopause, or even postpartum blues sometimes is treated successfully with larger-than-normal supplemental doses of vitamin B6.

HEART DISEASE. Low levels of vitamin B6 are found in patients who have suffered a heart attack; however, it is unknown whether a marginal deficiency of vitamin B6 is a cause or a result of the disease. Inadequate intake of vitamin B6 also might encourage the formation of atherosclerosis and increase the risk for developing premature heart disease, possibly because a deficiency of this vitamin results in elevated blood levels of the amino acid homocysteine.

Daily Recommended Intake

The RDA for vitamin B6 is based on protein intake. Measurements for the adult RDA are based on the assumption that the average daily protein intake is 100 grams; more of the vitamin would be needed if the protein intake was greater than this. Women on oral contraceptives, people exposed to radiation, patients with heart disease, and people on certain medications, such as amphetamines, chlorpromazine, and reserpine, need to increase the vitamin B6 content of their diets above the adult RDAs. Inadequate intake of vitamin B6 is common in adolescents, women, older adults, people on restricted diets, alcoholics, and people who consume diets high in sugar and fat.

The 1989 RDAs for vitamin B6 are:

	Vitamin B6 (mg)
INFANTS	
0 to 0.5 year	0.3
0.5 to 1 year	0.6
CHILDREN	
1 to 3 years	1.0
4 to 6 years	1.1
7 to 10 years	1.4
Males, 11 to 14 years	1.7
Females, 11 to 14 years	1.4
YOUNG ADULTS AND ADULTS	
Males, 15+ years	2.0
Females, 15 to 18 years	1.5
Females, 19+ years	1.6
Pregnant	2.2
Lactating	2.1

Sources in the Diet

The best dietary sources of vitamin B6 are protein-rich foods, such as extra-lean meat, wheatgerm, brewer's (nutritional) yeast, poultry, fish, soybeans, cooked dried beans and peas, and peanuts. Moderate sources include bananas, avocados, cabbage, cauliflower, potatoes, whole grain breads and cereals, and dried fruit. Significant amounts of vitamin B6 are lost during the processing and refining of flours. As much as 70 percent of the vitamin is lost when foods are frozen or when cooking water is discarded (Table 11).

Table 11
THE VITAMIN B6 CONTENT OF SELECTED FOODS

Food	Amount	Vitamin B6 (mg)
Banana	1 medium	.480
Avocado	½ medium	.420
Hamburger	3 ounces	.391
Chicken	3 ounces	.340
Fish	3 ounces	.289
Potato	1 medium	.200
Collard greens	½ cup	.170
Spinach, cooked	½ cup	.161
Rice, brown	½ cup	.127
Peas, green	½ cup	.110
Walnuts	8 to 10 halves	.109
Peanut butter	2 tbsp	.096
Wheat germ	1 tbsp	.055

Toxicity

Vitamin B6 is one of the few water-soluble vitamins that can be toxic to the nervous system when taken in large doses. Doses greater than 2,000mg/day can produce tingling sensations in the hands and feet, lack of muscle coordination, a stumbling gait, and degeneration of nerve tissue. Lower doses of 200mg might be toxic if taken daily for months or years. Most symptoms improve when supplementation is discontinued; however, some nerve damage might be permanent. Large doses of vitamin B6 might alter levels of amino acids in the blood. Vitamin B6 in doses exceeding 100 times the RDA or 200mg should be taken only with the supervision of a physician.

Nutrient-Nutrient Interactions

- Vitamin B6 requires vitamin B2 for its normal function in the body, including the conversion of tryptophan to niacin.

- Vitamin B6 deficiency results in reduced absorption and low blood and liver levels of vitamin B12.
- Vitamin C deficiency causes increased urinary excretion of vitamin B6 and vitamin B6 deficiency results in low blood levels of vitamin C.
- Vitamin B6 deficiency increases the urinary excretion of calcium and magnesium and reduces copper absorption.
- Vitamin B6 is involved in the distribution, transportation, and metabolism of selenium.

VITAMIN B12 (COBALAMIN, CYANOCOBALAMIN)

Overview

Cobalamin is the general name for vitamin B12 and reflects the inclusion of cobalt in the vitamin's structure. Cyanocobalamin, the most stable form of vitamin B12 and the main form of synthetic vitamin B12, has a cyanide group attached to the vitamin. The cyanide group is not found on the vitamin naturally, but is a consequence of processing. The amount of cyanide derived from this form of vitamin B12 is minimal and well below toxic levels.

A form of anemia that affected older adults and usually resulted in death within two to five years was identified in the 1800s and named pernicious anemia (meaning deadly or fatal). More than 70 years later researchers found that a daily intake of one pound of raw liver cured pernicious anemia, and investigators theorized that "intrinsic" and "extrinsic" factors were responsible for the disease. The extrinsic factor in liver was identified as vitamin B12 in the late 1940s.

Intrinsic factor is a substance in digestive juices that binds to vitamin B12 and assists in the absorption of the vitamin in the lower small intestine. Absorption decreases with age or with a deficiency of iron and vitamin B6, and increases during pregnancy. Unlike other water-soluble nutrients, vitamin B12 is stored in the liver, kidney, and other tissues, and symptoms of deficiency do not develop for five to six years despite poor dietary intake or inadequate secretion of intrinsic factor.

Functions

Vitamin B12 is necessary for normal processing of carbohydrate, protein, and fat in the body. It is important for the normal production of certain amino acids and fats and in the formation and maintenance of the nervous system. The formation of the insulation sheath around nerve cells, called the myelin sheath, requires vitamin B12. This sheath speeds the conduction of signals along nerve cells. The vitamin functions in the replication of the genetic code within each cell, and in this capacity vitamin B12 is essential for the replacement and maintenance of all cells in the body. Vitamin B12 and other B vitamins are essential in the formation of neurotransmitters, chemicals that facilitate communication between nerve cells. This function of vitamin B12 might play a role in preventing depression and other mood disorders.

Deficiency

A deficiency of vitamin B12 can result from poor dietary intake of the vitamin or inadequate secretion of intrinsic factor. In either case, anemia is the first clinical symptom. Vitamin B6 deficiency also is caused by intestinal disorders that impair vitamin B12 absorption, such as intestinal infections, or surgical removal of the portion of the small intestine where vitamin B12-intrinsic factor is absorbed or the portion of the stomach that secretes intrinsic factor.

Vitamin B12 deficiency affects the growth and repair of all body cells. Poor vitamin B12 intake or absorption results in faulty formation of nerve cells. Irreversible nerve damage results, including disorientation, numbness, tingling, dementia in seniors, moodiness, confusion, agitation, dimmed vision, delusions, hallucinations, or dizziness.

The improper replication of the genetic code that results from vitamin B12 deficiency causes poor formation of blood cells. Reduced numbers of red blood cells cause anemia and fatigue, and reduced numbers of white blood cells cause increased susceptibility to colds and disease. Reduced formation of blood cell fragments called platelets causes poor blood clotting and bruising. Poor cell formation in the digestive tract causes nausea, vomiting, loss of appetite, poor absorption of food, diarrhea, and increased likelihood of malnutrition. Faulty cell production in the skin causes dermatitis and changes in the lips and tongue. Vitamin B12 deficiency also might result in hypotension (low blood pressure).

ALZHEIMER'S DISEASE. Patients with Alzheimer's disease, a chronic and progressive brain disorder associated with memory loss, confusion, and nerve damage, also have low blood levels of vitamin B12. Whether the low vitamin levels are a cause or a result of the disease is unclear. Vitamin B12 deficiency is commonly found with dementia, a deterioration of intellectual faculties. Supplementation might improve mental functions if a deficiency is present, and in a few cases results in a complete cure.

ANEMIA. The classic deficiency symptom of vitamin B12 is either pernicious anemia or megaloblastic (macrocytic) anemia. As with iron deficiency anemia, both of these forms of anemia start with fatigue and poor concentration; however, under the microscope the red blood cells are larger, more fragile, and fewer in number than the small, pale red blood cells seen in iron deficiency samples. Macrocytic means "large cell." The condition is called pernicious anemia when the cause is a lack of intrinsic factor; it is called megaloblastic or macrocytic anemia when poor dietary intake of vitamin B12 is the cause.

DIABETES. The symptoms of vitamin B12 deficiency and the nerve disorders associated with diabetes are similar. Possible disturbances in vitamin B12 metabolism might be associated with diabetic neuropathy.

The body's ability to conserve and store the vitamin combined with minimal daily needs means that a deficiency takes years to develop. Deficiency more often results from poor absorption than from dietary lack. Vitamin B12 deficiency is usually found in mid to later life when the production of intrinsic factor declines, and injections or large oral doses of vitamin B12 are often necessary to correct the problem. Strict vegetarians—people who do not consume any foods of animal origin—and their children whose diets are composed entirely of breastmilk are at risk for vitamin B12 deficiency. Other vegetarian diets that contain milk, yogurt, cheese, or eggs supply adequate amounts of the vitamin. Dietary deficiency and low blood vitamin B12 levels are reported in several groups, including seniors and vegetarians. Although anemia is the classic symptom, low blood levels indicative of poor status are common despite the absence of anemia.

Daily Recommended Intake

The daily need for vitamin B12 is minimal, but essential. A diet that contains four or more servings a day of foods from animal origin contains between 7mcg and 30mcg of vitamin B12, or three to ten times the adult RDA.

The 1989 RDAs for vitamin B12 are:

	Vitamin B12 (mcg)
INFANTS	
0 to 0.5 year	0.3
0.5 to 1 year	0.5
CHILDREN	
1 to 3 years	0.7
4 to 6 years	1.0
7 to 10 years	1.4
YOUNG ADULTS AND ADULTS	
11+ years	2.0
Pregnant	2.2
Lactating	2.1

Sources in the Diet

Foods of animal origin or fermented vegetables, such as the fermented soybean product called miso, are the only sources of vitamin B12. The vitamin is produced only by bacteria and is not a natural component of plants. Vitamin B12 produced by bacteria in the intestines of animals is also absorbed. Extra-lean meats, poultry, fish, shellfish, milk, organ meats, cheese, and eggs are excellent dietary sources of the vitamin. Some of the vitamin is lost when food is cooked to temperatures above 100° C (Table 12).

Table 12
THE VITAMIN B12 CONTENT OF SELECTED FOODS

Food	Amount	Vitamin B12 (mcg)
Liver, beef	3 ounces	68.0
Clams, canned	½ cup	19.1
Oysters, canned	3½ ounces	18.0
Tuna	2 ounces	1.32
Yogurt	1 cup	1.06
Milk, nonfat	1 cup	.95
Halibut	3 ounces	.85
Egg	1 large	.77
Chicken	3 ounces	.36
Cheese, cheddar	1 ounce	.23

Toxicity

There are no known toxic effects in adults when the vitamin is consumed in amounts several times the RDA.

Nutrient-Nutrient Interactions

- Calcium is necessary for normal absorption of vitamin B12.
- A deficiency of either iron or vitamin B6 decreases the absorption of vitamin B12.
- A high intake of folic acid can mask the anemia caused by vitamin B12 deficiency.
- Vitamin E deficiency might impair the conversion of vitamin B12 to its active form.
- A deficiency of vitamin B6 results in reduced absorption and low blood and liver concentrations of vitamin B12.

FOLIC ACID (FOLACIN)

Overview

In 1941, a substance extracted from spinach leaves and named folic acid from the Latin word "folium" for leaf was found to be effective in the treatment of anemia. Folic acid, also called folacin, is a family of water-soluble compounds. The vitamin is absorbed from the small intestine and small amounts are stored in the liver and other tissues. Excess is excreted in the urine.

Functions

The main function of folic acid is to maintain the cells' genetic code and regulate cell division and the transfer of inherited traits from one cell to another. It is essential for the normal growth and maintenance of all cells. Folic acid is also involved in the production of neurotransmitters, such as serotonin, that regulate mood, sleep, and appetite.

NEURAL TUBE DEFECTS (NTD). Maternal folic acid intake is essential in preventing neural tube defects in infants. These defects occur within the first few weeks after conception (often before the mother even knows she is pregnant) when the tube that should eventually become the baby's spinal cord and brain does not close properly, leaving an open seam. If the opening occurs in the spine, the baby is born with a portion of the spinal cord exposed or, less commonly, covered only with skin. This neural tube defect is called spina bifida. If the open seam occurs at the top of the neural tube, as is the case with anencephalic babies, the brain never develops and the baby dies within a few hours of birth. Folic acid, either in food or supplements in doses of 400mcg to 800mcg (women with a history of NTD should take up to 4mg of folic acid daily) reduces the risk of NTD by up to 60 percent, especially if intake is optimal prior to and during the first trimester of pregnancy. Some studies indicate that folic acid also improves the birth weight and neurological development of newborns.

Deficiency

A deficiency of folic acid limits cell function and affects the growth and repair of all cells and tissues in the body. The tissues that have the fastest rate of cell replacement are affected first, including red blood cells, the digestive tract, the cervix and vagina, and the skin. Some studies show a link between low folic acid intake and increases in homocysteine levels, a risk factor for heart disease.

Symptoms of folic acid deficiency are macrocytic (megaloblastic) anemia, poor growth, digestive disorders, impaired nutrient absorption and malnutrition, diarrhea, loss of appetite, weight loss, weakness, apathy, sore tongue, headaches, heart palpitations, irritability, and behavioral disorders. Folic acid deficiency is common in patients, especially the elderly, suffering from depression and schizophrenia; folic acid supplementation daily might alleviate the symptoms of these psychiatric disorders.

CANCER. A folic acid deficiency causes damage to cells that resembles the initial stage of cancer and preliminary research shows low intake of folic acid might increase a woman's risk for developing cervical cancer. Women who take folic acid supplements show less precancerous cervical tissue as compared to women who consume a diet low in the vitamin. Folic acid might prevent the transformation of abnormal cells to cancer cells and might return damaged tissue to a healthy condition.

Folic acid is one of the most common vitamin deficiencies. Surveys show that the folic acid content of the American diet is half the recommended dietary intake. Stressful situations, including disease, alcohol consumption, tobacco use, and chronic use of medication add to the risk of developing a deficiency by increasing daily needs for the vitamin or reducing the absorption of the vitamin. There is some evidence that a high consumption of caffeinated beverages might increase folic acid-related chromosomal damage. Many major categories of drugs, including birth control pills, aspirin, and anticonvulsants, can produce a folic acid deficiency. A deficiency can develop within a few weeks to months of low dietary intake.

Daily Recommended Intake

Information on folic acid needs is limited and the latest RDAs are only estimates based on assumptions that adults require about 100mcg to 200mcg to maintain normal body functions and that approximately 25 percent to 50 percent of dietary intake is absorbed. RDAs for infants and children are based on body weight and the folic acid content of breastmilk. The small amount of folic acid stored in the liver is not adequate to meet the additional needs imposed by pregnancy, stress, lactation, ingestion of certain medications, or alcohol abuse. More information is necessary to determine more precise amounts of folic acid required for different age and sex groups. Previous RDA levels for folic acid were 400mcg and currently, the U.S. Public Health Service recommends this level of folic acid intake for all women from puberty to menopause.

The folic acid allowances in the 1989 edition of the RDAs are much lower than previous recommendations. Studies repeatedly showed that diets did not meet the previous allowances of 400mcg for adults to 800mcg for pregnant women, so the 1989 allowances were reduced based on the amount typically consumed by adults who show no clinical signs of deficiency. However, the new RDAs remain controversial as they do not consider marginal or subclinical status, the link between folic acid and neural tube defects, or the association between folic acid and the possible development of cancer. References in this book to the RDAs for folic acid refer to previous recommendations for higher intakes than the latest 1989 allowances.

The 1989 RDAs compared to previous RDAs for folic acid:

	Previous RDAs	1989 RDAs
INFANTS		
0 to 0.5 year	30	25
0.5 to 1 year	34	35
CHILDREN		
1 to 3 years	100	50
4 to 6 years	200	75
7 to 10 years	300	100
11 to 14 years	400	150
ADULTS		
Males, 15+ years	400	200
Females, 15+ years	400	180
Pregnant	800	400
Lactating	500	260–280

Sources in the Diet

The best dietary sources of folic acid are brewer's (nutritional) yeast, dark green leafy vegetables, and liver. Orange juice, avocado, beets, and broccoli are also good sources. Whereas romaine lettuce and other leaf lettuce are good sources, iceberg or head lettuce contains minimal amounts of folic acid.

The vitamin is easily lost when foods are improperly stored for too long or at too warm a temperature or are overcooked or reheated. The vitamin is also lost when the cooking water is discarded. Salads that contain dark green or leaf lettuce should be consumed daily to ensure adequate folic acid intake (Table 13).

Table 13
THE FOLIC ACID CONTENT OF SELECTED FOODS

Food	Amount	Folic Acid (mcg)
Brewer's (nutritional) yeast	1 tbsp	313
Liver, beef	3 ounces	123
Spinach, raw	1 cup	106
Spinach, cooked	½ cup	82
Orange juice	6 ounces	102
Lettuce, romaine	1 cup	98
Lettuce, iceberg	1 cup	0–20
Beets, cooked	½ cup	66

Table 13 (cont.)
THE FOLIC ACID CONTENT OF SELECTED FOODS

Food	Amount	Folic Acid (mcg)
Avocado	½ medium	59Broccoli, cooked
½ cup	44	
Wheat germ	2 tbsp	40
Beans, red, cooked	½ cup	34
Banana	1 medium	33
Brussels sprout, cooked	½ cup	28
Bread, whole wheat	1 slice	16
Bread, white	1 slice	10

Toxicity

Folic acid works closely with vitamin B12 in the maintenance and replication of the genetic code within each cell and the two vitamins share similar symptoms of deficiency. A diet high in folic acid or supplementation with the vitamin can cure the symptoms of anemia, but folic acid is ineffective against the more serious nerve damage that results from a vitamin B12 deficiency. Thus, folic acid could mask a vitamin B12 deficiency and nerve problems could progress undetected to irreversible stages. However, these cases are rare and usually result from very high supplemental doses of folic acid, i.e., 4mg. The amount of folic acid in vitamin preparations is limited by law to 400mcg for adults and 800mcg for pregnant women, as a precaution against this interaction between folic acid and vitamin B12.

Large doses of folic acid should not be taken unless the possibility of vitamin B12 deficiency has been first ruled out. A simple blood test would not be sufficient as the red blood cells will appear normal if folic acid intake is adequate. Strict vegetarians who consume large amounts of folic acid-rich foods and little or no vitamin B12 are at particular risk.

No toxic effects are known for folic acid even when doses 1,000 times the RDA are consumed; however, the vitamin might interfere with the effectiveness of anticonvulsant medications.

Nutrient-Nutrient Interactions

- Folic acid requires vitamin B12, niacin, and vitamin C to be converted to its biologically active form.
- Folic acid can mask an underlying vitamin B12 deficiency.

BIOTIN (VITAMIN B7)

Overview

The history of biotin is unique because this B vitamin was discovered several times and acquired several names prior to its final identification. It was originally discovered in 1901 and named "bios." Another group of researchers isolated a substance many years later that they called coenzyme R, and yet another group of investigators discovered "protective factor X" and "vitamin H." Eventually bios, biotin, coenzyme R, protective factor X, and vitamin H were identified as the same substance.

Biotin is water-soluble, absorbed in the small intestine, and excesses are excreted in the urine. Significant amounts are produced by bacteria in the intestines and are probably available for absorption as more biotin is excreted in the urine than is consumed in the diet.

Functions

Biotin is essential for numerous body processes that manufacture and break down fats, amino acids, and carbohydrates. The vitamin works closely with folic acid, pantothenic acid, and vitamin B12, and also might minimize the symptoms of a zinc deficiency.

Deficiency

A biotin deficiency is rare, even when a person consumes a diet low in the B vitamin. However, long-term consumption of large doses of raw egg whites, more than 15 to 20 raw eggs a day, can result in biotin deficiency. A protein in raw egg white called avidin binds to biotin in the intestine and prevents its absorption. Avidin is deactivated by cooking. An occasional raw egg in the diet will not produce a biotin deficiency.

Infants might develop deficiency symptoms from poor absorption of the vitamin. Some hospitalized patients on formulated tube or intravenous feedings also have developed a biotin deficiency. Symptoms include dermatitis, depression, conjunctivitis, progressive hair loss and color, elevated blood levels of cholesterol, anemia, loss of appetite, tingling and numbness in the hands and feet, nausea, lethargy, muscle pain, and enlargement of the liver.

Long-term use of antibiotics interferes with the production of biotin in the intestine and might increase the risk for deficiency.

Oxytetracycline and sulfonamides are two antibiotics that specifically reduce the growth of intestinal bacteria that produce biotin.

Daily Recommended Intake

The biotin content of the average American diet is estimated to be between 28mcg to 42mcg each day. Dietary intake combined with bacterial production in the intestine apparently is adequate to prevent deficiency symptoms.

The 1989 Safe and Adequate Intakes for biotin are:

	Biotin (mcg)
INFANTS	
0 to 0.5 year	10
0.5 to 1 year	15
CHILDREN AND ADULTS	
1 to 3 years	20
4 to 6 years	25
7 to 10 years	30
11+ years	30-100

Sources in the Diet

Good sources of biotin are organ meats such as kidney and liver, oatmeal, egg yolk, soybeans, cereals, clams, mushrooms, bananas, peanuts, and brewer's (nutritional) yeast (Table 14).

Table 14
THE BIOTIN CONTENT OF SELECTED FOODS

Food	Amount	Biotin (mcg)
Brewer's (nutritional) yeast	3$\frac{1}{2}$ ounces	85
Liver, beef	3 ounces	82
Almonds	1 ounce	23
Soybeans, cooked	$\frac{1}{2}$ cup	22
Clams, canned	$\frac{1}{2}$ cup	20
Peanut butter	2 tbsp	12
Egg, cooked	1 large	11
Salmon	3 ounces	10
Oat bran	$\frac{1}{3}$ cup	10

Table 14 (cont.)
THE BIOTIN CONTENT OF SELECTED FOODS

Food	Amount	Biotin (mcg)
Milk	1 cup	10
Oatmeal, cooked	1 cup	9
Rice, brown, cooked	½ cup	9
Chicken	3 ounces	9
Mushrooms, canned	½ cup	7
Banana	1 medium	6
Rice, white, cooked	½ cup	4

Toxicity

Biotin has no known toxic effects.

Nutrient-Nutrient Interactions

- Biotin works closely with folic acid, pantothenic acid, and vitamin B12.
- Biotin lessens the symptoms of a pantothenic acid and a zinc deficiency.

PANTOTHENIC ACID
(CALCIUM PANTOTHENATE, VITAMIN B3)

Overview

Pantothenic acid is a B vitamin named after the Greek word pantos, meaning "everywhere." The name reflects the vitamin's widespread appearance in plants and animals. Pantothenic acid is available commercially as calcium pantothenate. The B vitamin is water-soluble, absorbed from the intestine, and excesses are excreted in the urine. The body has a limited ability to store the vitamin.

Functions

Pantothenic acid is said to function at the "crossroads of metabolism." The vitamin is converted to a substance called coenzyme A, an important catalyst in the breakdown of fats, carbohydrates, and protein for energy. Pantothenic acid also functions in the production of fats, cholesterol, bile, vitamin D, red blood cells, and some hormones and neurotransmitters. The vitamin prevents graying of hair in some animals and stimulates wound healing.

Deficiency

A deficiency of pantothenic acid has not been reported in humans. A deficiency can be induced in laboratory animals and in volunteer subjects fed a highly refined synthetic diet complete in all nutrients except pantothenic acid and also given a medication that depletes the tissues of the vitamin. Under these severe conditions, animals and humans show a variety of symptoms including fatigue, cardiovascular and digestive problems, upper respiratory infections, dermatitis, burning sensations, lack of coordination, staggering gait, restlessness, and muscle cramps. Additional symptoms include irritability, poor wound healing, loss of appetite, indigestion, fainting, rapid pulse, increased susceptibility to infection, depression, and numbness and tingling in the hands and feet.

Daily Recommended Intake

The pantothenic acid content of the average American diet is between 4 and 10mg a day. This amount is assumed to be sufficient as no deficiency has been reported. Bacterial synthesis of the vitamin in the intestine that is available for absorption might be another source. Stressful situations, such as pregnancy and lactation, increase daily needs. However, there is not enough information to establish a specific recommended allowance for this B vitamin.

The 1989 Safe and Adequate Intakes for pantothenic acid are:

	Pantothenic Acid (mg)
INFANTS	
0 to 0.5 year	2
0.5 to 1 year	3
CHILDREN AND ADULTS	
4 to 6 years	3–4
7 to 10 years	4–5
11+ years	4–7

Sources in the Diet

Pantothenic acid is found in a wide variety of foods including liver, fish, chicken, cheese, whole grain breads and cereals, avocados, cauliflower, green peas, cooked dried beans and peas, nuts, dates, and potatoes. Significant amounts of pantothenic acid are lost in the milling and refining of grains. As this vitamin is not added in the "enrichment" process, refined flour, breads, rice, and noodles are a poor source of pantothenic acid. As much as 50 percent of the pantothenic acid is lost in the thawing and cooking of meat (Table 15).

Table 15
The Pantothenic Acid Content of Selected Foods

Food	Amount	Pantothenic Acid (mg)
Liver, beef	3 ounces	6.035
Egg	1 medium	1.100
Avocado	½ medium	1.100
Mushrooms, canned	½ cup	1.000
Milk	1 cup	.984
Chicken	3 ounces	.765
Soybeans, cooked	½ cup	.525
Peanut butter	2 tbsp	.476
Banana	1 medium	.450
Orange	1 medium	.450
Collard greens, cooked	½ cup	.425
Potato	1 medium	.400
Broccoli, cooked	½ cup	.315
Rice, brown, cooked	½ cup	.300
Rice, white, cooked	½ cup	.150
Cantaloupe	¼ melon	.300
Bread, whole wheat	1 slice	.184
Bread, white	1 slice	.092
Wheat germ	1 tbsp	.132

Toxicity

Large doses of pantothenic acid can be consumed with no serious toxic effects other than diarrhea. There is no known benefit to taking large doses of the vitamin other than a possible slight improvement in athletic performance.

Nutrient-Nutrient Interactions

- Pantothenic acid works with vitamin B1, vitamin B2, niacin, vitamin B6, and biotin in the breakdown of carbohydrates, protein, and fats for energy.
- Pantothenic acid is necessary for the production of vitamin D.
- Biotin lessens the symptoms of a pantothenic acid deficiency.

VITAMIN C
(L-ASCORBIC ACID, L-DEHYDROASCORBIC ACID)

Overview

Vitamin C cures the oldest known nutrient-deficiency disease: scurvy. In fact, ascorbic is the Latin word for "without scurvy." Prior to the discovery of vitamin C, scurvy was responsible for the death of one-half to two-thirds of the crew on prolonged ocean voyages where the diet consisted solely of cereals and meat. James Lind's recommendation to include limes or lemons (rich sources of vitamin C) in the daily menu was ignored at first by the British Navy, but eventually became the source of the nickname for British sailors—"limeys."

Vitamin C is a water-soluble vitamin that is easily absorbed in the intestine. Excesses of vitamin C are excreted in the urine. Humans are one of the few species that cannot manufacture vitamin C and must depend on the diet as their only source of the vitamin.

Functions

Vitamin C functions in the formation and maintenance of collagen, a protein that forms the basis for the most abundant tissue in the body: connective tissue. The shape and function of all tissues depend on collagen, which acts as a cementing substance between cells. Collagen is found in bones, the cornea of the eye, teeth, tendons, skin, and other tissues; is the supporting material in blood vessel walls; maintains the shape of the discs of the backbone; allows joints to move; and binds muscle cells together. Collagen, and therefore vitamin C, promotes the healing of wounds, bone fractures, bruises, hemorrhages, and bleeding gums; and forms a protective barrier between infections or disease and the surrounding healthy tissues.

ALLERGY. Vitamin C might reduce the bronchial constriction and impaired breathing that results from allergic reactions. The vitamin might improve lung function and white blood cell function, while decreasing hypersensitivity reactions and respiratory infections common in asthma and allergies. However, the research is contradictory for this role and recommendations cannot be made at this time.

ANTIOXIDANT. As the body's number one water-soluble antioxidant, vitamin C protects the watery areas of the body, such as the blood and the fluid inside and surrounding cells. It also possibly helps protect LDL cholesterol from damage caused by reactive oxygen fragments and other free radicals. Vitamin C also might reduce tissue damage associated with premature aging, cancer, heart disease, and rheumatoid arthritis.

BLOOD PRESSURE. Vitamin C might lower blood pressure in both mild hypertension (high blood pressure) and normal blood pressure. Vitamin C also might prevent, and even help treat, high blood pressure, a risk factor for heart disease and stroke.

CANCER. Vitamin C protects against cancer cell growth by destroying free radicals. The vitamin also inhibits the formation of potent cancer-causing substances called nitrosamines that are formed when nitrites, added to processed meats and found naturally in some foods, combine with other compounds in the stomach. A high intake of vitamin C might protect against the development or progression of oral, stomach, lung, cervical, rectal, liver, and esophageal cancers. The link between vitamin C and breast cancer remains controversial.

A study at the Department of Radiation Medicine, Massachusetts General Hospital in Boston indicates that cancer patients can withstand greater exposure to radiation treatment without increased side effects if they are first supplemented with high doses of vitamin C. (See page 187 for more information on vitamin C and cancer.)

CATARACTS. Vitamin C might inhibit the progression and encourage the regression of some types of cataracts in the eyes.

DIABETES. Adequate intake and maintenance of high blood levels of vitamin C might help regulate blood sugar. Low vitamin C levels in white blood cells are found in diabetics, indicating suppressed immunity.

FERTILITY. Limited evidence shows that vitamin C might improve male fertility by increasing sperm count and viability.

HEART DISEASE. Vitamin C helps regulate cholesterol production in the liver and conversion of cholesterol to bile for excretion. It also lowers

total blood cholesterol and LDL-cholesterol and increases HDL-cholesterol. These improvements are most often seen in individuals with
high cholesterol levels and/or a low tissue concentration of the vitamin. Vitamin C also maintains blood vessel walls; increases the production of prostacyclin, a prostaglandin that inhibits the clumping of
blood platelets and dilates blood vessels; and reduces risk for developing heart disease, atherosclerosis, and stroke. (See pages 195–196 for
more information on vitamin C and heart disease.)

IMMUNITY. Optimal intake of vitamin C might increase resistance to
colds and infection, especially during times of stress, such as vigorous exercise. Although vitamin C might not prevent infection, optimal intake of the vitamin at the first sign of infection might reduce
the severity and duration of a cold. (See pages 155–156 for more
information on vitamin C and immunity.)

SKIN PROTECTION. A vitamin C-rich diet or topical application of the
vitamin might protect against sun-induced damage to the skin associated with premature aging and skin cancer.

STRESS. Vitamin C is important in the formation of the stress hormones produced in the adrenal glands. Vitamin C is depleted from
these tissues and urinary excretion of the vitamin increases during
times of stress, which suggests an increased need for vitamin C during stressful times. Vitamin C also might benefit athletic performance by lowering working heart rate and the release of cortisol (a
stress hormone released from the adrenal glands).

Deficiency

The major symptoms of scurvy result from vitamin C's role in the formation of collagen. Poorly formed collagen results in small, pinpoint
hemorrhages under the skin; poor wound healing or breakdown of
old scars; spongy, bleeding gums; dry, scaly skin; damage to blood
vessels; swollen, tender joints and aching bones; gangrene; muscle
cramps; and loosened teeth. General weakness and lethargy, loss of
appetite, depression, swollen legs and arms, and shortness of breath
also are symptoms of scurvy.

Stomach disorders, such as gastritis and skin problems associated
with rheumatoid arthritis, might result from poor vitamin C intake.
Low intake of vitamin C can result in delayed healing, reduced resistance to colds and infections, and increased susceptibility to disease.

Severe vitamin C deficiency and scurvy are rare in the United
States; however, marginal deficiencies and poor dietary intake of vit-

amin C are common. Most large-scale national nutrition surveys in the United States report inadequate intake of vitamin C. Alcohol and tobacco, stress, limited food intake and poor intake of fruits and vegetables, chronic illness, and long-term use of some medications contribute to vitamin C deficiency. Bottle-fed infants should be given a vitamin C supplement or given vitamin C-rich fruit juice within the first six months; breastmilk contains adequate amounts of the vitamin if the mother's diet is adequate.

Daily Recommended Intake

Scurvy is prevented when the dietary intake of vitamin C is approximately 10mg a day. Tissue stores are saturated at 100mg to 120mg a day and the antioxidant functions of vitamin C are enhanced at intakes of 150mg or more, the potential total body pool is at least 1,500mg. Daily needs increase above the adult RDA during physical and emotional stress such as fever, infection, elevated environmental temperatures, or burns; illness such as congestive heart failure, kidney and liver disease, gastrointestinal disturbances, and cancer; alcohol and tobacco use; or use of medications such as birth control pills.

The 1989 RDAs acknowledge the negative effect tobacco use has on vitamin C status and recommend that people who use tobacco consume at least 100mg of vitamin C each day. However, several studies report that an even higher vitamin C intake, i.e., at least 200mg, is needed to maintain normal vitamin C levels and counteract some of the harmful effects of cigarette smoking.

The 1989 RDAs for vitamin C are:

	Vitamin C (mg)
INFANTS	
0.0 to 0.5 year	30
0.5 to 1.0 year	35
CHILDREN	
1 to 3 years	40
4 to 10 years	45
11 to 14 years	50
YOUNG ADULTS AND ADULTS	
15+ years	60
Pregnant	70
Lactating, 1st 6 mo.	95
Lactating, 2nd 6 mo.	90

Sources in the Diet

The best sources of vitamin C are fresh fruits and vegetables. Poor sources of vitamin C include milk, meat, eggs, poultry, fish, cereals and bread, and nuts. Freezing has little effect on vitamin C content, so frozen vegetables are an excellent source of the vitamin. Some vitamin C is lost when fruits and vegetables are heated during the canning process and more vitamin C is lost if canning water is discarded.

The vitamin is easily lost when foods are handled or prepared improperly. Aging, bruising, storing at temperatures above 40° F, overwashing, cooking too long, discarding cooking water, and reheating or holding foods at room temperature or higher destroys the vitamin. Baking soda added to vegetables to retain their color destroys vitamin C. Slicing or chopping vegetables exposes a greater surface area to air and light and more of the vitamin is lost. For example, French fries contain less vitamin C than a baked potato and vegetables cut and exposed to air at a salad bar lose substantial amounts of vitamin C.

To maximize vitamin C intake, purchase only the amount of food that can be used within a few days. Fruits and vegetables should be sun-ripened, chilled and used immediately after picking, eaten raw or cooked for a short time in a minimum amount of water, and only enough should be cooked for immediate consumption (Table 16).

Table 16
THE VITAMIN C CONTENT OF SELECTED FOODS

Food	Amount	Vitamin C (mg)
Orange juice	6 ounces	90
Brussels sprouts	¹/₂ cup	68
Strawberries	¹/₂ cup	66
Orange	1 medium	66
Broccoli	¹/₂ cup	52
Collard greens	¹/₂ cup	44
Cantaloupe	¹/₄	32
Tomato juice	6 ounces	30
Cabbage	¹/₂ cup	24
Asparagus	¹/₂ cup	19
Green peas	¹/₂ cup	17
Potato	1 small	15
Lima beans	¹/₂ cup	15
Pineapple	¹/₂ cup	15
French fried potatoes	8	10
Mashed potatoes	¹/₂ cup	10
Corn on the cob	1 small	7
Banana	1 medium	6
Carrots	¹/₂ cup	5

Toxicity

Vitamin C is water-soluble and, since excesses are excreted in the urine, large amounts of the vitamin can be consumed without risk for toxicity. However, some toxic effects might be experienced when doses greater than one gram are consumed regularly. Megadoses of vitamin C might reduce the absorption or utilization of selenium and copper and might produce a conditioning effect that results in mild, temporary symptoms of deficiency when supplementation is stopped. Vitamin C might aggravate kidney stone formation, but only in patients with kidney disease. Excess intake of vitamin C might give a false positive test for diabetes and interfere with test results for hemoglobin. Mega-doses of vitamin C can cause nausea, stomach cramping, diarrhea, vomiting, and increased susceptibility to colds and infections, especially in children.

Nutrient-Nutrient Interactions

- Vitamin C is necessary for the conversion of folic acid to its potent or biologically active form.
- Vitamin C is important in the conversion of tryptophan to the hormone-like substance serotonin, which regulates sleep, pain, depression, and other behaviors.
- A deficiency of vitamin C is associated with increased urinary excretion of vitamin B6 and a vitamin B6 deficiency results in low blood levels of vitamin C.
- Vitamin C enhances the absorption of iron when both are consumed in the same meal.
- Vitamin C has a protective function against the toxic effects of cadmium.
- Toxic symptoms caused by high doses of copper, vanadium, cobalt, mercury, and selenium are reduced by vitamin C.
- Large doses of vitamin C might lower blood levels of copper and selenium.
- Calcium or manganese supplementation might decrease urinary excretion of vitamin C.
- Vitamin C supplementation might increase absorption of manganese.

VITAMIN-LIKE FACTORS (PHYTOCHEMICALS, CHOLINE, INOSITOL, LIPOIC ACID, UBIQUINONE)

Several naturally-occurring substances in foods have been investigated for their use in the body. Some have no known functions. Others are essential to animals but do not appear to be necessary for humans. Still others are necessary for health but are manufactured in the body and dietary requirements, if any, are unknown.

Phytochemicals

Phytochemicals (phyto is the Greek word for "plant") are plants' natural protection against disease, sun damage, fungus, and bugs. Many of these chemicals also reduce disease risk and stimulate immunity in people. Every carrot stick, every sprig of parsley, every spear of broccoli is literally a bumper crop of disease-preventing chemicals.

Take for example the bioflavonoids, including rutin, the flavonones—herperidins, erioctrin, naringen, and naringenin; the flavones; and the flavonols. These phytochemicals, which are found in citrus fruits, vegetables, and tea, reduce blood clots associated with stroke and inhibit the oxidation of LDL that turns harmless cholesterol in the blood into the sticky glue that clogs artery walls. They also stimulate the immune system, have antioxidant capabilities, and might strengthen blood vessel walls. In fact, the low incidence of heart disease in France might be caused by the high bioflavonoid content of the red wine consumed in that country.

Other phytochemicals in vegetables prevent or slow cancer growth. Broccoli is rich in sulforaphane—a compound that extradites cancer-causing compounds from cells and is linked to a reduced risk for breast cancer. Tomatoes contain three chemicals— p-coumaric acid, lycopene, and chloragenic acid—that prevent the formation of carcinogens. Cabbage is loaded with phenethyl isothiocyanate (PEITC) that inhibits the growth of lung cancer. Ellagic acid in strawberries and grapes neutralizes carcinogens that otherwise attack the cells' DNA and initiate abnormal cell growth. Genistein in soybeans discourage the initiation and progression of cancer. The hundreds of carotenoids, of which beta carotene is only one, also have anti-cancer capabilities. The list is endless and is growing almost daily as researchers uncover more about these non-nutrients.

Other phytochemicals might protect us against heart disease. Phytosterols, including beta sitosterol, stigmasterol, and campesterol, are found in wheatgerm, seeds, nuts, and legumes. These compounds are plants' equivalent to cholesterol, except they reduce, rather than promote, colon cancer risk and possibly heart disease. Plant sterols or other phytochemicals may be the reason why blood cholesterol levels drop 40 percent in animals fed diets high in mushrooms.

While a clove of garlic supplies next to nothing when it comes to vitamins and minerals, it is a phytochemical gold mine. From its sulfur-containing compounds such as allicin and ajoene to the saponins and phenolic compounds, garlic has been linked to the prevention of cancer, heart disease, the common cold, and more. Thirty phyto- chemicals alone have been isolated that help prevent cancer.

In short, the health-enhancing effects of the phytochemicals are one of the best arguments in favor of food over supplements, since only wholesome, minimally processed foods, especially fresh fruits, vegetables, whole grains, and legumes, supply these compounds in the proper ratio and amounts.

Choline

Choline is an essential nutrient for some animals and recent evidence shows it might be essential for brain development, liver function, and the prevention of cancer in humans. The human body can make choline with the help of vitamin B12, folic acid, and an amino acid called methionine, although not always in sufficient amounts to meet daily needs.

Choline functions in the production and transportation of fats from the liver and thus aids in the prevention of fat accumulation in this organ. Choline is also used in the formation of phospholipids, such as lecithin, and in the structure of cell membranes. As a compo- nent of the nerve chemical acetylcholine, choline is necessary for normal nerve and brain function. Levels of this nerve regulator increase in proportion to dietary intake of choline. Pharmacological doses of choline have been experimentally used with varying success in the treatment of Huntington's disease, tardive dyskinesia, disor- ders of the nervous system such as Alzheimer's disease related to low levels of acetylcholine in brain or nerve tissue, learning disabilities, impaired language development, and delays in motor function.

No recommended daily intakes or toxicity levels have been estab- lished for choline. The average daily diet supplies between 400 and 900mg of choline. This amount is apparently adequate to maintain health, but should not be considered a dietary requirement. However, as people cut back on their consumption of eggs in an effort to lower cholesterol intake, they also have significantly reduced their intake of choline. Unless other dietary sources of this compound are found, marginal intake could result. Deficiency symptoms might develop when intake falls below 500mg daily.

The best dietary sources of choline are eggs, liver and other organ meats, extra-lean meat, brewer's (nutritional) yeast, wheatgerm, soy- beans, peanuts, and green peas. Supplemental lecithin capsules and granules contain approximately 35 percent choline, as phosphatidyl- choline (Table 17).

Table 17
THE CHOLINE CONTENT OF SELECTED FOODS

Food	Amount	Choline (mg)
Brewer's (nutritional)		
yeast	3½ ounces	275.0
Egg	1 large	238.4
Egg, yolk	1 large	238.0
Egg nog	1 cup	48.0
Milkshake	1 cup	30

Inositol

Inositol was a recognized component of food for years before it was accepted as a vitamin in 1940. Its status, however, is controversial. The body and intestinal bacteria can make inositol, but whether or not synthesis meets daily needs is unclear.

Inositol is found in the brain and nerve, muscle, skeletal, reproductive, and heart tissues. It is a component of cell membranes and functions in nerve transmission and the regulation of certain enzymes. It also might function in the manufacture, transportation, and function of fats.

Inositol deficiency in animals produces fat accumulation in the liver, nerve disorders similar to those observed in diabetics, and intestinal problems. Inositol might have a therapeutic function in the treatment of nerve disorders associated with diabetes. The metabolism of inositol is altered in chronic renal failure and multiple sclerosis, but increased dietary intake has not proven beneficial. Claims that inositol cures baldness were based on a few animal studies and have no relevance to hereditary hair loss in humans.

No deficiency or toxicity has been identified for inositol and this is unlikely as the substance is found in a variety of foods. Dietary intake averages approximately 1,000mg a day. Inositol also is added to infant non-cow's milk formulas as a preventive measure.

Lipoic Acid

Lipoic acid is a fat-soluble compound produced in the body and not considered a dietary essential for health. It is not a vitamin. Lipoic acid works with vitamin B1, vitamin B2, niacin, and pantothenic acid in the breakdown of carbohydrates, protein, and fats for energy. Dietary sources include liver and brewer's (nutritional) yeast.

Ubiquinone (Coenzyme Q)

Ubiquinone is named for its ubiquitous (widespread) distribution in plants and animals. It is a fat-soluble substance produced in the body and present in all cells, where it functions in the production of energy from carbohydrates. Ubiquinone is an antioxidant that protects the blood vessels from oxidative damage and the heart and brain from damage caused by ischemia (reduced blood supply).

Ubiquinone chemically resembles vitamin E, but possesses only 20 percent of the antioxidant activity of its vitamin counterpart. Despite its relatively low antioxidant potency, ubiquinone shows protective capabilities for the heart and blood vessels. Low levels of this compound are found in patients suffering from congestive heart failure, while increased concentrations of ubiquinone reduce the damage to the heart and brain caused by limited or blocked oxygen supply.

Apparently, damaged tissue with high levels of free radicals acts as a chemical messenger to encourage the formation of antioxidants, such as ubiquinone. Consequently the increased concentration of antioxidants in the tissue helps counteract free-radical activity and reduce the severity of further damage. Tissue levels of ubiquinone decrease with age and sedentary lifestyle, which supports the free-radical theory of aging; while longevity and aerobic exercise is associated with increased tissue levels of this compound.

Ubiquinone concentrations in the tissue can be increased by supplementation. In addition, oral intake of this compound inhibits the synthesis of cholesterol in the liver, thus potentially reducing blood cholesterol levels and the risk of developing atherosclerosis. One study showed supplementation with ubiquinone in glaucoma patients reduced the cardiovascular side effects without interfering with the lowering of pressure within the eye of the beta-blocker medications. However, ubiquinone is not a vitamin and no deficiencies or toxicities have been identified.

NON-VITAMINS (LAETRILE, PANGAMIC ACID)

Laetrile

A biochemist named Ernst Krebs announced in 1952 he had developed a new drug that cured cancer. He called the drug laetrile and a few years later reclassified it as a vitamin (vitamin B17). Krebs and his son produced and promoted the substance as a cancer preventative and cure, and claimed the Food and Drug Administration (FDA) and the medical association had joined efforts to keep the public away from this wonder drug.

Laetrile, or amygdalin, is obtained from apricot pits or almond kernels. Extensive testing of laetrile by the National Cancer Institute and other reputable organizations has found no benefits from its use in cancer prevention or treatment. In addition, laetrile does not meet the criteria to be called a vitamin as it has no known metabolic function and its removal from the diet does not produce deficiency symptoms. Laetrile contains 6 percent cyanide, is highly toxic, and potentially lethal. However, laetrile's greatest harm is that people with potentially curable cancer abandon conventional treatments and take laetrile until it is too late to benefit from effective therapy.

Pangamic Acid

Pangamic acid mistakenly has been called a vitamin (vitamin B15). This substance is not essential to health, nor has a need, deficiency, or level of safe consumption been identified. Pangamic acid falsely has been credited with numerous functions. Claims are unfounded that pangamic acid will cure fatigue, cancer, alcoholism, schizophrenia, heart disease, aging, senility, diabetes, hypertension, glaucoma, drug addiction, cirrhosis, hepatitis, jaundice, dermatitis, sciatica, brain dysfunction, autism, gangrene, sexual problems, or allergies.

Pangamic acid was originally obtained from apricot pits, but commercial products can contain anything. Analysis of pangamic acid samples reveals a variety of ingredients and no products sold commercially have been found by the Food and Drug Administration (FDA) to contain the substance alleged to be the original formula. The term vitamin B15 is meaningless and is used to describe anything the manufacturer wishes to include in the product.

CHAPTER 4

The Minerals

The human body reduced to its simplest form is a small pile of ashes. The carbon, hydrogen, oxygen, and nitrogen from protein-rich tissues and carbohydrate or fat stores have dissolved into the air or evaporated as water leaving only the minerals. These ashes, weighing approximately five pounds, might be small in size, but they play vital roles in all body tissues.

Minerals are involved in a variety of functions. They provide structure to bones and participate in muscle contraction, blood formation, building protein, energy production, and numerous other body processes. Some minerals, such as sodium, potassium, and calcium, have electrical "charges" that act something like a magnet to attach to other electrically charged substances and form complex molecules, conduct electrical impulses along nerves, or transport substances in and out of the cells.

In the blood and other fluids, minerals regulate the pH balance of the body and the fluid pressure between cells and the blood. Minerals also bind to proteins and other organic substances and are found in red blood cells, all cell membranes, hormones, and enzymes—the catalysts of all bodily processes.

There are 22 minerals essential to human health and these nutrients are divided into two categories: major minerals and trace minerals. Major minerals are present in the body in amounts greater than a teaspoon, while a trace mineral totals less than a teaspoon. The terms "major" and "trace" do not reflect the importance of a mineral in maintaining optimal health, as a deficiency of either major or trace minerals produces equally harmful effects.

The major minerals include the following:

calcium	potassium
chloride	sodium
magnesium	sulfur
phosphorus	

The trace minerals include:

boron	molybdenum
chromium	nickel
cobalt	selenium
copper	silicon
fluoride	tin
iodine	vanadium
iron	zinc
manganese	

There are also trace amounts of aluminum, arsenic, barium, bismuth, bromine, cadmium, gallium, gold, lithium, silver, strontium, and other minerals in the body, but little is known about how, or if, these minerals affect health and maintenance of normal bodily processes.

In this chapter, the minerals are discussed individually, but should not be considered separate with respect to their absorption, function, or requirements. Minerals work either together or against each other. Some minerals compete for absorption, so a large intake of one mineral can produce a deficiency of another. This is especially true of the trace minerals, such as copper, iron, and zinc. In other cases, some minerals enhance the absorption of other minerals. For example, the proper proportion of calcium, magnesium, and phosphorus in the diet enhances the absorption and use of all three minerals. Absorption is also dependent on body needs; a person who is deficient in a mineral will absorb more of it than someone who is adequately nourished.

BORON

Overview

Boron was discovered in the early 1900s and has been considered an essential trace mineral for plants since the early 1920s. Evidence of an essential role in humans was first identified in the mid-1980s.

Functions

Boron apparently is essential for normal calcium and bone metabolism and, therefore, might prevent bone loss associated with osteoporosis. The potential effects boron might have on the development of muscle mass and male hormone levels remains controversial.

Deficiency

Poor dietary intake of boron causes bone changes similar to those noted in osteoporotic women. Boron deficiency results in decreased blood levels of ionized calcium and calcitonin, elevated levels of total calcium and urinary excretion of calcium, and in animals causes depressed growth rates.

Boron and magnesium metabolism also might be related, since a combined deficiency of these two minerals exacerbates the osteoporotic condition, suppresses bone anabolism, and results in decreased magnesium concentrations in bone. In contrast, boron supplementation elevates serum concentrations of beta-estradiol and testosterone and produces changes consistent with the prevention of calcium loss and bone demineralization.

Daily Recommended Intake

The information on boron is limited and no dietary recommendations have been established. Current intakes range from 1.5 to 7mg, but whether these intakes are optimal is unknown. Studies showing benefits in the prevention of osteoporosis have used 3mg of boron.

Sources in the Diet

Good dietary sources of boron include fresh fruits and vegetables, and nuts. Meat and fish are poor sources.

Toxicity

Excessive intake of boron, i.e., 150mg per liter of water or more, can cause nausea, diarrhea, skin rashes, and fatigue. Limited research on animals shows that excessive boron intake also might suppress growth and immunity.

Nutrient-Nutrient Interactions

- Boron works with calcium, magnesium, and vitamin D in bone metabolism, growth, and development.

CALCIUM

Overview

Calcium is the most abundant mineral and the fifth most abundant substance in the body after carbon, hydrogen, oxygen, and nitrogen. The average healthy male body contains about two to three pounds of calcium; the average healthy female body contains approximately two pounds. Of this calcium, 99 percent is located in the bones and teeth. The other 1 percent is in the blood and other body fluids and within all cells where it aids in the regulation of numerous body processes.

The mineral is absorbed in the small intestine with the help of vitamin D. Between 10 percent and 40 percent of dietary intake is absorbed, although women after menopause absorb as little as 7 percent of dietary intake. More calcium is absorbed when a person is deficient in the mineral; when intake is marginal; or when lactose (milk sugar) and adequate, but not excessive, amounts of protein, magnesium, phosphorus, and vitamin D are present.

Calcium absorption is reduced with excessive intake of substances called oxalates and phytates that are found in foods such as spinach and unleavened whole wheat products; intake of alcohol, coffee, sugar, or drugs such as tetracycline, diuretics, and aluminum-containing antacids; or stress. People who exercise infrequently or who are bedridden absorb less and excrete more calcium and are more prone to bone disorders than are active people.

Functions

BONES AND TEETH. The primary function of calcium is in the development and maintenance of healthy bones and teeth. A constant supply of the mineral is required throughout life, especially during periods of growth, such as childhood, pregnancy, and lactation.

Calcium is found in two different forms in the bones. One form of calcium is bound tightly within the bone and is not easily removed. A second form of calcium can be easily removed from bone to aid in maintaining normal blood calcium levels. This exchangeable portion of calcium is a reserve that builds up when the diet is adequate in calcium. Calcium is removed from the less mobile portion of bone only when the calcium reserves are exhausted and dietary intake is poor. This can result in osteoporosis.

As with most tissues, bones are constantly being reformed. They are not static tissue. Throughout life, bones lose and gain calcium daily, which results in constant "remodeling" of bone tissue. In children, the gain in calcium outweighs the loss, and bone tissue increases in size and hardness. In later years or when dietary intake is poor, calcium loss might outweigh calcium gain and the bones become less dense and more susceptible to fracture. In the healthy adult who consumes an optimal diet, the process of bone mainte-nance is in balance with approximately equal amounts of calcium entering and leaving the bones each day. The "wives' tale" that a woman loses a tooth for each child is not true, as little calcium is lost from teeth even during times of calcium deprivation.

BLOOD CLOTTING. Calcium is necessary for the normal blood clotting mechanisms that begin the process of wound healing.

BLOOD PRESSURE. Adequate intake of calcium helps maintain normal blood pressure. In countries where the intake of calcium-rich milk products is high, the incidence of hypertension is low. Calcium sup-plementation aids in the maintenance of normal blood pressure and increased calcium intake helps lower blood pressure in hyperten-sives. (See page 244 for more information on calcium and hyperten-sion.)

CANCER. Calcium and vitamin D might offer some protection against cancer of the colon. People with colon cancer consume less calcium and vitamin D compared to cancer-free persons. Low intake of cal-cium and vitamin D might increase the risk of developing breast can-cer; however, this research is limited and inconclusive.

DIABETES. Many diabetics have increased levels of calcium in many of their tissues. These elevated levels might disturb the metabolism of calcium and its interaction with body processes. Complications com-mon in diabetes, such as heart disease and cataracts, might be related to abnormal calcium metabolism.

ENZYMES AND HORMONES. Calcium is essential for the production and activity of numerous enzymes and hormones that regulate digestion, energy and fat metabolism, and the production of saliva.

HEART DISEASE. Increased calcium intake, whether from supplements or from fermented milk products such as yogurt, might lower blood cholesterol levels and reduce the risk for developing premature heart disease. The balance between calcium and magnesium is important in the prevention of heart disease. Heart disease rates increase when too much calcium is consumed in relation to magnesium.

MEMBRANES. Calcium aids in the transport of nutrients and other substances across cell membranes. The mineral also helps maintain all cell membranes and aids in the maintenance of connective tissue, the "glue" that holds body cells together.

MUSCLE CONTRACTION. Calcium and magnesium work together in the normal contraction of muscles, including the heartbeat. The normal balance between calcium, sodium, potassium, and magnesium maintains muscle tone.

NERVE TRANSMISSION. Calcium is essential for normal transmission of electrical impulses along nerves. The nerves become hypersensitive when blood calcium levels drop below normal and tetany (painful spasms of the muscles) can result. Calcium also aids in the release of neurotransmitters, the chemicals that transmit messages from one nerve cell to another.

PERIODONTAL DISEASE. Diseases of the gums are called periodontal diseases. Calcium supplementation or increased dietary intake of the mineral to 1,000 to 2,000mg a day might reduce the incidence and progression of periodontal disorders. In contrast, a diet low in calcium might encourage the development of periodontal disease.

Deficiency

HYPERTENSION. Abnormally low levels of calcium inside and outside cells, reduced intake of calcium, and a low ratio of calcium to sodium are linked to increased risk for developing high blood pressure (hypertension). Increased intake of the mineral often alleviates or improves the condition.

OSTEOPOROSIS. Osteoporosis is the classic deficiency symptom of prolonged poor intake of calcium. Inadequate intake of calcium results in removal of calcium from the bone ("osteo" means bone, "porosis" means porous). The first bones to be affected are the backbone and jaw. (See page 266 for more information on calcium and osteoporosis.)

TETANY. Very low levels of calcium in the blood can increase the sensitivity of the nerves and result in muscle spasms such as leg cramps, a condition called tetany. Pregnant women who consume inadequate calcium or excess phosphorus are at greatest risk for developing tetany.

Daily Recommended Intake

Establishment of a Recommended Dietary Allowance is difficult as people can adapt to a wide range of calcium intakes. Some people in other parts of the world consume 200mg of calcium daily and appear healthy. In the United States, the current adult RDA of 800mg might not be adequate to prevent osteoporosis and evidence suggests that daily intakes should be increased to 1,000 to 1,200mg for premenopausal women and 1,500 to 1,700mg for postmenopausal women not taking estrogen. The daily need for calcium also increases to at least 1,200mg during pregnancy and lactation. Calcium intake above the RDA during periods of rapid growth i.e. childhood, adolescence, and even young adulthood increases bone mass and reduces the risk of osteoporosis later in life.

The 1989 RDAs for calcium are:

	Calcium (mg)
INFANTS	
0 to 0.5 year	400
0.5 to 1 year	600
CHILDREN AND ADULTS	
1 to 10 years	800
11 to 24 years	1,200
25+ years	800
Pregnant	1,200
Lactating	1,200

Sources in the Diet

Milk products, such as low-fat and nonfat milk, low-fat cheese, and low-fat yogurt are good dietary sources of calcium. They also contain lactose or milk sugar, which improves calcium absorption. Vitamin

D-fortified milk is the only reliable dietary source of vitamin D, a nutrient essential for calcium absorption. Fatty selections within the dairy group, such as butter, sour cream, and cream cheese, are poor sources of calcium. Other good sources include dark green leafy vegetables, broccoli, canned fish with the bones, cottage cheese, and cooked dried beans and peas (Table 18).

Table 18
THE CALCIUM CONTENT OF SELECTED FOODS

Food	Amount	Calcium(mg)
Yogurt, plain	1 cup	415
Sardines	3 ounces	372
Milk, nonfat	1 cup	302
Milk, nonfat, instant	$^1/_3$ cup	279
Cheese, cheddar	1 ounce	204
Salmon, canned with bones	3 ounces	167
Tofu	1 cake	154
Cottage cheese, uncreamed	1 cup	146
Oysters	$^1/_2$ cup	113
Mustard greens, cooked	$^1/_2$ cup	97
Orange	1 medium	54
Broccoli, cooked	$^1/_2$ cup	50
Navy beans, cooked	$^1/_2$ cup	48
Apricots, dried	$^1/_2$ cup	44
Whole wheat bread	1 slice	24

Toxicity

Excessive intake of calcium, more than several grams each day, might raise blood levels of calcium above the normal range and increase the risk for calcium deposition into soft tissues, such as the kidneys or heart. However, research does not support the theory that calcium causes kidney stones. Large intakes of calcium might reduce zinc and iron absorption, impair vitamin K metabolism, and encourage loss of calcium from bone.

In regards to calcium supplements, a recent study found that "natural" calcium supplements, such as oyster shell and bone meal sources, often contain lead at levels exceeding the amount considered safe for children. Lead exposure can result in lower IQs and impaired nervous system development in young children. Other supplemental sources, such as calcium carbonate or calcium citrate, are safer, less toxic sources of the mineral.

Nutrient-Nutrient Interactions

- Calcium, magnesium, zinc, fluoride, and phosphorus work together in the formation and maintenance of bones and teeth.
- The ratios of calcium to phosphorus and calcium to magnesium are important in the absorption, use, and excretion of these minerals.
- Calcium requires vitamin D for absorption; consequently, a vitamin D deficiency results in reduced calcium absorption.
- Calcium competes with zinc, manganese, magnesium, copper, and iron for absorption in the intestine, and a high intake of any one of these minerals could reduce the absorption of the others.
- Calcium might counteract the effects of sodium chloride in the development of hypertension. The interaction of calcium with other electrolytes, such as sodium, potassium, and magnesium, can affect blood pressure.
- Heart disease rates increase when too much calcium in relation to magnesium is consumed.
- Calcium absorption is reduced in the presence of excess dietary protein, fat, or phosphorus.
- While calcium usually reduces aluminum and lead absorption, calcium citrate might increase aluminum absorption from dietary sources.

CHROMIUM

Overview

The average body contains about 600mcg of chromium with the highest concentration occurring during infancy.

Functions

BLOOD SUGAR. The main function of chromium is as a component of glucose tolerance factor (GTF), a substance that works with insulin to facilitate the uptake of blood sugar (glucose) into the cells. Chromium maintains normal blood sugar levels by regulating insulin; consequently, optimal chromium intake reduces the amount of insulin needed to sustain normal blood sugar. The chromium-insulin combination also stimulates the synthesis of protein.

HEART DISEASE. Optimal chromium intake might help protect against heart attack in high-risk populations, such as diabetics and patients with atherosclerosis. Chromium improves the blood fat profile by reducing total blood cholesterol and LDL cholesterol and increasing HDL cholesterol levels. Whether or not chromium supplementation can reverse atherosclerosis is unknown.

WEIGHT LOSS. Chromium, as supplemental chromium picolinate, might increase lean body mass and decrease body fat and weight. However, additional research is needed to confirm these preliminary results.

Deficiency

DIABETES. Poor dietary intake of chromium might contribute to maturity-onset diabetes by impairing GTF function and increasing insulin levels. Elevated insulin levels, in turn, increase urinary loss of chromium, exacerbating the chromium deficiency and contributing to the development of diabetes. Chromium supplementation might prevent diabetes by improving glucose tolerance, reducing insulin levels, and decreasing the amount of insulin needed to maintain normal blood sugar levels. The greatest benefit from supplementation is seen in the most severely deficient individuals; chromium does not improve glucose and insulin function in individuals well-nourished in the nutrient.

Other symptoms of chromium deficiency also resemble diabetes. In both conditions, the person experiences numbness and tingling in the toes and fingers, an increase in blood sugar, nerve disorders in the arms and legs, glucose intolerance, and reduced muscle coordination. In many people, these symptoms disappear when chromium intake is increased. (See pages 210–211 for more information on chromium and diabetes.)

HYPOGLYCEMIA. Hypoglycemia is the opposite of diabetes. Instead of the elevated blood sugar (hyperglycemia) characteristic of diabetes, hypoglycemics experience low blood sugar. Hypoglycemia is not a disease, but a symptom of an abnormality in the body's use of sugar and is found in diabetes as well as other conditions. Reactive hypoglycemia occurs after consumption of a meal high in carbohydrates when blood sugar drops below normal levels as a result of insulin. Limited evidence shows that supplementation with 200mcg of chromium might improve the symptoms of hypoglycemia in some persons.

HEART DISEASE. Poor dietary intake of chromium might be associated with elevated blood cholesterol levels and increased risk for developing heart disease. (See page 197 for more information on chromium and heart disease.)

In the United States, blood and tissue levels of chromium decrease as a person ages; at the same time, the risk for developing diabetes and heart disease increases. In contrast, people in non-industrialized countries have chromium levels two to three times higher than most Americans, their chromium status does not decline with age, and these degenerative diseases are infrequent to nonexistent.

As many as 90 percent of all American diets are low in chromium. Even well-designed diets contain only 25mcg/1,000 calories. At this level of intake, it would take 8,000 calories each day to obtain the upper dietary limit considered safe and adequate. A person who consumes 2,000 calories or less, or who consumes a diet high in refined white breads and rice and processed or convenience foods, and low in whole grain breads and cereals and other nutrient-dense foods would not meet even the lower level of intake for chromium. In addition, a diet that contains high amounts of sugar or strenuous exercises increases urinary loss of chromium and might contribute to a chromium deficiency.

Daily Recommended Intake

There is limited information on chromium requirements for humans.
The 1989 Safe and Adequate Ranges for chromium are:

	Chromium (mcg)
INFANTS	
0 to 0.5 year	10–40
0.5 to 1 year	20–60
CHILDREN	
1 to 3 years	20–80
4 to 6 years	30–120
Children and Adults 7+ years	50–200

Sources in the Diet

The best dietary source of chromium is brewer's (nutritional) yeast grown on a chromium-rich medium. Other good sources include whole grain breads and cereals, pork kidney, molasses, extra-lean meats, cheeses, spices, and herbs (Table 19). Little information exists on the chromium content of vegetables. Refined and processed foods are low in the mineral.

Cooking acidic foods in stainless steel cookware such as a steel wok or cast iron pan causes chromium to leach into the food and provides a source of dietary chromium. Hard tap water can supply between 1 percent and 70 percent of the daily intake. Inorganic chromium, such as chromic chloride, is not as well absorbed as the form of chromium found in foods, nutritional yeast, and supplemental chromium picolinate.

Table 19
THE CHROMIUM CONTENT OF SELECTED FOODS

Food	Amount	Chromium(mcg)
Brewer's (nutritional) yeast	1 ounce	168
Corn on the cob	1 ear	52
Beef, round, cooked	3½ ounces	44
Buckwheat, raw	½ cup	38
Apple	1 medium	36
Sweet potato	1 medium	36
Egg	1 medium	26
Tomato	1 medium	24
American cheese	1 slice	14
All bran cereal	1 cup	14
Mozzarella cheese	1 ounce	11
Puffed rice cereal	1 cup	10
Orange juice	1 cup	9.6
Cheddar cheese	1 ounce	9
Molasses	2 tbsp	4.4
Whole wheat cereal, raw	1 cup	3
Wheat germ	2 tbsp	1.4
Sugar	2 tbsp	0

Toxicity

Excess intake or tissue accumulation of chromium can inhibit, rather than enhance, the effectiveness of insulin. At very high levels, chromium might encourage the growth of cancer.

Nutrient-Nutrient Interactions

- Chromium combines with the B vitamin niacin to form glucose tolerance factor (GTF).
- Diets high in simple sugars increase the loss of chromium.

COBALT

Functions

The only known function of cobalt is as a constituent of vitamin B12. In this capacity, cobalt aids in the formation of normal red blood cells, maintenance of nerve tissue, and normal formation of cells.

Deficiency

A deficiency of cobalt is equivalent to a deficiency of vitamin B12 and can cause anemia, nerve disorders, and abnormalities in cell formation. Strict vegetarians who do not consume foods of animal origin can develop vitamin B12 and cobalt deficiencies within three to six years of poor dietary intake.

Daily Recommended Intake

The dietary intake of cobalt is based on the body's need for vitamin B12, or 2mcg of vitamin B12 each day. There is no known need for cobalt alone. There are no RDAs or Estimated Safe and Adequate ranges for cobalt.

Sources in the Diet

Information is limited on the dietary sources of cobalt as consumption of the mineral alone is thought to be of little importance. Organ meats, such as liver and kidneys, oysters, and clams are excellent sources of cobalt and muscle meats are good dietary sources because these foods supply the mineral as part of vitamin B12. Vegetables, fruits, and other foods of plant origin contain cobalt, but as these sources do not provide the mineral as part of vitamin B12 it is of little use.

Toxicity

Toxicity is rare; however, large doses of inorganic cobalt (cobalt not combined with vitamin B12) might stimulate thyroid and bone marrow function, resulting in excess production of red blood cells (polycythemia). Cobalt is used as an anti-foaming agent in the processing of some beer. Consumption of large amounts of this beer could cause polycythemia and heart disorders.

Nutrient-Nutrient Interactions

See the section on vitamin B12, page 61.

COPPER

Overview

This essential trace mineral is found in all tissues, but is most concentrated in the brain, heart, kidney, and liver. The copper concentration in bones and muscles is moderate to low, but because these tissues comprise a large portion of the body, one-half of the total copper content of the body is found here. Only about 30 percent of dietary intake is absorbed.

Functions

Copper facilitates the activity of several enzymes and in this capacity is involved in the development and maintenance of the cardiovascular system, including the heart, arteries, and other blood vessels, the skeletal system, and the structure and function of the nervous system, including the brain. Copper helps maintain myelin, the insulating sheath that surrounds nerve cells and aids in nerve transmission, and helps regulate neurotransmitter levels in the brain. Copper also is important in the development and maintenance of red blood cells (and their protein hemoglobin) and normal hair and skin color.

Copper is a component of the antioxidant enzyme superoxide dismutase and might protect cell membranes from potential damage by highly reactive oxygen fragments. In this antioxidant role, copper might function to prevent the development of cancer; however, the link between copper and cancer remains unclear. (See pages 150–153 for more information on antioxidants.)

Copper releases iron from storage and increases the intestinal absorption of iron, aids in the formation of connective tissue, breaks down fats in fat tissue, and is necessary for the normal functioning of insulin. Copper also aids in the conversion of dietary protein, carbohydrate, and fat to energy; and contributes to the synthesis of hormone-like compounds called prostaglandins that regulate a variety of body functions including heartbeat, blood pressure, and wound healing.

HEART DISEASE. How copper affects heart disease risk is controversial. Some research shows that adequate intake of copper decreases heart attack risk, while diets low in copper might increase heart attack risk factors such as blood clot formation, weakened connective tissue in the heart, and increased cholesterol levels. On the other hand, some studies report that patients with heart disease have higher blood levels of copper than healthy people. Elevated copper levels might promote heart disease by increasing the damaging oxidation of LDL cholesterol and decreasing the effectiveness of the antioxidant selenium. Consequently, copper may be an example of how delicate the balance is between too little and too much when it comes to minerals.

Deficiency

A clinical deficiency of copper is rare, but has been observed in children with severe protein malnutrition, chronic diarrhea or other malabsorption problems, or iron-deficiency anemia. Marginal copper deficiencies might be more common and are found in patients consuming hospital diets. Copper is stored in the liver, so a deficiency develops slowly even in the presence of a low-copper diet. Because copper is necessary for the normal development and maintenance of blood, bone, nerves, connective tissue, and other tissues, a deficiency of this essential trace mineral can cause a variety of disorders.

ANEMIA. As blood levels of copper drop, iron absorption also decreases, red blood cell production is inhibited, and anemia develops. Supplementation with both iron and copper is required in the treatment of this form of anemia.

HAIR AND SKIN. A copper deficiency causes loss of color from the skin and hair. This results from poor formation of melanin, the copper-dependent pigment that gives color to hair and contributes to a suntan.

HEART DISEASE. Copper deficiency causes extensive damage to the heart and arteries, abnormal electrocardiograms, increased risk of heart attack, and is associated with high blood pressure and the formation of blood clots. (See page 197 for more information on copper and heart disease.)

MENKES' SYNDROME. Menkes' syndrome is a genetic defect in copper absorption. Infants show stunted growth, defective skin pigmentation, kinky or steely hair, abnormal development of the arteries and bones, and progressive mental deterioration. Premature death is typical.

NERVOUS SYSTEM. Impaired energy production and reduced enzyme activity that results from a copper deficiency interferes with the proper functioning of the central nervous system. This impairment causes poor concentration, numbness and tingling, and a variety of nervous system disorders.

RESISTANCE TO INFECTION. A low copper intake can result in a reduction in white blood cells and increased susceptibility to colds, infections, and disease. The ratio of zinc intake to copper intake also influences the immune system and resistance to infection; a person is more susceptible to disease when copper intake is high and zinc intake is low.

SCOLIOSIS. Scoliosis is a condition that can strike young people, especially girls, and women. It results in defects in muscular growth, connective tissue formation, and skeletal development. The cause of scoliosis has not been determined. Studies on skeletal defects in animals show a relationship between the severity of spinal abnormalities and the degree of dietary copper restriction; an increased intake of copper reduces the risk for developing scoliosis.

Copper might aid in the treatment of scoliosis by its role in the development of connective tissue that provides the framework for normal bone development. This preliminary information does not prove that copper deficiency causes scoliosis, but does suggest that diet plays a role in the development of the disorder.

TISSUE FORMATION. A copper deficiency results in poor formation of collagen, the protein component of connective tissue. Connective tissue provides the framework for numerous other tissues and faulty formation results in bone deformities, damaged blood vessels, reduced resiliency of skin and other internal and external linings of the body, and heart failure.

Daily Recommended Intake

Typical diets in the United States provide between 0.8mg and 3.0mg of copper daily.

The 1989 Safe and Adequate Ranges for copper are:

	Copper (mg)
INFANTS	
0 to 0.5 year	0.4–0.6
0.5 to 1 year	0.6–0.7
CHILDREN	
1 to 3 years	0.7–1.0
4 to 6 years	1.0–1.5
7 to 10 years	1.0–2.0
11+ years	1.5–2.5
ADULTS	1.5–3.0

Sources in the Diet

Copper is found in a wide variety of unprocessed foods including whole grain breads and cereals, shellfish, nuts, organ meats, poultry, cooked dried beans and peas, and dark green leafy vegetables (Table 20). Milk and milk products are poor sources of the mineral. Drinking water that runs through copper pipes can contribute substantial amounts of the mineral to the diet.

Table 20
THE COPPER CONTENT OF SELECTED FOODS

Food	Amount	Copper (mg)
Oysters	6 medium	14.2
Lobster	1 cup	2.45
Liver, cooked	3 ounces	2.4
Avocado	1 half	0.5
Potato, baked	1 medium	0.36
Soybeans, cooked	½ cup	0.3
Banana	1 medium	0.26
Fish, cooked	3 ounces	0.16
Chicken, meat only	3½ ounces	0.14
Spinach, cooked	½ cup	0.13
Peas, green, cooked	½ cup	0.12
Bread, whole wheat	1 slice	0.06
Carrots, cooked	½ cup	0.06
Cheddar cheese	1 ounce	0.03
Cottage cheese	½ cup	0.01

Toxicity

Copper toxicity is rare. Patients with ulcerative colitis might accumulate copper in the tissues. This excess of copper might aggravate the symptoms of the intestinal disorder, including impaired healing and reduced resistance to infection. Daily intakes of more than 20mg can cause nausea and vomiting. Some research shows an increased risk of heart disease when copper levels in drinking water are high.

Wilson's disease is an inherited disorder characterized by excessive accumulation of copper in the tissues, liver disease, mental retardation, tremor, and loss of coordination. Copper deposits in the cornea of the eye produce an apparently harmless ring configuration. Treatment of Wilson's disease includes a low-copper diet and the medication penicillamine that binds to copper and increases its excretion.

Nutrient-Nutrient Interactions

- The balance between iron, zinc, and copper is important in the absorption and use of both minerals. Excessive intake of one mineral might result in a secondary deficiency of the other nutrient, or increased risk for developing heart disease, high blood pressure, increased susceptibility to infection, or a variety of disorders.
- Cadmium, molybdenum, and sulfate alter copper absorption.
- Copper facilitates the absorption and use of iron.
- Excessive calcium intake inhibits the absorption of copper.
- Blood levels of copper are elevated when there is a niacin deficiency, although the significance of this association is unknown.
- Copper and vitamin C work together in the formation of collagen.

THE ELECTROLYTES: SODIUM, POTASSIUM, AND CHLORIDE

Overview

Sodium, potassium, and chloride are so closely related in the body that they should be discussed together. These three elements are distributed throughout all body fluids, including the blood, lymph, the fluid between cells, and the fluid within each cell (intracellular fluid). Sodium and chloride are primarily found in fluids that surround cells and potassium is primarily found in fluids within cells. They are called "the electrolytes" because they carry an electrical charge when dissolved in body fluids and, thus, help regulate nerve transmission and many cell membrane functions.

The blood and other fluids require a narrow range of sodium concentration. When a person consumes a salty meal, the blood concentration of sodium increases, which stimulates thirst and more water is consumed to dilute the blood back to normal sodium levels. The extra water and sodium are then excreted by the kidneys. Water retention in many cases is a result of not drinking enough water to allow the kidneys to excrete excess fluid and sodium.

The blood becomes too diluted if blood levels of sodium drop and water is replaced without sodium, the lack of sodium outside the cells (extracellular) allows water to move from the blood into the cells. Symptoms of water intoxication develop, such as headache, muscular weakness, and poor memory.

Functions

Sodium, potassium, and chloride function to maintain the normal balance and distribution of fluids throughout the body. They also function in the maintenance of the normal pH balance, and with calcium and magnesium in the maintenance of normal muscle contraction and relaxation, and nerve transmission.

Sodium contributes to hypertension by raising blood pressure. "Salt-sensitive" people (30 percent of the general population and 40 percent to 50 percent of hypertensives) can reduce their blood pressure and risk of hypertension by restricting sodium intake.

Potassium also helps prevent and treat hypertension by regulating normal blood pressure, maintaining proper calcium balance, and minimizing the pressure-raising effects of a sodium-rich diet. Inadequate potassium intake increases blood pressure in those with normal and borderline hypertensive blood pressure. An increase of potassium-rich foods in the diets of hypertensives reduces blood pressure and often lessens the need for antihypertensive medications.

The ratio of potassium to sodium also might be important in the development of hypertension. An increase in potassium and a decrease in sodium in the American diet might provide the proper ratio between these two elements that would prevent hypertension.

In addition to its role in blood pressure regulation, potassium is important in the regulation of the heartbeat. The reduction in blood levels of potassium and abnormal blood sugar levels characteristic of people on very-low-calorie diets might be alleviated with potassium supplements.

Chloride is a component of hydrochloric acid or stomach acid and so aids in the digestion of foods. Excessive vomiting causes loss of chloride from the stomach, which upsets the pH balance of the body, causing a range of disorders from dehydration to coma.

A chlorine compound is used to kill harmful bacteria in public water supplies that would otherwise spread disease. The addition of chlorine to water is an important public health measure and has eliminated numerous waterborne diseases, such as typhoid fever. The related compound, chloride, in the diet is harmless.

Deficiency

SODIUM. Sodium deficiency is uncommon and usually is a result of starvation or severe fasting, vomiting, perspiration, or diarrhea. In the rare occurrence of sodium deficiency, fluids move from the blood into the cells, which results in muscle weakness and twitching, poor concentration and memory loss, dehydration, and loss of appetite. A liter of perspiration contains only one gram of sodium. Therefore, it is much more important to replace fluids than to take sodium tablets when dehydrated, as more water than sodium is lost in perspiration.

POTASSIUM. Potassium deficiency can occur with chronic diarrhea, vomiting, diabetic acidosis, kidney disease, or prolonged use of laxatives or diuretics. Symptoms of a potassium deficiency include slowed growth, bone fragility, paralysis, sterility, muscle weakness, mental apathy and confusion, kidney damage, and damage to the heart.

Sudden death that can occur during fasting, anorexia nervosa, or starvation is often a result of heart failure caused by potassium deficiency. Dehydration is dangerous because the potassium deficiency that occurs numbs the person's desire for water. Excessive use of laxatives and diuretics, vomiting and diarrhea, or chronic low intake of water combined with profuse perspiration can lead to dehydration and potassium deficiency.

CHLORIDE. A chloride deficiency upsets the body's pH balance, called alkalosis. This imbalance between acid and alkaline produces vomiting, sweating, and diarrhea. Other symptoms of chloride deficiency include muscle weakness, loss of appetite, lethargy, and, in infants, "failure to thrive." Deficiency is uncommon as the element is consumed in salt (sodium chloride).

Daily Recommended Intake

SODIUM. Sodium intake reflects habit, taste, and custom, not need. A daily intake of between 200mg and 500mg maintains fluid balance in the body; however, daily sodium intakes vary between 2,300mg and 20,000mg. No RDA has been established for sodium. In general, sodium intake should be reduced to no more than 2,000mg a day, the equivalent of one teaspoon of salt.

The 1989 Estimated Minimum Requirements of Healthy People for sodium are:

	Sodium (mg)
INFANTS	
0.0 to 0.5 year	120
0.5 to 1 year	200
CHILDREN AND ADULTS	
1 year	225
2 to 5 years	300
6 to 9 years	400
10+ years	500

POTASSIUM. The typical adult intake of potassium is between 800mg and 1,500mg.

The 1989 Estimated Minimum Requirements of Healthy People for potassium are:

	Potassium (mg)
INFANTS	
0.0 to 0.5 year	500
0.5 to 1 year	700
CHILDREN AND ADULTS	
1 year	1,000
2 to 5 years	1,400
6 to 9 years	1,600
10+ years	2,000

CHLORIDE. Interest in the nutritional requirements of chloride have been minimal because the element is so easily obtained from the diet.

The 1989 Estimated Minimum Requirements of Healthy People for chloride are:

	Chloride (mg)
INFANTS	
0.0 to 0.5 year	180
0.5 to 1 year	300
CHILDREN AND ADULTS	
1 year	350
2 to 5 years	500
6 to 9 years	600
10+ years	750

Sources in the Diet

SODIUM AND CHLORIDE. Sodium and chloride are in most foods, but by far the largest amounts are in table salt. A pinch of salt contains 267mg of sodium; a teaspoon of salt sprinkled on a meal provides more than 2,000mg of sodium. Processed and convenience foods, olives, pickles, sauerkraut, catsup, sandwich meats, beef broth, soy sauce, baking powder, monosodium glutamate (MSG), and numerous food additives contain large amounts of sodium (Table 21). Meat, chicken, fish, grains, vegetables, fruits, nuts, milk and milk products, and seeds contain moderate amounts of sodium and chloride. A diet of unprocessed, natural foods with no added salt would provide more than the daily recommendation for sodium and chloride.

POTASSIUM. Potassium is found in a variety of foods including fruits, vegetables, meat, milk, and grains. Extra-lean meats contain 300 to 500mg of potassium per serving. Potatoes, avocados, bananas, apricots, orange juice, and other dried or fresh fruits or cooked dried beans and peas are excellent sources of potassium (Table 21).

Table 21
THE SODIUM AND POTASSIUM CONTENTS OF SELECTED FOODS

Food	Amount	Sodium(mg)	Potassium(mg)
Asparagus	5 spears	2	278
Avocado	½ medium	4	604
Bacon	2 slices	440	90
Banana	1 medium	2	550

Table 21 (cont.)
THE SODIUM AND POTASSIUM CONTENTS OF SELECTED FOODS

Food	Amount	Sodium(mg)	Potassium(mg)
Beans, red cooked	²/₃ cup	3	340
Beef broth	1 serving	784	107
Bouillon	1 cube	960	0
Bread, whole wheat	1 slice	121	63
Cantaloupe	¹/₄ melon	12	251
Carrots, raw	1 large	47	341
Cheeseburger	1	823	303
Crackers, saltines	2	66	7
Egg	1 medium	59	62
Fish, no added salt	3 ounce	70	380
French Fries, no added salt	Small order	170	361
Ham, cured	3 ounces	860	332
Lettuce, romaine	3 ¹/₂ ounces	9	264
Meat, poultry,	3 ounces	100	221
Milk, nonfat	1 cup	128	408
Olives	2 large	150	5
Orange	1 medium	2	300
Peanuts, roasted	2¹/₂ ounces	2	740
Peanuts, salted	2¹/₂ ounces	460	700
Peas, fresh	¹/₂ cup	9	380
Peas, frozen	¹/₂ cup	100	160
Peas, canned	¹/₂ cup	230	180
Pickles	1 large	1,428	200
Pie, apple	1 piece	482	128
Potato, baked	medium	6	755
butter	2 tsp	81	2
salt	1 tsp	2,000	0
Pudding, chocolate	¹/₂ cup	161	168
Salad dressing	1 tbsp	120	5
Soup, freeze-dried	1 pkg	1,350	131
Soup, creamed, canned	1 cup	996	166
Soup, chicken (low-sodium)	1 cup	48	149
Soup, chicken	1 cup	754	40

Toxicity

SODIUM. Diets in the United States contain excessive amounts of sodium—as much as 15 times the recommended daily intake. A diet high in sodium is linked to hypertension, and restriction of sodium lowers blood pressure in many people with hypertension. There are no known benefits to excessive sodium intake and consumption of a low-sodium diet throughout life is not only harmless, but might prevent the development of hypertension.

POTASSIUM. Dietary intake of potassium in excess of 18,000mg can cause high concentrations of the element in the blood, disturbances in heart and kidney function, and alterations in fluid balance. Blood levels of potassium can escalate as a result of excessive intake of salt substitutes that contain potassium, kidney failure, acidosis, major infections, hemorrhages in the gastrointestinal tract, and severe breakdown of muscle.

Nutrient-Nutrient Interactions

- Potassium supplementation in patients with hypertension might increase magnesium requirements. Potassium levels decrease in response to a magnesium deficiency, while adequate magnesium levels help maintain potassium balance.
- Sodium's effect on raising blood pressure intensifies when calcium intake is low.
- Sodium increases and potassium decreases urinary loss of calcium.

FLUORIDE

Overview

The average body contains approximately 2.6 grams of fluoride, and the largest accumulation is in the bones and teeth.

Functions

DENTAL. The main function of fluoride is to protect developing and mature teeth from decay. One milligram of fluoride for every liter of water (1 part fluoride for every million parts water or 1ppm) reduces dental cavities by 70 percent. Fluoride's effects are especially pronounced if fluoride ingestion is started during the early years when teeth are still forming.

BONE. Bones are more stable and resistant to degeneration and osteoporosis when the diet is adequate in fluoride. Some elderly patients show a reduction in urinary excretion of calcium, improved bone strength, and a reduction in the symptoms of osteoporosis when their intake of fluoride is adequate. However, fluoride supplementation might increase the number of hairline fractures in bone, and the use of this mineral in the treatment of osteoporosis remains controversial.

Fluoride also might aid in wound healing and enhance iron absorption.

Deficiency

DENTAL. The incidence of dental caries is high in areas of the United States where the water is not fluoridated and fluoride intake is low.

Daily Recommended Intake

No RDAs have been established for fluoride. However, it is recommended that water supplies be fortified with the mineral to a level of 1ppm to provide an adult with 1.5 to 4.0mg daily. The average daily intake of fluoride is between 0.2mg and 4.4mg.

The 1989 Estimated Safe and Adequate Ranges for fluoride are:

	Fluoride (mg)
INFANTS	
0 to 0.5 year	0.1–0.5
0.5 to 1 year	0.2–1.0
CHILDREN AND ADOLESCENTS	
1 to 3 years	0.5–1.5
4 to 6 years	1.0–2.5
7+ years	1.5–2.5
Adults	1.5–4.0

Sources in the Diet

The best dietary source of fluoride is fluoridated water. The fluoride content of food depends on the fluoride content of the soil in which the food is grown. Other sources of fluoride include unintentional ingestion of fluoridated toothpaste or use of fluoridated water in food processing. A cup of tea provides 0.3mg of fluoride. Bottled fluoridated water or fluoride tablets can be used by people who live in areas where the water is not fluoridated. Topical application of fluoride to the teeth is not as effective in preventing cavities as is ingested fluoride.

Toxicity

Mottling, pitting, and dulling of the teeth has been observed in areas where fluoride is a natural ingredient in the water at levels of 2ppm to 6ppm. Intakes greater than 8ppm can cause fluorosis of the bones that produces arthritis-like symptoms. Fatal poisoning can occur if fluoride is ingested in amounts greater than 2,500 times the recommended intake. Chronic ingestion of 50mg/day can occur with some forms of air or environmental pollution and results in bone and tooth deformities. The levels used in the fluoridation of water pose no harmful effects to health and greatly reduce the incidence of tooth decay and possibly periodontal disease.

Nutrient-Nutrient Interactions

- Fluoride works with calcium, phosphorus, magnesium, and vitamin D in the formation and maintenance of healthy bones and teeth.

IODINE

Overview

More than 60 percent of the approximately 20 to 30mg of iodine in the body is found in the thyroid gland. The remaining 40 percent is distributed throughout the body, especially in the ovaries, muscles, and blood. Besides dietary intake, iodine also can be absorbed through the skin.

Functions

The only known function of iodine is as a component of the thyroid hormones. These hormones regulate the rate of metabolism, growth, reproduction, nerve and muscle function, the synthesis of proteins, the growth of skin and hair, and the use of oxygen by cells. One of these hormones, thyroxin, regulates the rate at which the body uses energy from food and thus is an important regulator of body weight.

IF SOME IS GOOD, IS MORE BETTER?

Many nutrients are found in the body within narrow ranges of concentration. Fluctuations from this normal range, either up or down, can result in disorders that have a wide range of effects on body function. For example, vitamins A or D are essential nutrients, but if their concentrations in the body rise above or fall below acceptable limits, deficiency or toxicity symptoms develop. For this reason, the oversimplified view that "if a little is good, more is better," or its opposite, "if high doses are bad, small doses also must be bad" can be dangerous.

Consider the reasoning behind the following beliefs:

- Some fiber is good for you, so you should eat as much fiber as possible.
- Too much sugar is bad for you, so you should not eat any sugar.
- Chlorine is a poison, so we should not consume any salt because it contains the related compound chloride.
- High doses of fluoride can cause mottling of teeth, so we should not drink fluoridated water.
- Protein is an essential nutrient, so we should supplement the diet with protein powders.

The simple black and white nature of these statements makes them easy to believe; however, the reasoning implied in these beliefs leads people to the wrong conclusions. Moderate intake of fiber is wise to prevent heart disease, hypertension, and cancer, but excessive intake of fiber can result in mineral deficiencies and gastrointestinal upsets. It is true that a diet high in sugar is linked to malnutrition or obesity, but moderate intake of sugar in conjunction with a nutritious diet of whole grain breads, fresh fruits and vegetables, extra-lean meats or dried beans, and nonfat milk products is harmless.

Deficiency

Poor iodine intake is associated with the development of endemic or simple goiter, a condition called hypothyroidism. During an iodine deficiency, the activity of the thyroid hormones remains normal until the body stores of the mineral are exhausted. A center in the brain called the pituitary gland recognizes the lack of iodine and diminished thyroid gland function and signals to the thyroid gland to increase its activity. The thyroid gland enlarges or swells as a result of this increased activity and the swelling that occurs at the front of the neck is called a goiter. Young women between the ages of 12 and 18 years old and boys between the ages of 9 and 13 years old living in areas where the iodine content of the soil is poor are the most prone for developing goiter. Iodine deficiency during pregnancy causes cretinism: extreme and irreversible mental and physical retardation.

Substances in foods called goitrogens also can cause goiter. Goitrogens are natural inhibitors of the thyroid gland and are found in raw cabbage, turnips, peanuts, cauliflower, rutabagas, mustard seeds, soybeans, and cassava. Prolonged consumption of large amounts of these raw foods when the diet is low in iodine could produce goiter; cooking deactivates these compounds. Some drugs act as goitrogens, such as thiourea, thiouracil, sulfonamide, and disulfiram.

Goiter can be prevented and treated with the inclusion of adequate amounts of iodine in the diet. A person who consumes a low-iodine diet and who lives in an area of the country where the soil is low in this mineral should consume iodized salt. A person who must severely restrict the intake of salt should consider iodine supplements, unless fresh saltwater fish is included frequently in the weekly diet.

Daily Recommended Intake

The 1989 RDAs for iodine are:

	Iodine (mcg)
INFANTS	
0 to 0.5 year	40
0.5 to 1 year	50
Children	
1 to 3 years	70
4 to 6 years	90
7 to 10 years	120
ADOLESCENTS AND ADULTS 11+ YEARS	150
Pregnant	175
Lactating	200

Sources in the Diet

Fresh saltwater shellfish and seafood, iodized salt, and foods grown on iodine-rich soil are good sources of the mineral. The iodine content of milk depends on the iodine in the cows' diets. A teaspoon of iodized salt contains 420mcg of iodine. Half of the salt sold in the United States is iodized. Many of the "natural" brands of sea salt do not contain iodine. Some bakeries use iodine as a dough stabilizer and a slice of this bread contains as much as 150mcg of iodine. Milk processed in equipment cleaned with related compounds called iodates also contributes to the daily intake. Iodine comes in a variety of forms and its presence in foods is difficult to measure (Table 22).

Table 22
THE IODINE CONTENT OF SELECTED FOODS

Food	Amount	Iodine(mcg)
Salt, iodized	1 tsp	400
Morton Light Salt substitute	1 tsp	400
Nutritional yeast	3½ ounces	110
Milk, evaporated, skim	4 fluid ounces	54
Milk, evaporated	4 fluid ounces	52
Egg, whole	1 large	26
Cheddar cheese	1 ounce	12
Cream cheese	1 ounce	9
Chicken, luncheon meat	1.9 ounces	4
Tuna	1.9 ounces	4
Turkey, luncheon meat	1.9 ounces	4
Almonds	1 ounce	4
Egg, white	white of 1 large	1

Toxicity

Doses greater than 25 times the recommended daily intake can produce "iodide goiter," a hyperactive, enlarged goiter, which is similar to the effect noted in an iodine deficiency. It does not appear that intakes of iodine below 25 times the RDA is a public health concern.

Hyperthyroidism or Graves' disease is an overactive thyroid. Hyperthyroidism is not a result of overconsumption of iodine, but rather develops as a result of disruption in the regulatory mechanisms that control thyroid hormone function. The person is anxious, nervous, loses weight, has an increased metabolic rate, cannot tolerate heat, and the eyeballs protrude.

Nutrient-Nutrient Interactions

- There is no evidence at this time that iodine interacts with other nutrients.

IRON

Overview

The adult body contains $1/2$ to 1 teaspoon of iron, with more than 65 percent of that iron used in hemoglobin, enzymes, and other functions. The remaining 35 percent is stored for future use.

Functions

EXERCISE. Animal studies show that adequate iron intake increases endurance capacity three-fold and increases voluntary physical activity. Many athletes have marginal or inadequate iron intake, which can impair their exercise performance by decreasing hemoglobin levels and the amount of oxygen delivered to the muscles, impair muscle contractions and strength, decrease enzyme activity, and increase post-exercise recovery times.

IMMUNITY. Iron strengthens the immune system and increases resistance to colds, infections, and disease.

OXYGEN TRANSPORTATION. Iron is the oxygen-carrying component of the blood. Four particles (atoms) of iron are bound to each protein molecule, called hemoglobin, in each red blood cell. When the blood passes through blood vessels in the lungs, oxygen binds to iron and is carried to all the tissues of the body. After releasing oxygen to the tissues, iron binds to the cellular waste product carbon dioxide and carries it to the lungs for exhalation.

An iron-containing molecule within each cell, called myoglobin, has a similar function to hemoglobin. Myoglobin transports oxygen within the cell to all the cellular components for use in the conversion of substances to energy and for all normal cell activities. Therefore, iron is the main determinant of how much oxygen reaches and is used by all body tissues, including the brain, muscles, heart, and liver.

Deficiency

While as few as 8 percent of women are anemic, as many as 80 percent of exercising women and 20 percent of premenopausal women in general are iron deficient. Routine blood tests for iron status, such as the hemoglobin and hematocrit tests, reflect only a woman's risk for anemia, the final stage of iron deficiency. Long before the onset of anemia, the tissue stores of iron have slowly drained, leaving a woman feeling tired and irritable. Her concentration and exercise ability is "not up to par," and her immune system is affected, placing her at higher risk for developing and fighting colds and infections.

People at risk for developing iron deficiency anemia include infants, children less than two years old, teenage girls, pregnant women, premenopausal women, women using intrauterine devices (IUDs), people who avoid eating red meat, the elderly, and female endurance athletes. Pregnant teenagers are at very high risk. It is estimated that between 10 percent and 80 percent of people in these categories are iron deficient. However, everyone is a possible candidate for deficiency.

Poor dietary intake and increased losses of iron are primary reasons for the development of a deficiency. Menstruating females compared to men require almost twice the iron to replace monthly losses. In addition, females frequently follow weight-loss diets and consume less food and less iron than do males. The average well-balanced diet in the United States supplies 6mg of iron/1,000 calories. It would take 2,500 calories to meet the RDA for women, but the average intake is 1,600 calories or less.

ANEMIA. Iron deficiency anemia is the classic symptom of poor iron intake. It is the most common form of anemia, and might be the most prevalent nutrient deficiency in the United States. Anemia is the final stage of iron deficiency. Prior to a reduction in red blood cells, the tissue stores have been depleted, mental capacity has diminished, hyperglycemia might be present, growth might be impaired, and other symptoms of marginal iron deficiency have developed. (See page 172 for more information on anemia.)

FOOD CRAVINGS. Cravings for nonfood items, such as ice, clay, or starch, is common in iron deficiency. This condition is called pica and it is easily remedied by increasing iron intake.

HEART DISEASE. Iron deficiency has an adverse effect on the heart. An electrocardiogram (EKG), a measurement of heart function, shows irregularities in heartbeat and function in people who are iron-deficient. These abnormalities disappear when the person is supplemented with iron.

MENTAL SKILLS. Iron can be found in almost every part of the brain and is used throughout life, but iron uptake is highest during periods of rapid brain growth, such as infancy and childhood. Infants with iron-deficiency anemia or marginal iron status have impaired mental and motor development and appear more unhappy, tense, fearful, or withdrawn than infants with adequate iron intake. However, treatment with iron supplements can improve development in iron-deficient infants.

Children who were anemic as infants or are currently iron-deficient do not perform as well in school or on intelligence tests as do children born to well-nourished mothers or who consume adequate amounts of iron in early life. The iron-deficient children also show impairment in attention span, learning and memory, and hand-eye coordination and might be hyperactive. These symptoms appear prior to signs of iron deficiency anemia and can be treated with iron supplements.

Iron deficiency might affect job performance, mood, and memory, and increased intake of iron might improve an iron-deficient adult's ability to work effectively and efficiently. Iron status also might affect electroencephalograms (EEG), a measure of brain activity, in older persons. One study showed that higher iron intakes are associated with EEGs in seniors similar to those of younger persons.

Daily Recommended Intake

The 1989 RDAs for iron were reduced to 15mg for women and 10mg for men to achieve a target iron store in the tissues of 300mg. However, research shows that some groups such as menstruating women, require twice the recommended amounts of iron to reach optimal iron stores; yet many women consume as little as 8mg of iron daily.

It is impossible for a woman during pregnancy and lactation to consume enough food to meet her iron requirement and a supplement that contains 30mg or more of elemental iron is usually recommended by a physician. Although the current RDAs are probably adequate to prevent clinical iron deficiency, they fall short for groups with increased iron losses and subsequent increased iron needs.

Most cases of iron deficiency go undetected because routine blood tests for iron status that measure hemoglobin or hematocrit levels only indicate anemia, the final stage of iron deficiency. More sensitive tests for tissue iron levels, such as serum ferritin, total iron binding capacity, or a combination of measurements can indicate mild to moderate deficiencies (Table 23). Dietary questionnaires are not always effective in screening the risk for iron deficiency.

TABLE 23
TESTS FOR IRON DEFICIENCY AND
IRON-DEFICIENCY ANEMIA

SERUM FERRITIN
Normal values—40 to 160mcg/l
Iron depletion—20mcg/l
Iron-deficiency anemia—12mcg/l

IRON BINDING CAPACITY
Normal values—300 to 360mcg/dl
(TIBC): Iron depletion—360mcg/dl
Iron-deficiency anemia—410mcg/dl

TRANSFERRIN SATURATION
Normal value—20 percent to 50 percent
Iron depletion—30 percent
Iron-deficiency anemia —< 10 percent

HEMOGLOBIN
Normal value—12 to 16g/dl
Iron-deficiency anemia —< 12g/dl

HEMATOCRIT
Normal value—37 percent to 47 percent
Iron-deficiency anemia—< 37 percent

The 1989 RDAs for iron are:

	Iron (mg)
INFANTS	
0 to 0.5 year	6
0.5 to 1 year	10
CHILDREN	
1 to 10 years	10
YOUNG ADULTS AND ADULTS	
Males	
11 to 18 years	12
19+ years	10
Females	
11 to 50 years	15
51+ years	10
Pregnant	30
Lactating	15

Sources in the Diet

Excellent sources of iron include organ meats, extra-lean red meats, dried fruits, cooked dried beans and peas, dark green leafy vegetables, fish, poultry, prune juice, and oysters. Good sources include whole grain breads and cereals, green peas, strawberries, tomato juice, Brussels sprouts, winter squash, blackberries, nuts, and broccoli. (Table 24)

The iron in supplements and fortified foods is poorly absorbed, but does contribute to daily needs. High-dose iron supplements, i.e., 30mg or more, can cause side effects such as nausea, constipation, or diarrhea, in some persons. However, a recent study at the University of Oslo, Norway reports that even low-dose iron supplements of 18 to 20mg daily can improve iron status without the adverse effects experienced with higher intakes.

Table 24
THE IRON CONTENT OF SELECTED FOODS

Food	Amount	Iron (mg)
Liver, cooked	3 ounces	7.5
Oysters, raw	½ cup	6.6
Heart, beef, cooked	3 ounces	5.0
Dried apricots	½ cup	3.6
Molasses, blackstrap	1 tbsp	3.2
Beef, ground, cooked	3 ounces	3.0
Raisins	½ cup	2.6
Navy beans, cooked	½ cup	2.6
Spinach, cooked	½ cup	2.4
Lima beans, cooked	½ cup	2.4
Split peas, cooked	½ cup	2.1
Chicken meat only	3½ ounces	1.4
Potato, baked	1 medium	1.1
Whole wheat bread	1 slice	0.8
Banana	1 medium	0.8
Avocado	½ medium	0.7
Broccoli, cooked	½ cup	0.7
Orange	1 medium	0.6
Apple	1 medium	0.4
Milk	1 cup	0.1
Cheese	1 ounce	0.05

The way in which a food is prepared will affect its iron content. Acidic foods, such as spaghetti sauce and tomato-based soups, cooked in cast-iron cookware can increase the iron content of the meal 300-fold. Foods should be cooked for a short amount of time in a minimum amount of water to maximize iron intake. Iron leaches from food during prolonged cooking and is lost if the cooking water is discarded.

The iron in meats is called heme iron and it is better absorbed than the nonheme iron in vegetables, fruits, beans, and whole grain items. The iron in foods of plant origin is better absorbed if it is eaten at the same meal with a small amount of meat (heme iron) or vitamin C-rich foods. For example, only about 2 percent of the iron in nuts is absorbed if they are eaten alone. When nuts are consumed in a meal with chicken, which contains heme iron, and a salad that contains vitamin C, iron absorption increases to 7 percent to 10 percent.

For infants, breast milk is a better source of absorbable iron than is cow's milk. Research at the University of New Mexico School of Medicine indicates that iron absorption, regardless of iron source, increases when tissue stores are depleted and decreases as iron stores reach optimal levels.

Toxicity

Under normal circumstances, iron intake is regulated by need, so dietary excesses are not absorbed. Accumulation of iron is possible, however, as the body cannot quickly excrete excesses once they are absorbed. Controversy about high iron levels erupted in 1992 when a well-publicized study from Finland reported that men with high serum ferritin (above 200mcg/dl) and elevated LDL-cholesterol were four times as likely to die from heart attacks as men with lower iron and LDL levels.

The study, however, showed a correlation, not a cause-and-effect relationship, between iron and heart attack. It is just as likely that the high iron levels reflect some other, as yet unidentified, factor that increases heart attack risk. For example, excess iron in the body might combine with oxygen to form free radicals, which would increase damage to fatty parts of cells and initiate atherosclerosis and heart disease. Optimal intake of antioxidants might counteract these reactions between free-floating iron and free radicals.

Another confounding issue is hemochromatosis, a genetic disorder mostly occurring in males that causes excessive iron accumulation into soft tissue and results in heart problems and other abnormalities. The high incidence of heart attacks, therefore, could be a result of genetics, not diet.

Even if the iron-heart disease link is accurate, these findings have no bearing on women or men consuming normal iron intakes. Iron overload is extremely rare in women, since they typically have serum ferritin levels between 20mcg to 120mcg, considerably lower than the 200mcg associated with heart attack risk in the Finland study. In addition, dietary intake of iron in the Finnish men was as high as 64mg daily (with an average of 19mg, or almost double the recommended level of 10mg).

The Finnish study sparked additional research into a possible iron-heart disease link. Although the final word is not yet in and large supplemental doses of iron should not be taken without physician supervision, recent studies do not support the findings in the Finland study that iron, under normal circumstances, increases heart disease risk.

High tissue stores and dietary intakes of iron also have been linked with an increased risk of cancer in both animals and humans. Research on colon cancer in human populations suggests that excessive iron intake might be involved in the initiation and promotion stages of cancer development. While most of the body's iron is safely attached to proteins, if intake is excessive, the extra iron not bound to proteins in the body might participate in the development of free radicals, intensifying their damage to cells and contributing to cancer.

The research is confounded by the fact that high circulating iron levels are not always linked to iron intake and, thus, might reflect other abnormalities in iron metabolism, not diet per se. At this time, the research on iron and cancer is inconclusive and has no implications for groups such as infants, children, adolescents, women of childbearing age, pregnant women, and seniors that are often in danger of inadequate, not excessive, iron intake.

Nutrient-Nutrient Interactions

- Vitamin C increases the absorption of iron.
- Vitamin B6 is necessary for the formation of the iron-containing protein in red blood cells called hemoglobin.
- Excess consumption of calcium, copper, or magnesium carbonate could reduce the absorption of iron.
- Iron competes with calcium, manganese, and zinc for absorption in the intestine and excess intake of one of these minerals could produce a deficiency of the others.
- Vitamin E may reduce the possible harmful effects of excess iron.

MAGNESIUM

Overview

More than half of the body's magnesium is in bone, one-fourth is in muscle, and the remainder is in body fluids and soft tissues, such as the heart and kidneys. The relatively large stores of magnesium in the bone provide a reservoir that can be used to ensure an adequate blood supply of the mineral to the rest of the tissues when dietary intake is poor.

Functions

Magnesium is one of the most abundant minerals in soft tissues. It helps convert carbohydrates, protein, and fats to energy, manufacture proteins, synthesize the genetic material within each cell, and remove excess toxic substances, such as ammonia, from the body. Magnesium also functions in muscle relaxation and contraction, nerve transmission, the prevention of tooth decay, and the prevention of heart disease and arrhythmias (irregular heartbeat).

Magnesium and calcium have similar functions and can either encourage or antagonize each other. For example, excess intake of magnesium inhibits bone formation. The balance between these two minerals is reflected in their role in muscle contraction: calcium stimulates muscles and magnesium relaxes muscles. An excess intake of calcium produces symptoms that resemble magnesium deficiency.

HEART DISEASE. There is a high incidence of sudden death from heart attack in areas where people consume soft water; heart attack risk declines in hard water areas. The high concentration of magnesium in hard water might be responsible for these statistics as people dying from heart disease have unusually low levels of magnesium in their heart tissue. Adequate or high magnesium intake not only reduces the risk of heart disease, but also increases survival rates after a heart attack.

Inadequate magnesium intake might increase heart disease risk by weakening the heart's defenses to free-radical damage. Two animal studies show that magnesium decreases the risk of atherosclerosis by reducing the accumulation of cholesterol in artery walls, even when the diet is high in cholesterol.

An association exists in the balance between calcium and magnesium and the incidence of heart attack. Calcium and magnesium help regulate the constriction and relaxation of blood vessels. If too much calcium is present this balance might be affected, the arteries might constrict more than they relax, and the blood and oxygen supply to the heart might be reduced. Prolonged constriction of the coronary arteries (blood vessels that supply the heart with blood and oxygen) could result in heart attack.

Magnesium might reduce the pain and cramping of intermittent clau-dication, a condition caused by reduced blood flow to the legs. Magne-sium levels are low in the muscles of patients with this disorder. Magne-sium supplementation increases muscle concentrations of the mineral, reduces pain and cramping, and allows patients to walk without pain. (See pages 198–199 for more information on magnesium and heart disease.)

HYPERTENSION. Magnesium might prevent and treat hypertension by reducing resistance in the blood vessels, which lowers the pressure within the blood vessels. Low levels of magnesium are associated with increased sodium and decreased potassium levels in the body, all of which contribute to rising blood pressure. Additionally, a dis-turbance in the calcium-magnesium balance during pregnancy might play a role in hypertension that accompanies pre-eclampsia.

PREMENSTRUAL SYNDROME. Blood levels of magnesium are low in women with Premenstrual Syndrome. Some women who experience headache, dizziness, and craving for sweets sometimes respond to magnesium supplementation, whereas those with breast tenderness or other symptoms do not.

Deficiency

Poor magnesium intake affects all tissues, especially tissues of the heart, nerves, and kidneys. Heart failure caused by irregular heartbeat is linked to insufficient intake of magnesium. Other symptoms of mag-nesium deficiency include loss of appetite, growth failure, muscle spasms, depression, hypertension, muscle weakness, convulsions, con-fusion, personality changes, nausea, lack of coordination, and gas-trointestinal disorders. Loss of hair, swollen gums, and damage to the arteries resembling atherosclerosis are also symptoms of advanced magnesium deficiency. Deficiency symptoms can result from poor dietary intake, excessive vomiting or diarrhea, long-term use of diuret-ics, alcohol abuse, kidney disease, diabetes, or protein malnutrition.

Magnesium deficiency might contribute to respiratory disorders, such as asthma and apnea (pauses in breathing that can be life-threatening). Many infants with apnea have magnesium-deficient mothers and supplementing these infant reduces the recurrence of apneic episodes. Magnesium might open up airways, increase lung volume, and reduce wheezing of asthmatics.

Clinical deficiencies are rare, but marginal deficiencies might be more common. Many Americans do not consume the RDAs for mag-nesium and it is suspected that even the RDAs might not be optimal for many people. Lifestyle factors, such as physical or emotional stress, further increase the need for magnesium.

Daily Recommended Intake

Magnesium's complex interrelationship with other nutrients, such as calcium, protein, phosphorus, lactose, potassium, and calories, makes the establishment of RDAs difficult. A typical diet in the United States provides 120mg of magnesium for every 1,000 calories and appears to prevent clinical deficiencies. This minimal amount will be inadequate to meet the increased demands of stress, disease, athletic activities, or poor absorption. The RDAs for children are only estimates based on the magnesium content of human milk and cow's milk.

Current RDA levels have been challenged by some researchers who feel higher intakes might be needed to prevent disorders, such as heart disease. One review of magnesium concluded that many people require as much as 6 to 8mg/kg body weight/day (or 368 to 613mg for a 135-pound person). In addition, limited evidence shows that magnesium is best absorbed when consumed in frequent, moderate doses of less than 100mg per meal. The 1989 RDAs reduced magnesium recommendations, despite evidence showing the importance of maintaining the calcium to magnesium ratio.

The 1989 RDAs compared to previous RDAs for magnesium:

Magnesium (mg)	Previous RDA	1989 RDA
INFANTS		
0 to 0.5 year	50	40
0.5 to 1 year	70	60
CHILDREN		
1 to 3 years	150	80
4 to 6 years	200	120
7 to 10 years	250	170
YOUNG ADULT MALES		
11 to 14 years	350	270
15 to 18 years	400	400
YOUNG ADULT FEMALES		
11 to 14 years	300	280
15 to 18 years	300	300
ADULTS		
Males 19+	350	350
Females 19+	300	280
Pregnant	450	320
Lactating	450	260–280

Sources in the Diet

The magnesium content of foods is variable. Good sources of magnesium include nuts, cooked dried beans and peas, whole grain breads and cereals, soybeans, dark green leafy vegetables, and seafood (Table 25). Milk supplies about 22 percent of the magnesium in the American diet. Limited evidence shows that supplemental magnesium citrate is more quickly and effectively used by the body than is magnesium oxide.

Table 25
THE MAGNESIUM CONTENT OF SELECTED FOODS

Food	Amount	Magnesium (mg)
Peanuts	¼ cup	63
Banana	1 medium	58
Beet greens	1 cup	58
Avocado	½	56
Peanut butter	2 tbsp	56
Cashews	9 medium	52
Milk, low-fat	1 cup	40
Wheat germ	2 tbsp	40
Brewer's (nutritional) yeast	2 tbsp	36
Collard greens	1 cup	31
Oysters	6 medium	27
Haddock, baked	3 ounce	20
Bread, whole wheat	1 slice	19
Bread, white	1 slice	5

Toxicity

The kidneys are efficient at excreting excess magnesium and it is unlikely that the mineral will accumulate to toxic levels. High levels of magnesium can develop in patients with kidney failure and in elderly people whose kidney functions are reduced.

Symptoms of magnesium toxicity include weakness, lethargy, drowsiness, and difficulty breathing. High intake of magnesium might impair absorption and use of calcium. Magnesium intake above 600mg can cause loose stools or diarrhea.

Nutrient-Nutrient Interactions

- All chemical reactions that involve vitamin B1 also require magnesium.

- Magnesium supplementation might prevent the deposition of oxalate stones in the kidneys during vitamin B6 deficiency.
- Magnesium, calcium, and phosphorus function together in bone formation, muscle contraction, and nerve transmission.
- High intake of calcium might impair absorption of magnesium.
- High intake of sugars, such as glucose and sucrose, might increase urinary loss of magnesium.
- Magnesium and potassium are closely related; if magnesium levels are low, potassium will decrease, while magnesium supplementation reduces potassium loss.

MANGANESE

Overview

Information on manganese is limited, since the first report of a manganese deficiency occurred as recently as 1972.

Functions

The known functions of manganese are not specific and other minerals, such as magnesium, apparently can function in its place. Manganese participates in the formation of connective tissues, fats and cholesterol, bones, blood clotting factors, and proteins. It is also important in the digestion of proteins. Manganese might function as an antioxidant in some body processes. Manganese plays an important role in the metabolism of carbohydrates by helping transport glucose in the body.

Deficiency

Inadequate intake of manganese is associated with impaired fertility, growth retardation, birth defects, bone malformations, seizures, and general weakness.

Daily Recommended Intake

Average intake of manganese ranges from 2 to 9mg/day. This intake prevents known clinical deficiency symptoms, but it is unknown whether it also prevents a marginal deficiency.

The 1989 Estimated Safe and Adequate Ranges for manganese are:

	Manganese (mg)
INFANTS	
0 to 0.5 year	0.3–0.6
0.5 to 1 year	0.6–1.0
CHILDREN	
1 to 3 years	1.0–1.5
4 to 6 years	1.5–2.0
7 to 10 years	2.0–3.0
ADOLESCENTS AND	
ADULTS 11+	2.5–5.0

Sources in the Diet

Excellent sources of manganese include spinach, tea, whole grain breads and cereals, raisins, blueberries, wheat bran, pineapple, cooked dried beans and peas, and nuts. Moderate amounts are obtained from dark green leafy vegetables and dried fruits (Table 26).

Table 26
THE MANGANESE CONTENT OF SELECTED FOODS

Food	Amount	Manganese (mg)
Tea	1 cup	.4–2.7
Raisins	1 small box	.201
Spinach, cooked	½ cup	.128
Carrots, cooked	½ cup	.120
Broccoli, cooked	½ cup	.119
Orange	1 medium	.052
Green peas	½ cup	.051
Wheat bran	1 cup	.048
Apple	1 medium	.046
Milk	1 cup	.046
Chicken, meat only	3½ ounces	.021

Toxicity

Excessive dietary intake of manganese could interfere with iron absorption and result in iron-deficiency anemia.

Nutrient-Nutrient Interactions

- Calcium, iron, copper, manganese, and zinc compete for absorption in the small intestine and high intake of one of these minerals reduces the absorption of the others.
- Manganese functions with vitamin K in the formation of blood clotting factors.

MOLYBDENUM

Overview

All tissues contain small amounts of molybdenum, with the largest amounts found in the liver, kidney, bone, and skin. These concentrations are sensitive to dietary intake and increase or decrease by raising or lowering the amount consumed in the diet.

Functions

Molybdenum is a component of the enzyme xanthine oxidase that aids in the formation of uric acid (a normal breakdown product of metabolism), is important in the mobilization of iron from storage, and is necessary for normal growth and development.

Deficiency

A deficiency of molybdenum causes stunted growth, anemia, loss of appetite, weight loss, and shortened life span in animals. Deficiency symptoms have not been reported in humans.

Daily Recommended Intake

The estimated average daily intake in the United States is between 45mcg and 500mcg.

The 1989 Estimated Safe and Adequate ranges for molybdenum are:

	Molybdenum (mcg)
INFANTS	
0 to 0.5 year	15–30
0.5 to 1 year	20–40
CHILDREN	
1 to 3 years	25–50
4 to 6 years	30–75
7 to 10 years	50–150
ADOLESCENTS AND	
ADULTS 11+ years	75–250

Sources in the Diet

The molybdenum content of vegetables, fruits, and grains depends on the content of the soil in which they are grown. Plants grown on molybdenum-rich soil can contain as much as 500 times the molybdenum as plants grown on depleted soil. Hard tap water is a good source of the mineral. Extra-lean meat, whole grain breads and cereals, cooked dried beans and peas, dark green leafy vegetables, and organ meats are good dietary sources.

Toxicity

Toxicity symptoms vary between species of animal and age groups in humans and depend on the form of molybdenum consumed. Prolonged intake of more than 10mg is associated with goutlike symptoms, such as pain and swelling of the joints in humans.

Nutrient-Nutrient Interactions

- Excessive intake of copper might interfere with the absorption of molybdenum.

- Molybdenum works with vitamin B2 in the conversion of food to energy.
- Molybdenum is important in iron metabolism.

PHOSPHORUS

Overview

Phosphorus is second only to calcium as the most abundant mineral in the body; the average body contains approximately 1 to 1½ pounds. Phosphorus is essential to life but receives little attention as it is found in all foods of plant and animal origin, and a deficiency is rare to nonexistent in humans. More than 80 percent of the body's phosphorus is in bones and teeth. The other 20 percent is active in many metabolic processes and is found in every cell in the body.

Functions

A complete review of the roles of phosphorus in the body would require a list of all body processes. In addition to its contribution to the structure and function of bones and teeth, phosphorus also is a component of all soft tissues, including kidney, heart, brain, and muscles; is a substance fundamental to growth, maintenance, and repair of all body tissues; and is a part of the genetic code in all cells. Phosphorus is also necessary for the conversion of dietary carbohydrate, protein, and fat to energy and is a component of cell membranes. The mineral helps maintain the pH balance in the blood; is a component of many proteins, such as casein in milk; and helps activate the B vitamins. Phosphorus is also a component of the storage form of energy in the body and facilitates the absorption of nutrients such as glucose, which is the form of sugar found in the blood and used for energy in the body.

Deficiency

Excessive intake of phosphorus is much more common than a deficiency of the mineral. Long-term and excessive use of anticonvulsant medications or of antacids containing aluminum hydroxide reduces absorption of phosphorus and might result in deficiency symptoms. Patients placed on formula diets low in phosphorus are also at risk for developing phosphorus deficiency.

Phosphorus deficiency has been observed in animals, but is rare in humans, except in the case of prolonged intake of high doses of nonabsorbable antacids. Because of this mineral's widespread function in the body, a deficiency would result in serious consequences to numerous organs and tissues, including the nerves, muscles, skeleton, blood and kidneys. Symptoms include weakness, anorexia (loss of appetite), bone pain and demineralization, anemia, destruction of the muscles and heart (cardiomyopathy), osteomalacia or rickets, tetany, and even death.

Daily Recommended Intake

The Recommended Dietary Allowances for phosphorus are arbitrary and are based on an estimate of the best ratio (1:1) for calcium and phosphorus. The average American diet contains 1,500 to 1,600mg, or twice the adult RDA for phosphorus, and the ratio of calcium to phosphorus is often as low as 1:2.

The 1989 RDAs for phosphorus are:

	Phosphorus (mg)
INFANTS	
0 to 0.5 year	300
0.5 to 1 year	500
CHILDREN AND ADULTS	
1 to 10 years	800
11 to 24 years	1,200
25+ years	800
Pregnant	1,200
Lactating	1,200

Sources in the Diet

Protein-rich foods, such as meat, organ meats, fish, poultry, and eggs, are good sources of phosphorus. Milk is a good source of both calcium and phosphorus, as it provides the two minerals in the best ratio. Fortified milk also contains vitamin D, which improves phosphorus and calcium absorption. Phosphorus is present as phytic acid in unleavened whole grain breads and cereals, but it is unclear how well this form of phosphorus is absorbed. Food additives contribute as much as 30 percent of dietary phosphorus. Soft drinks contain as much as 500mg of phosphoric acid per serving and can contribute to excessive phosphorus intake if consumed regularly (Table 27).

Table 27
THE PHOSPHORUS CONTENT OF SELECTED FOODS

Food	Amount	Phosphorus (mg)
Liver	3 ounces	405
Yogurt, low-fat	1 cup	326
Chicken	3½ ounces	266
Milk, nonfat	1 cup	247
Haddock	3 ounces	210
Tuna, canned	3½ ounces	188
Soybeans, cooked	½ cup	166
Hamburger	3 ounces	159
Peanut butter	2 tbsp	122
Egg	1 large	90
Bread, whole wheat	1 slice	57
Broccoli, cooked	½ cup	48
Orange	1 medium	33
Banana	1 medium	27
Carrots, cooked	½ cup	24

Toxicity

Overconsumption of phosphorus might occur in people who consume diets high in meat, convenience foods, and soft drinks and low in calcium-containing foods such as nonfat milk and dark green leafy vegetables. The effects of this imbalance in the ratio of calcium to phosphorus can contribute to faulty bone maintenance and osteoporosis.

Nutrient-Nutrient Interactions

- Phosphorus works with the B vitamins in energy metabolism.
- Vitamin D increases phosphorus absorption.
- The functions of calcium, magnesium, and phosphorus are closely related and disturbances in one mineral affect the other.

SELENIUM

Overview

In the 1960s, selenium was identified as an essential mineral. The highest concentrations of selenium are found in the liver, kidney, heart, and spleen.

Functions

The most important known function of selenium is as a component of the antioxidant enzyme glutathione peroxidase. This selenium-dependent enzyme protects red blood cells and cell membranes from damage by highly reactive oxygen fragments called free radicals. Selenium also works closely with, and in some cases can replace, the antioxidant vitamin E. It is also important for normal development of the fetus during pregnancy.

CANCER. Leukemia and cancers of the colon, rectum, ovaries, and lung are less likely to develop in people who consume a selenium-rich diet. However, selenium has not been shown to be effective in reducing the risk of breast cancer. Some evidence also shows that selenium might enhance the effectiveness of the immune system and the body's natural defense system that combats the development of infection and diseases, such as cancer. (See page 189 for more information on selenium and cancer.)

HEART DISEASE. The heart muscle is exposed to high levels of the most common form of free radicals: oxygen fragments. Selenium works with other antioxidants to reduce the free-radical damage that might initiate the early stages of heart disease.

IMMUNITY. Selenium enhances the activity of immune system cells such as macrophages, assists in detoxifying the body of heavy metals that suppress the immune system and reduce macrophage activity, and stimulates the release of lymphocytes, a type of white blood cell that fights infections. Some evidence shows that daily selenium intakes up to 400mcg significantly improve immune function. Selenium might benefit the elderly by stimulating compromised immune responses and returning immune function to levels typically seen in younger populations.

MOOD. Selenium supplements at approximately twice the RDA level might improve mood, anxiety, depression, and fatigue in some persons. Additional research is needed to determine how selenium affects mood, and if mood changes reflect a marginal deficiency.

RHEUMATOID ARTHRITIS. Selenium, as a component of the antioxidant enzyme glutathione peroxidase, reduces the quantity of damaging compounds, such as hydrogen peroxide, that initiate or promote inflammation associated with rheumatoid arthritis. Selenium also is involved in the production of hormone-like substances called prostaglandins that regulate the inflammation process. Selenium supplements improved symptoms in 40 percent of arthritis patients in one study.

SKIN. Selenium protects the skin from the damaging effects of ultraviolet (UV) light. Animals fed a high-selenium diet and then exposed to UV rays show reduced sunburn damage, such as inflammation and skin discoloration, and are less likely to develop skin cancer tumors than are UV-exposed animals consuming a non-supplemented diet.

Deficiency

BIRTH DEFECTS. A selenium deficiency during pregnancy could have irreversible effects on the baby's development and growth, and have detrimental effects on the formation of the immune system.

CANCER. People with low blood levels of selenium are at increased risk for developing cancer. Healthy people have the highest selenium concentrations in their blood and people with cancer, such as cancers of the ovaries, pancreas, cervix, and uterus, have the lowest concentrations. These blood levels reflect dietary intake; as selenium intake drops, the risk for developing cancer increases.

DOWN'S SYNDROME. Patients with Down's syndrome have low blood levels of selenium, which might contribute to the free-radical damage to nerves characteristic of this condition. (See pages 150–153 for more information on free radicals and antioxidant nutrients.)

FIBROCYSTIC BREAST DISEASE (FBD). FBD is a condition characterized by painful breast lumps. Women with low blood levels of selenium might have a higher risk for developing FBD than do healthy women.

HEART DISEASE. People at risk for heart disease who have low levels of selenium in their blood might benefit from selenium supplementation. People who consume selenium-poor diets have weakened and damaged hearts, a condition called cardiomyopathy, which may be the reason for their increased risk of premature heart attacks. A form of heart disease, called Keshan's disease that affects primarily children, is effectively treated with selenium supplementation. (See page 199 for more information on selenium and heart disease.)

LIVER DISEASE. Persons with chronic liver disorders, including both alcohol- and non-alcohol-induced liver disease, have low levels of selenium in their blood and livers as compared to people with healthy liver function.

Other symptoms of selenium deficiency include muscle weakness and tenderness, anemia, and damage to the pancreas.

Daily Recommended Intake

The 1989 RDAs for selenium are:

	Selenium (mcg)
INFANTS	
0 to 0.5 year	10
0.5 to 1 year	15
CHILDREN	
1 to 6 years	20
7 to 10 years	30
ADOLESCENTS AND ADULTS	
Males 11 to 14 years	40
15 to 18 years	50
19+ years	70
Females 11 to 14 years	45
15 to 18 years	50
19+ years	55
Pregnant	65
Lactating	75

Sources in the Diet

The selenium content of food is dependent on the selenium content of the soil in which the food is grown and can vary 200-fold. Grains, such as whole wheat, brown rice, and oatmeal are excellent sources if the grain was grown on selenium-rich soil. Poultry, low-fat milk products, extra-lean meat, organ meats, and fish are also good sources (Table 28). Some of the selenium content is lost when foods are washed, cooked, stored improperly, or processed or refined.

Table 28
THE AVERAGE SELENIUM CONTENT OF FOOD TYPES

Food Type	*Amount*	*Selenium (mcg)*
Organ meats	4 ounces	149.6
Seafood	4 ounces	37.9
Lean meat and chicken	4 ounces	22.7

Table 28 (cont.)
THE AVERAGE SELENIUM CONTENT OF FOOD TYPES

Food Type	Amount	Selenium (mcg)
Whole grain cereals and bread	1 serving	12.3
Low-fat milk products	1 serving	3.6
Vegetables	1 serving	1.6
Fruit	1 serving	0.5
Sugar	1 tsp	0.2

Selenium-rich areas around the country are Montana, Utah, South Dakota, Wyoming and parts of New Mexico, Colorado and Tennessee. In these states, the plants eaten by animals and humans alike are selenium-rich, making the grains, vegetables and meat from those states good sources of selenium. The soil in most midwestern states has intermediate amounts of selenium, while levels in southern states and on both coasts are lower. Fortunately, grains contribute the most selenium from plant sources to the diet and the durum wheat used to make pasta is grown in the selenium-rich areas of the country.

Organic and inorganic sources of selenium function differently in the body. Selenium yeasts, an organic source of selenomethionine, raise selenium levels in the blood; but the inorganic sodium selenate and selenite are more effective at increasing activity of the antioxidant enzyme glutathione peroxidase.

Toxicity

Selenium can be toxic when consumed in amounts greater than 600mcg to 750mcg. Children are the most susceptible to toxicity. For example, children raised in selenium-rich areas of the country have a higher incidence of tooth decay and tooth loss. Large doses of either the inorganic forms of selenium or nutritional yeast fortified with inorganic selenium might cause cancer. Other symptoms of selenium toxicity include hair loss, white streaking of the fingernails, tenderness and swelling of the fingers, fatigue, nausea, and vomiting.

Doses two to three times the RDA appear to be harmless. The organic forms of selenium, such as selenomethionine and selenocysteine, are better absorbed and less likely to cause toxic symptoms than the inorganic forms of the mineral, such as sodium selenite and selenate. The organic forms of selenium are available in selenium-rich nutritional yeast, whole grain products, and some supplements.

Nutrient-Nutrient Interactions

- Selenium and vitamin E work closely as antioxidants in preventing damage to cell membranes and possibly in the prevention of cancer. The anti-cancer effects of selenium are enhanced in the presence of vitamin E and a deficiency of the vitamin might reduce the effectiveness of selenium.
- Large doses of vitamin C interfere with the absorption and use of inorganic selenium, such as sodium selenite.

SULFUR

Overview

Sulfur is a component of all body tissues, especially those tissues that contain high amounts of protein such as hair, muscles, and skin. Insulin, the hormone that regulates blood sugar, also contains sulfur. Most of the sulfur in the body is bound to the sulfur-containing amino acids: methionine, cystine, and cysteine, which are building blocks of protein. Sulfur also is a component of vitamin B1 and biotin.

Functions

Sulfur gives proteins their characteristic differences in shape, i.e., it makes hair curly, is involved in the formation of bile acids important for fat digestion and absorption, is a constituent of bones and teeth, activates certain enzymes, and helps regulate blood clotting. Sulfur helps in the conversion of proteins, carbohydrates, and fats to energy because it is a component of vitamin B1, biotin, and pantothenic acid; helps regulate blood sugar by being a constituent of the hormone insulin; and is a component of collagen, a protein in the connective tissue that holds cells together.

Deficiency

A deficiency of sulfur is unknown, although it is conceivable that a diet very low in protein would be inadequate in sulfur and could produce a deficiency. The protein deficiency, however, would be of greatest concern and the sulfur deficiency would be cured with increased protein intake.

Daily Recommended Intake

No Recommended Dietary Allowances or Safe and Adequate ranges have been established for sulfur. The American diet is high in protein and supplies adequate amounts of sulfur.

Sources in the Diet

Meat, organ meats, poultry, fish, eggs, cooked dried beans and peas, milk, and milk products are good sources of protein and sulfur.

Toxicity

No toxicity symptoms have been reported for sulfur. Excesses are excreted in the urine.

Nutrient-Nutrient Interactions

- The poisonous effects of arsenic are a result of its ability to bind to the sulfur portion of amino acids and inactivate them.
- Sulfur is a component of vitamin B1, biotin, and the active form of pantothenic acid called co-enzyme A.

ZINC

Functions

Zinc is a component of numerous enzymes in the body and functions in the detoxification of alcohol in the liver, the mineralization of bone, the digestion of protein, and the conversion of calorie-containing nutrients to energy. Zinc intake of the mother helps ensure a healthy birth weight for the newborn, an important factor in reducing risk of infant illness and death. It also functions in the production of proteins, the proper functioning of insulin in the regulation of blood sugar, the maintenance of the genetic code, normal taste, wound healing, and the maintenance of normal blood levels of vitamin A and use of the vitamin by the tissues.

Zinc is important in the maintenance of normal blood cholesterol levels, normal growth and development, the production of hormone-like substances called prostaglandins that regulate numerous body processes including blood pressure and heart rate, and the normal functioning of the oil glands of the skin. Several studies show that zinc has some antioxidant activity, such as detoxifying free radical-promoting metals and protecting some substances needed for enzyme activity from free-radical damage.

ANOREXIA NERVOSA. Although the onset might be related to social pressures, the progression of anorexia might be partially attributed to altered taste perception and metabolic upsets. Zinc improves taste perception and weight gain in patients with anorexia, whereas depressed zinc status might be a sustaining factor for abnormal eating behaviors.

CANCER. Zinc might aid in the prevention and treatment of cancer. The effect of zinc on the immune system strengthens the body's defense against abnormal cell growth associated with cancer development. This essential trace mineral is also important in normal cell growth and development, which would aid in the prevention of any disease associated with abnormal cell growth. Zinc improves taste perception in cancer patients undergoing radiation therapy and aids in the maintenance of normal weight and nutrient intake during treatment.

HEALTHY BABIES. Zinc is essential for a baby's development from conception to delivery. Zinc levels of the mother are linked to proper formation of the palate and lip, brains, eyes, heart, lungs, and urogenital system in the baby. It also plays an important role in growth, bone development, birth weight, and the completion of full-term pregnancy. Zinc might help prevent neural tube defects, strengthen infant immunity, and reduce infant mortality.

IMMUNITY. Zinc has a beneficial effect on the immune system and the body's natural defense against colds, infection, and disease. Zinc also increases levels of some antibodies and immune cells, such as T-lymphocytes. Zinc also inhibits the growth of disease-causing bacteria and, in moderate doses, might reduce tooth decay caused by bacteria in the mouth. Zinc also might reduce some of the symptoms of the common cold.

Deficiency

Symptoms of a zinc deficiency include anemia, slowed growth, reduced taste perception, poor appetite, birth defects, impaired nerve conduction and nerve damage, poor healing of wounds, sterility, poor alcohol tolerance, spontaneous abortion, delayed sexual maturation, glucose intolerance, mental disorders, dermatitis, and hair loss. Inadequate zinc intake might contribute to atherosclerosis by increasing blood vessel vulnerablity to damage and by reducing antioxidant defenses. Even mild deficiencies of zinc result in slowed growth, poor wound healing, delayed maturation, and inflammatory bowel disorders.

Pregnant women are at a high risk for zinc deficiency, which could increase the likelihood of having a low-birth-weight infant, impairing fetal development, or reducing infant survival rates. Children who consume a low-zinc diet are shorter and exhibit mild mental impairment as compared to children who consume a zinc-rich diet. Vegetarians also have low levels of zinc in the blood and vegetarian children tend to be short for their age, although it is not clear if zinc is the causative factor.

Several dietary factors affect zinc absorption and can contribute to a zinc deficiency. A high-fiber diet that contains excessive amounts of phytates in unleavened whole grain products contributes to a zinc deficiency, especially when the diet is already low in zinc. Phytates bind to zinc and reduce absorption of the mineral. Leavening agents, such as baker's yeast used in most breads, deactivate phytates. Overconsumption of foods or supplements fortified with iron or copper, but not zinc, can produce a secondary deficiency of the latter.

Zinc deficiency is frequently reported in preschool children, hospital patients, low-income families, and elderly populations. Athletes and vegetarians also might be at risk for marginal zinc intake. Extralean meat is the best dietary source of zinc and anyone who avoids eating red meat, while consuming refined grains and convenience foods, could be at risk for zinc deficiency.

Daily Recommended Intake

Healthy adult men require about 12.5mg of zinc daily and it is assumed that non-pregnant women require somewhat less because of their lower body weights. A well-balanced diet contains between 10mg and 15mg of zinc per day. Some studies show that zinc requirements are greater than the RDAs during the last half of pregnancy. Stomach acid is importance for proper absorption of zinc; any health condition or medication that lowers stomach acid might limit the availability of zinc.

The 1989 RDAs for zinc are:

	Zinc (mg)
INFANTS	
0 to 1 year	5
CHILDREN	
1 to 10 years	10
ADOLESCENTS AND ADULTS	
Males 11+ years	15
Females 11+ years	12
Pregnant	15
Lactating (1st 6 mo.)	19
(2nd 6 mo.)	16

Sources in the Diet

Oysters, extra-lean meat, poultry, fish, and organ meats are the best dietary sources of zinc and the most available to the body; even including three ounces of extra-lean meat in the diet can significantly improve zinc status. Whole grain breads and cereals are good sources of zinc (Table 29). The zinc in breast milk is better absorbed than the zinc in infant formula or cow's milk.

Table 29
THE ZINC CONTENT OF SELECTED FOODS

Food	Amount	Zinc (mg)
Oysters	6 medium	124.9
Turkey, dark meat only	3 ounces	3.7
Liver, cooked	3 ounces	3.3
Lima beans, cooked	½ cup	2.7
Pork, lean, cooked	3 ounces	2.6
Wheat germ	2 tbsp	1.8
Turkey, light meat only	3 ounces	1.8
Yogurt, plain	1 cup	1.3
Almonds	¼ cup	1.2
Milk, nonfat	1 cup	0.9
Potato, baked	1 medium	0.4
Lentils, cooked	½ cup	0.18
Spinach, cooked	½ cup	0.17
Orange juice	6 ounces	0.13

Toxicity

Zinc is relatively nontoxic in doses up to 45mg/day, after which it might impair copper absorption unless copper intake also is increased. Zinc in quantities 10 to 30 times the RDA for several months results in diminished blood levels of copper.

Zinc in doses greater than 150mg might interfere with normal immune function, thus reducing the body's defense against disease. Long-term ingestion of 80 to 150mg of zinc might lower HDL-cholesterol and, thus, increase risk for heart disease.

Zinc sulfate supplements in amounts exceeding two grams a day can cause nausea, stomach upset, and vomiting. Zinc intakes up to 100mg are safe if the diet is comprised of low bioavailable zinc, such as the zinc in foods of plant origin, and foods high in fiber and phytates.

Nutrient-Nutrient Interactions

- High intakes of zinc can inhibit copper absorption and result in copper deficiency.
- High dietary intake of zinc might reduce iron absorption and encourage iron depletion from body storage.
- Adequate zinc intake might aid in vitamin D and calcium metabolism and reduce bone loss associated with marginal calcium intake.
- Zinc assists in the transportation of vitamin A in the blood.
- Zinc deficiency increases the amount of dietary vitamin E necessary to maintain normal blood and tissue levels of this fat-soluble vitamin.

ADDITIONAL TRACE MINERALS (Aluminum, Arsenic, Cadmium, Lead, Mercury, Nickel, Silicon, Tin, Vanadium)

Aluminum, arsenic, cadmium, lead, mercury, nickel, silicon, tin, and vanadium are trace minerals found in the tissues of humans. The biological usefulness of these minerals is poorly understood and some of these minerals are toxic.

Aluminum

Aluminum, once thought to be a harmless mineral, might be related to serious bone and brain disorders. A high intake of aluminum affects the absorption and use of calcium, phosphorus, magnesium, selenium, and fluoride and might be implicated in the development of bone deterioration. Muscle weakness and aching also is related to aluminum intake.

Abnormal levels of aluminum in the body are associated with nerve damage and brain disorders, such as Alzheimer's disease. Alzheimer's disease affects people in their middle to later years and is characterized by progressive and irreversible loss of memory and body function. Rats injected with aluminum learn at a slower rate and deposit aluminum in their brains in a pattern that resembles Alzheimer's patients. Whether the accumulation of aluminum is the cause or a result of Alzheimer's disease is unclear.

Sources of aluminum include food additives (such as sodium aluminum phosphate used as an emulsifier in processed cheese, cake mixes, frozen dough, pancake mixes, and self-rising flours), table salt (contains sodium silicon aluminate or aluminum calcium silicate to retard clumping), and white flour (contains potassium alum to whiten the flour). Acidic foods, such as spaghetti sauce, cooked in aluminum pans dissolve the mineral into the food and increase the aluminum content of the diet. The mineral leaches from aluminum coffee pots into the coffee; the newer the pot or the longer the brewing time, the higher the aluminum content of the beverage.

Aluminum-containing antacids, antiperspirants, and other products add to the daily intake of aluminum. Antacids average 35 to 208mg of aluminum per dose; heavy users of antacids can ingest up to 5,000mg. Hemorrhoidal preparations, vaginal douches, and lipstick also contain aluminum.

Arsenic

Arsenic is found throughout the body. Animal studies show that arsenic is essential for growth, development, and reproduction, possibly because of its role in the metabolism of methionine, an amino acid involved in growth. The requirement for arsenic might be as low as 12mcg daily. Estimated daily intakes are approximately 140mcg, an amount far below toxic levels, which are estimated at greater than 250mcg/day. Foods that contain arsenic include fish, grains, and cereals.

Cadmium

Cadmium is not excreted from the body and can accumulate over time to toxic levels. The estimated daily intake is 13mcg to 24mcg, of which very little is absorbed. Excessive intake occurs when soft water leaches cadmium from pipes. Cigarette smoke, air pollution, and the air near zinc refineries also provide a source of cadmium. Symptoms of cadmium toxicity include anemia, muscle wastage, hypertension, and liver and kidney damage.

Lead

Lead is a toxic metal that produces nerve damage, anemia, muscle wastage, lethargy, and mental impairment. Lead is ingested from a variety of sources including fresh and canned food, water, lead-based paint, plants grown in soil contaminated with lead, lead-glazed pottery, and air pollution. Adequate intake of calcium, iron, zinc, copper, and vitamin C might help prevent and might even treat the symptoms of lead exposure.

Mercury

Mercury salts are used in medicine, agriculture, and industry, and accumulation of toxic levels is possible. Mercury alters the shape and function of proteins, such as hormones, antibodies, hemoglobin in red blood cells, and all enzymes. The consequences of mercury toxicity are widespread. Ingestion of a toxic dose of mercury causes immediate gastrointestinal disturbances, including a metallic taste in the mouth, thirst, nausea, vomiting, pain in the abdomen, and bloody diarrhea. A common first aid for mercury poisoning is to drink a protein-rich beverage such as milk. The mercury acts on the protein in the milk rather than the proteins that line the mouth, throat, stomach, and intestine. Vomiting is induced to remove the mercury and milk.

The body accumulates mercury in the kidneys, nerves, blood, liver, bone marrow, spleen, brain, heart, skin, and muscles. The developing infant is very susceptible to mercury toxicity during pregnancy. Some fish, such as tuna, are high in mercury and should be consumed in moderation, especially during pregnancy and breast-feeding.

Many people in the United States have dental fillings that contain mercury amalgams and the stability of this mercury has been questioned. Some evidence shows that mercury in the mouth might dissolve and over time migrate into the blood. This source of mercury might suppress the immune system and the body's natural defense against infection and disease.

Nickel

No established role for nickel has been identified, although the mineral is found in association with the genetic code within each cell and might help activate certain enzymes. Nickel is probably involved in the activity of hormones, cell membranes, and enzymes. Low blood levels of nickel are observed in people with vitamin B6 deficiency, cirrhosis of the liver, and kidney failure. The significance of these low blood levels is not known. In contrast, elevated blood levels of nickel are associated with the development of cancer, heart attack, thyroid disorders, psoriasis, and eczema. However, the intestinal tract absorbs very little of the ingested nickel, so toxicities are rare.

The average daily intake of nickel is between 0.17mg and 0.70mg and the best dietary sources include whole grain breads and cereals, chocolate, peas, fruits, vegetables, nuts, and cooked dried beans and peas. A diet high in meat and other foods of animal origin and fat might be low in nickel.

Silicon

Silicon's primary function is in the development and maintenance of bone, and a silicon deficiency causes weak and malformed bones of the arms, legs, and head. Silicon is primarily located in areas of active growth inside bones where it might be involved in the growth of bone crystals and the calcification of bone. Silicon also is important in the formation of cartilage and connective tissue, the protein webwork in bone in which calcium is embedded. Silicon levels are high in people with atherosclerosis, but it is not known whether or not the mineral is related to the development or progression of cardiovascular disease.

Animals fed a silicon-deficient diet show abnormal bone formation and weakened fibrous tissues. However, there is no documentation of similar deficiency symptoms in humans.

The daily diet contains ample amounts of silicon and the mineral is well absorbed. However, fiber, molybdenum, magnesium, and fluoride alter silicon absorption. Low intakes of calcium might increase silicon requirements. Dietary sources include whole grain breads and cereals, root vegetables, and cooked dried beans and peas.

Tin

Tin is essential for some species and functions in normal growth and development, but no essential role has been identified in humans.

High intakes of tin might destroy red blood cells. Elevated tissue and blood levels of tin can be a result of leakage of the metal into canned foods. Tin absorption is poor and it is not clear how much of the daily intake of 1.5 to 3.5mg actually crosses the intestinal lining and enters the blood.

Vanadium

Vanadium is essential for some animals and a deficiency can cause growth retardation, bone deformities, spontaneous abortion, and infertility. However, no role for vanadium has been proven in humans.

The average human body contains 20mg of vanadium located in the blood, organ tissues, and bones (where it is stored long-term). This trace mineral is probably involved in building bones and teeth, cholesterol metabolism, red blood cell growth, iodine metabolism, thyroid function, and hormone production. Preliminary reports show that vanadium might protect against the development of breast cancer, slow the growth of tumors, and improve glucose metabolism of diabetics.

Daily intake of vanadium is estimated at 15mcg to 30mcg, well above the 10mcg researchers estimate the human body requires. Seafood, cereals, mushrooms, parsley, corn, soy, gelatin, dill, and liver are good sources of vanadium. However, processed or refined foods contain higher levels of vanadium. This additional vanadium is probably from stainless steel processing equipment and might not be a form usable by humans. Airborne vanadium entering the body through the lungs is another major source of the nutrient.

Little information exists on vanadium toxicity. If the mineral is toxic, the tissues probably most susceptible to damage would be the nerves, kidneys, liver, and blood-building tissues such as spleen and bone marrow. Toxicity symptoms in animals include stunted growth, loss of appetite, and diarrhea.

SECTION 2

VITAMINS AND MINERALS IN THE PREVENTION AND TREATMENT OF DISEASE

CHAPTER 5

Vitamins, Minerals, and Disease

INTRODUCTION

Modern history of nutrition begins with disease. The novelty and excitement of nutrition started at the turn of the century with the discovery of the first vitamin and its cure of a deficiency disease. In these early stages of research, vitamins and minerals were only investigated for their roles in curing specific diseases. The attempts were successful and common diseases that crippled, blinded, or killed, such as scurvy and pellagra, were miraculously erased. Clinical vitamin and mineral deficiency diseases were discovered and a "well-balanced" diet was believed to be one that prevented the onset of overt disease. Today, clinical nutrient deficiency diseases are uncommon in the United States and when they do occur they are usually a result of long-term medication use or another disease that limits food intake or nutrient use.

As the science of nutrition continues to develop and more sophisticated techniques for assessing nutritional status are discovered, the association between nutrients and disease expands beyond the realm of overt clinical deficiencies. Many conditions once thought to be the natural consequence of aging are now considered the result of lifelong poor eating habits.

For example, a strong relationship exists between marginal dietary intake of vitamins and minerals and the development, progress, and cure of chronic disorders such as infectious diseases, disorders of the stomach and intestine, bone diseases, heart and blood vessel diseases, diseases of the liver, and cancer. Marginal vitamin and mineral intake is also related to wound healing, stress, the healing of burns, the strength of the immune system, and the aging process. (See pages 13–16 for more information on marginal nutrient deficiencies.) In addition, overconsumption of foods high in fat or sugar results in obesity and disorders related to obesity.

The science of nutrition expanded beyond just the prevention of physical diseases with the discovery of a relationship between the intake of specific nutrients and behavior, intelligence, and mental health. For example, women were told for years that the changes in their emotions and bodies experienced the week before menstruation were "all in their heads." Marginal nutrient deficiencies have been associated with these symptoms and increased intake of certain vitamins and minerals, such as vitamin B6 and magnesium, might lessen the severity and frequency of premenstrual symptoms in some women. It appears that the "balanced diet" once thought to be a solution to clinical nutrient deficiency diseases is actually one that meets the unique nutrient needs of each individual for optimal health of both body and mind.

In less than a century, the study of vitamins and minerals has grown from a small focus on clinical nutrient deficiencies to include the role of nutrients in the prevention and treatment of chronic disease, the dietary and pharmacological role of vitamins and minerals in behavior and intelligence, and the function of nutrients in fundamental metabolic systems, such as the antioxidant and immune systems that affect the very basis of life and health.

THE ANTIOXIDANTS

Research on the antioxidants has expanded and diversified in this decade. In the past five years alone, more research has been published on vitamin C, beta carotene, and vitamin E, and their antioxidant functions than at any other time in research history. These vitamins, along with the antioxidant minerals, such as selenium, copper, zinc, and manganese, have been strongly linked to the prevention (and possibly treatment) of numerous diseases from heart disease and cancer to cataracts and arthritis, and also to the regulation of the immune system and the prevention of premature aging.

Free Radicals

The story of antioxidants begins with free radicals. Free radicals are highly reactive compounds formed by radiation; found in air pollution, ozone, and cigarette smoke; consumed in rancid fats; and produced during the normal breakdown of proteins in the body and generated during the breakdown of certain medications. Fragments of oxygen, such as peroxides and superoxides, are the most commonly identified free radicals.

All substances are formed by the chemical bonding of two or more elements. Stable bonds are created when electrically charged portions of an element, called electrons, pair up. Free radicals are unstable and reactive because they have an unpaired or "extra" electrical charge that causes them to seek out other substances in the body to bond with in order to neutralize themselves. When free radicals bond with an electron from a stable compound, another electron becomes unpaired and another free radical is created. A chain reaction begins and thousands of free-radical reactions can occur within seconds of the first reaction and severely harm the body unless the extra free radical is deactivated.

The fatty membranes that surround cells are the prime targets for free-radical attack. The shape and function of the fats in membranes are changed when a free radical attacks them. The damaged membrane is no longer able to transport nutrients, oxygen, and water into the cell or regulate the removal of waste products. Extensive free-radical damage can cause the membrane to rupture and release its cellular components. These cellular components can further damage the surrounding tissues.

Free radicals also attack nucleic acids that comprise the genetic code within each cell. Nucleic acids regulate normal cell formation and the growth and repair of damaged or aging tissues. The damage caused by free radicals has been linked to premature aging. Although why a body ages is only partially understood, all theories agree that at some point the body's cells become unable to replenish their components and as one cell dies, other cells dependent on the dying cell also are lost. The accumulation of cellular debris within a cell also is associated with aging. Finally, the cells' inability to correctly replenish necessary proteins because of damage to the genetic code is common in aging. Free radicals contribute to all of these processes.

Free-radical damage also is associated with age-related diseases. Free-radical damage to chromosomes and nucleic acids might initiate the growth of abnormal cells, which is the first step in the development of cancer. Free radicals also are associated with the promotion phase of cancer, where already mutated cells are encouraged to grow.

The initial stages of atherosclerosis and heart disease, where the lining of the arteries are damaged and cholesterol begins to accumulate in the damaged area, are thought to be caused by free-radical attack to the cell membranes of the tissues that line the blood vessels. Free radicals also attack low-density lipoprotein cholesterol (LDLs) in the blood and these "oxidized" LDLs are the types of fat most likely to accumulate in arteries, blocking blood flow and resulting in atherosclerosis. Free-radical damage to the heart tissue following open-heart surgery further damages an already weakened tissue and interferes with recovery and prognosis.

Free radicals also are associated with inflammation, drug-induced damage to organs, suppression of immunity and increased susceptibility to infection and disease, and increasing the symptoms of other disorders, such as muscular dystrophy, arthritis, and Parkinson's disease. In addition, diseased tissues are more susceptible to free-radical damage, so damage escalates during illness.

Antioxidants: The Body's Anti-Free Radical System

Oxygen might have its harmful side but it is still the most important "nutrient" for life; a person can survive for only a few moments without it. The body has developed a complex antioxidant system to defend itself from oxygen fragments and other free radicals. An antioxidant is any compound that fights against (anti) the destructive effects of free-radical oxidants. This antioxidant system is comprised of enzymes, vitamins, minerals, and other substances produced in the body or obtained from the diet. Antioxidants act as scavengers and prevent the formation of free radicals or bind to and neutralize these reactive substances before they damage tissues.

Many nutrients, such as selenium, copper, manganese, and zinc, are considered antioxidants because they work in conjunction with an antioxidant enzyme and are necessary for the enzyme to function properly. Antioxidant enzymes protect the body by using free radicals in reactions that change them to less harmful compounds. The antioxidant enzyme is not produced or is ineffective when the diet does not supply adequate amounts of the related mineral. For example, selenium is essential for the production of the enzyme glutathione peroxidase that protects red blood cells and cell membranes from free-radical damage. Copper and manganese are components of the antioxidant enzyme superoxide dismutase (also called SOD) that protects cell membranes and cell contents.

Other nutrients, such as vitamin C, vitamin E, and beta carotene, function as antioxidants independent of an enzyme. Vitamin C is water-soluble, so it reduces free-radical damage in the watery areas of the body, such as the bloodstream, lymph fluids, and the fluid between and within cells. The fat-soluble vitamin E is the first line of defense against damage to fatty cell membranes. It is the most effective free-radical scavenger in the cell membranes, i.e., only one vitamin E molecule can disarm up to 1,000 free radicals. Beta carotene also protects the fatty parts of cell membranes, as well as preventing free radicals from forming.

Individual antioxidants work as a team to defend the body against free radicals. For example, vitamin C can restore vitamin E when it is damaged. Selenium and vitamin E assist each other in protecting cell membranes from free-radical attack. In essence, selenium destroys any free radicals that are missed by vitamin E. More information is needed on how free radicals affect tissues and the functions of antioxidants in inhibiting free-radical activity. The evidence shows, however, that a low-fat, high-antioxidant diet might aid in the prevention of some diseases and premature aging. During conditions that expose the body to high amounts of free radicals, such as exposure to air pollution, radiation, and herbicides; poor diet; cigarette smoke; high dietary intake of vegetable oils; and the inflammatory diseases, the need for antioxidant nutrients is even higher than normal.

The body's need for the antioxidant nutrients might vary from the RDAs depending on the disease, the site, and possibly the severity or duration of the condition. For example, even sub-RDA levels of vitamin E prevent hemolytic anemia, but full RDA levels are required to maintain optimal blood levels, and intakes far in excess of the current RDAs and typical dietary intakes might be needed to protect against heart disease and cancer.

VITAMINS, MINERALS, AND THE IMMUNE SYSTEM

The body is under constant attack. Air, food, water, other people, and all aspects of the environment expose a person to bacteria, viruses, and other microscopic organisms. Some of these microorganisms are useful to the body and help maintain health. For example, a bacteria called Lactobacillus acidophilus found in some yogurt can live in the small intestine and reduces the risk for developing gastrointestinal disorders or possibly high blood cholesterol levels. Other microorganisms, however, promote infection and disease.

One of three things can happen when a microorganism, such as a bacteria, invades the body:

1. the bacteria can die;
2. the bacteria can cause the body's defense system, called the

immune response, to activate even though there are no obvious signs of disease or infection; or

3. the microorganism can survive, multiply, and produce observable signs of infection or disease that even can result in illness or death to the infected person.

Swelling, inflammation, and increased body temperature are symptoms of infection. Diseases related to invasion of the body by microorganisms include infections associated with acquired immune deficiency disease (AIDS), herpes simplex, and possibly cancer.

The immune system is the body's defense against invasion by foreign substances, such as microorganisms. It is a complex network of specialized tissues, organs, cells, and chemicals whose primary purpose is to recognize and destroy a foreign invader. The lymph nodes and vessels, spleen, bone marrow, thymus gland, and tonsils are examples of organs and tissues that participate in the immune system. The cells and secretions of the immune system include specialized white blood cells called T-lymphocytes and B lymphocytes, a chemical called interferon produced by T-lymphocytes, chemicals called antibodies produced by B lymphocytes, and scavenger cells (monocytes and macrophages) that engulf and destroy microorganisms and other foreign substances. In addition, the skin and mucous membranes that line all internal and external surfaces of the body form a natural barrier against invasion by unwanted substances.

A well-functioning immune system recognizes unwanted microorganisms, abnormal and potentially cancerous cells, or any foreign substance in the body and destroys them, thus preventing the development of infection and disease. In contrast, the body's defenses are weak and a variety of disorders are possible when the immune system is not functioning at its best.

Poor nutrition is one of the most frequent reasons that the immune system malfunctions. The immune response is affected very early during marginal or inadequate intake of nutrients. How severely the immune system is damaged depends on which vitamin or mineral is deficient and to what extent it is missing from the diet, the presence of an infection that might further challenge the system, and age. The very young and the very old often are at an increased risk for compromised immune systems, but these conditions are more likely due to diet and lifestyle than to natural consequences of age. For example, breast-feeding during infancy provides passive immunity, while optimal intake of key nutrients in the elderly improves immune function.

All immune system processes are affected during malnutrition; the size, structure, and composition of the immune system organs are altered, the white blood cells are reduced in number and strength, and the chemicals produced by these cells are altered. Low intake of one or more vitamins and minerals with or without generalized malnutrition reduces a person's ability to fight off infection and increases the risk for developing immune-related diseases. In contrast, optimal intake of vitamins and minerals and consumption of a low-fat diet enhances the immune system and reduces the risk for developing diseases or infections (Table 30).

Immunity and the Antioxidants

The antioxidant nutrients—vitamin E, beta carotene, and vitamin C—are important in maintaining optimal immune function. These vitamins prevent damage to immune cells and tissues caused by free radicals. Researchers theorize that free radicals weaken the immune system making it vulnerable to attack.

Vitamin A stimulates the immune system and decreases the risk of infections. A research review at the University of Queensland Medical School in Australia showed that adequate vitamin A intake in children reduces the death rate by a third and resulted in a 70 percent decrease in deaths from respiratory diseases. This vitamin also reduces the severity of and complications associated with measles. Beta carotene enhances immunity by increasing T- and B-lymphocyte activity, protecting macrophages, and facilitating communication between immune system cells. Beta carotene also lessens the damage to the immune system associated with exposure to ultraviolet radiation in sunlight or x-rays.

Even marginal dietary intake of vitamin C can have far-reaching effects on a person's resistance to infection and disease. Two or more servings daily of vitamin C-rich foods, such as orange juice, strawberries, and Brussels sprouts, strengthens the immune system by increasing the production of B- and T-cells and other white blood cells. This antioxidant also increases white blood cells' ability to destroy disease-causing microorganisms and increases the production of interferon. In contrast, white blood cell formation and wound healing are suppressed when vitamin C intake is suboptimal.

Vitamin E is an essential component of all cell membranes, including the outer cell membrane and the membranes that surround the cell's nucleus (which houses the genetic material) and the cell's power house centers called mitochondria. Vitamin E and other antioxidants prevent free-radical damage to, and help maintain the normal structure and function of immune cells and tissues. Vitamin E improves T-lymphocyte function and, if applied directly to the skin, can prevent the immune suppression caused by as little as 30 minutes exposure to UV light in sunlight.

While even marginal deficiencies of one or more of these nutrients can compromise the body's defense system, typical American diets often are low in the antioxidants. In addition, diet alone might not be enough. William Pryor, Boyd Professor of Chemistry and Biochemistry at Louisiana State University, suspects that at least 100IU of vitamin E is needed daily to see improvements in immune function. Diet alone cannot supply this much vitamin E, suggesting supplements might be necessary.

Immunity and Other Vitamins and Minerals

Several other vitamins are essential to optimal immune function. A deficiency of vitamin B6 can reduce lymphocyte numbers, impair antibody production, and might contribute to immune suppression associated with aging and HIV infection, while increasing dietary intake of this vitamin improves immune function. Inadequate vitamin D intake impairs immunity, while a vitamin D-rich diet corrects this impairment.

Zinc is essential for antibody production, normal thymus gland function, and the effectiveness of specialized T-lymphocytes called helper cells. Optimal zinc intake restores compromised immune functions and reduces susceptibility to infections. A copper deficiency might impair immunity and increase the risk for, and prolong the duration of, infections, especially in premature infants.

Iron also affects immunity. Adequate iron intake results in fewer infections in infants, while iron deficiency in people of all ages impairs lymphocytes activity and decreases interleukin production. Adequate selenium intake stimulates the release of lymphocytes, increases natural killer cell activity, and protects the body from toxic metals that suppress the immune system. Additional vitamins and trace minerals that might strengthen the immune response include folic acid, pantothenic acid, magnesium, nickel, and tin.

The immune system can be strengthened or stimulated to an optimal level, beyond which further attempts to activate this system sometimes have an adverse effect. While moderate doses of some nutrients stimulate the body's defense system, larger doses impair the immune response. For example, some evidence shows that vitamin C in doses greater than several grams a day, zinc in doses greater than

150mg/day, and excessive copper intake might interfere with the immune response and place a person at increased risk for developing disease or infection.

Other compounds in foods, besides vitamins and minerals, also might keep a cold at bay. Garlic, for example, contains substances that inhibit the growth of bacteria and might stimulate the immune system. Although no optimal dose has been identified, including one to three cloves in the daily diet might turn on your immune system without turning off your friends.

Finally, diet is only one of several factors that can improve or suppress immunity. For example, moderate, regular exercise decreases the risk of infectious illnesses and might prevent age-related declines in immune function. Social support for people attempting to lose weight helps increase the number of lymphocytes and improves immune function. A generally healthy lifestyle, i.e., not smoking, sleeping 7 to 8 hours per night, eating breakfast, and avoiding excessive mental stress, also improves immune function and a person's resistance to disease and infection.

Table 30
VITAMIN/MINERAL-RICH SNACKS THAT BOOST YOUR IMMUNE SYSTEM

Here are a few simple ways to include at least five servings a day of fresh fruits and vegetables:

- Fresh strawberries, blueberries or blackberries
- Fresh kiwi dunked in yogurt flavored with shredded orange peel, poppy seeds and cinnamon
- A tortilla filled with shredded carrots, zucchini, low-fat cheese and salsa
- A cup of vegetable soup
- Fresh fruit stirred into vanilla yogurt
- Unsweetened fruit juice frozen in ice cube trays
- Mix unsweetened fruit juice concentrate with gelatin and chill to form a "jellied" juice snack
- Fresh fruit and nonfat milk smoothie
- One-half honeydew melon filled with nonfat yogurt
- One-half papaya filled with cottage cheese
- A spinach salad
- Carrots dunked in peanut butter
- Three bean salad with low-fat dressing
- A sweet potato, cut into chunks
- Crisp vegetables dunked in curried nonfat yogurt dip
- Nonfat milk blended with fresh fruit, wheat germ and a tablespoon of frozen orange concentrate
- A glass of fresh-squeezed orange juice

SIFTING FACT FROM FALLACY

Nutrition, the study of nourishment, is the "new kid on the block" in the scientific community. The word "vitamin" was first used in 1911 and essential minerals were still being discovered in the 1970s, whereas other sciences such as medicine, physics, and astronomy have been active for centuries. The expanding role of vitamins and minerals in the prevention and treatment of disease has created more questions than answers, and this limited supply of accurate information, coupled with the enthusiasm and interest in nutrition, leaves gaps that are often filled with inaccurate information and confusion. This chapter attempts to clarify many of the confusing issues related to vitamins, minerals, and disease by presenting the most reliable information based on current research.

ACNE

Overview

Acne is an inflammatory disease of the oil-producing (sebaceous) glands of the skin. There are many types of acne, but acne vulgaris is the most common; it usually begins during puberty and rarely lasts beyond the 25th year.

Nutrition and Acne

Certain foods have been blamed as the cause of acne and it has been suggested that chocolate, soft drinks, sugar, greasy foods, nuts, milk, salt, or iodine should be eliminated from the diets of children with acne. None of these foods, however, have been shown in scientific studies to increase the symptoms of acne. Poor nutrition will affect the body's immune system and increase the likelihood of the child developing a number of disorders or infections, but the addition of a small amount of chocolate to an otherwise healthy diet will not cause acne. A child might show allergic-like symptoms to certain foods that cause skin disruptions. Elimination of the food from the diet will not produce immediate relief from symptoms and it can take up to two months before results are seen.

Stress, and its associated increase in certain hormones, is related to the development and severity of acne. Relaxation, in the form of vacations or recreation, usually relieves some or all of the symptoms of acne. Sunshine and swimming are also relaxing and the sun inhibits bacterial growth, while the water cleanses the skin.

VITAMIN A. The synthetic form of vitamin A called retinoic acid (Retin-A) has been confused with the vitamin for the treatment of acne. There is no evidence that supplemental doses of vitamin A (retinol or beta carotene) is an effective treatment for acne and consumption of large doses of this fat-soluble vitamin can cause toxic symptoms, such as joint pain, nausea, itching, cracking and drying of the lips and skin, hair loss, and cracks at the corners of the mouth, especially in children. An individual should not self-medicate with retinoic acid without the advice and supervision of a pharmacist or physician.

ZINC. Zinc supplementation might be effective in the treatment of acne. Zinc maintains normal blood levels of vitamin A and aids in the normal functioning of the oil-producing glands of the skin. These functions, combined with the typical adolescent diet low in zinc, could explain why zinc is sometimes effective in the treatment of this disorder. Some people show fewer skin blemishes and their skins are less oily when zinc supplements are added to their diets.

Dietary Recommendations

The best dietary approach to the prevention or treatment of acne is to consume a low-fat, high-fiber, nutrient-dense diet optimal in all vitamins and minerals and low in sugars and refined and convenience foods. The diet should contain a variety of fruits, vegetables, whole grain breads and cereals, cooked dried beans and peas, low-fat or nonfat milk products, and extra-lean meats, chicken, and fish and should contain ample amounts of zinc-rich foods. (See page 141 for dietary sources of zinc.)

The most important prevention and treatment for acne is thorough daily cleansing of the skin to keep it free from dirt and oil. Antibiotics, such as tetracycline, reduce the number of bacteria that break down the plugged oils and these medications are effective in the treatment of acne for some people. Retinoic acid is available by prescription and might help prevent the formation of or release the plug of oils or reduce the formation of excess oils in acne. Benzoyl peroxide is also used in the treatment of this skin disorder. The blemishes should never be squeezed or poked, as this will cause more scarring than the acne. Regular exercise, effective stress management, avoidance of alcohol and tobacco, and moderate exposure to sunshine are also important for health and the prevention and treatment of acne.

ACRODERMATITIS ENTEROPATHICA

Overview

Acrodermatitis enteropathica is an inherited zinc-deficiency disorder in infants characterized by loss of hair, dermatitis, diarrhea, psychological disturbances, and a chronic condition called "failure to thrive." The parents and family members of the infant have low blood levels of zinc. The cause of acrodermatitis enteropathica is unknown; however, a defect in the body's ability to absorb zinc has been suggested.

Nutrition and Acrodermatitis Enteropathica

Acrodermatitis enteropathica was first noted in infants fed cow's milk. All symptoms of the disorder disappeared when the infants were placed on breast milk. The zinc in cow's milk is poorly absorbed, whereas the zinc in breast milk is easily digested and absorbed by the infant's developing gastrointestinal tract. Moderate-dose supplementation with zinc usually reverses all symptoms of this disorder and returns the infant to health.

ACQUIRED IMMUNODEFICIENCY SYNDROME (AIDS)

Overview

Acquired immunodeficiency syndrome (AIDS) is a devastating, progressive disease caused by the human immunodeficiency virus (HIV). AIDS is characterized by suppression of the immune response, the body's natural defense system against disease and infection, and a high incidence of a type of cancer called Kaposi's sarcoma. The person does not die from AIDS, but from secondary infections, such as pneumonia or cancer. The HIV-infected person often does not succumb to a final infection for ten years or more after exposure to the virus.(See pages 153–157 for more information on the immune system.)

Nutrition and AIDS

Nutrition is important throughout all the stages of HIV infection and AIDS, including even whether or not a person contracts the virus. For example, people who consume suboptimal levels of nutrients, have a suppressed immune system and, if exposed to the virus that causes AIDS, have an increased risk of contracting the virus, while optimal nutrition and strong immune function can help resist infection.

Malnutrition is common in AIDS patients. Signs of malnutrition are observed in patients in both the early and advanced stages of the disease and poor dietary intake probably interferes with treatment or encourages the progression of the disease. In fact, seven out of ten people with HIV infection are deficient in at least one vitamin or mineral, a compounding risk factor for impaired immune function.

Studies show many AIDS patients consume a diet adequate in nutrients or take vitamin and mineral supplements, but nonetheless have deficiencies, possibly as a result of altered metabolism. Limited evidence shows that HIV-infected individuals require an intake above RDA levels for vitamins A, E, B6, and B12, and zinc to maintain normal blood concentrations of those nutrients.

Many AIDS patients show severe muscle and tissue wastage and an increase in infections and tumors that result from suppressed immunity and weight loss. The condition is called the HIV wasting syndrome and might result from loss of appetite, increased nutrient requirements, altered ability to process nutrients, and decreased absorption of nutrients. Long-term low intake of certain vitamins and minerals might contribute to an already weakened immune system, which further increases the patient's risk for opportunistic infections that cause or increase the symptoms of AIDS. The severity of malnutrition is directly related to mortality rate; consequently, consuming optimal levels of all vitamins, minerals, and other essential nutrients is critical to prolonging the onset of disease and death.

Information is limited on specific nutrients and their association or impact on the prevention and treatment of AIDS. Blood levels of the antioxidant nutrients, including vitamins A, C, and E, beta carotene, selenium, and zinc, are often low in AIDS patients and these deficiencies might contribute to a poorly functioning immune system and increased susceptibility to disease. HIV-infected patients with the highest blood levels of these antioxidants have a slowed progression to AIDS. Deficiencies of fatty acids, such as eicosapentaenoic acid (EPA) and gamma linolenic acid (GLA) might contribute to the development of AIDS and Kaposi's sarcoma; however, this is purely speculative at this time.

ZINC. Low serum zinc levels in patients with AIDS has been noted and correlated to the severity of the disease and immunocompetence.

The most common cause of zinc deficiency is poor dietary intake. Several complications of AIDS alter appetite and reduce dietary intake, including nausea, vomiting, digestive malabsorption, and alterations in zinc metabolism. In addition, frequent infections associated with AIDS drain serum zinc concentrations, which can remain low even after the infection has been successfully treated. Finally, a substance called tumor necrosis factor (TNF) is elevated in AIDS patients, is correlated with the severity of the disease, and might contribute to zinc deficiency. In contrast, optimal dietary intake of zinc might inhibit the action of TNF and improve immune responses.

Zinc is an essential component of numerous metabolic processes associated with the susceptibility to, progression, and severity of AIDS. Zinc is a co-factor for more than 200 enzymes essential in protein synthesis, energy metabolism, DNA and RNA production, and other fundamental processes. For example, as a co-factor for enzymes in protein metabolism, zinc is essential for normal levels of certain transport proteins, including albumin, transferrin, and prealbumin. Other nutrients dependent on these transport proteins, such as vitamin A, are affected by zinc deficiency even when dietary intakes are adequate. Blood protein levels decrease when zinc intake is low and probably reflects altered DNA and RNA activity, impaired protein synthesis, increased protein degradation, and other mechanisms. Low zinc intake could contribute to hypoalbuminemia, which often develops in AIDS patients.

Zinc is essential in the maintenance of the immune system, especially normal T-cell function, maturation, and differentiation. Dietary intake of zinc increases the number of circulating T-cells, while zinc deficiency decreases T-cell function. Zinc deficiency also causes thymic and lymph node atrophy and might have harmful effects on replicating cells, such as those involved in certain immune processes. Zinc deficiency also is associated with numerous abnormalities common to AIDS patients, including anorexia, gastrointestinal malfunction, diarrhea, and central nervous system malfunction.

Zinc has not been shown to inhibit the replication or action of retroviruses, such as HIV. However, it might inhibit the replication of other viruses, including herpes simplex type 2, and is effective in the treatment of virus-related disorders, such as herpetic keratitis.

Zinc's functions in immunity, protein synthesis, and other metabolic processes strongly suggests it is an important factor in the pathogenesis of AIDS, and might be responsible for many of the secondary conditions associated with HIV infection. Consequently, zinc supplements might be an important adjunct therapy to currently used agents.

Dietary Recommendations

Research on nutrition and AIDS is far from complete. The following theories await further studies for confirmation, and while some can reduce susceptibility to HIV infection or slow the inevitable progression to AIDS, none prevent AIDS.

1. Optimal intake of the antioxidant nutrients vitamin A, beta carotene, vitamin C, vitamin E, selenium, and zinc enhance immune function and might lengthen the time between infection and the onset of AIDS.
2. Deficiencies of vitamins B1 and B12 are common in AIDS patients, whereas adequate intake might prevent neurological changes associated with the advanced stages of these conditions.
3. Researchers at SUNY Health Science Center at Brooklyn, New York found that dementia associated with AIDS was effectively treated in one patient within two months of vitamin B12 supplementation.
4. Levels of glutathione, a substance formed in the body and a component of the antioxidant enzyme glutathione peroxidase, are low in HIV-infected patients. Researchers suspect this deficiency might suppress immunity and speed the progression of AIDS.

Until further information is available on dietary requirements for the prevention and treatment of AIDS, the best dietary advice is to consume a low-fat, high-fiber, nutrient-dense diet, which is optimal in all vitamins and minerals and low in sugars and refined and convenience foods. The diet should contain a variety of fruits, vegetables, whole grain breads and cereals, cooked dried beans and peas, low-fat or non-fat milk products, and extra-lean meats, chicken, and fish. Calorie intake should be adequate to maintain normal body weight. In addition, a multiple vitamin-mineral supplement that supplies at least 100 percent of the RDA for all vitamins and minerals including magnesium, selenium, and zinc, and an extra dose of the antioxidant nutrients, vitamin C (250mg daily), vitamin E (200IU to 400IU daily), and beta carotene (15mg daily) should be considered. Regular exercise, effective stress management, avoidance of alcohol and tobacco also are important considerations in the prevention and treatment of AIDS.

ALLERGIES

Overview

Food allergy is an adverse reaction to a food that results in the activation of the immune system. For an adverse reaction to be labeled a food allergy, it must be proven that the person reacts to a specific food, the symptoms must recur two or more times when the food is consumed (preferably without the patient knowing he or she is ingesting the suspected food), and changes in the immune system must be observed.

More commonly, people misdiagnose food intolerances as food allergies. People can have a "simple" intolerance to a food that results from a genetic defect in an enzyme or other metabolic peculiarities not related to the allergic response. An example is lactose intolerance, where a person is missing a digestive enzyme (lactase) that aids in the breakdown and absorption of lactose or milk sugar. The bloating, flatulence, diarrhea, and discomfort that results from drinking milk is not an allergic response, but is a result of the accumulation of gas and fluids from the presence of undigested sugar in the intestine.

Pseudointolerances to food also are mistaken for food allergies. Personal preferences against or avoidance of a food or foods results in the person avoiding the food because it "does not agree with him or her." Dislike for a food is not a food allergy, and avoidance of an entire food group can result in vitamin and mineral deficiencies.

Up to one-third of the adults in the United States avoid a food because of a related adverse reaction, such as headaches, nausea, vomiting, skin irritations, or indigestion. Although these might be allergic symptoms, more than likely they are signs of food intolerance, pseudointolerance, or other psychological associations with food. In fact, less than 5 percent of people who claim they have a food allergy actually test positive when exposed to the offending food under controlled conditions.

The development of food allergies depends on individual variation in heredity, intestinal absorption of nutrients, immune response, and exposure to foods. Food allergies are most common in premature infants and in children two years old and under when the immature digestive tract allows semi-digested food particles to pass into the blood stream. Breast-feeding for the first 6 to 12 months of a child's life reduces the incidence of food allergies in the newborn.

Food allergies are more likely to develop in children of allergic parents than in children with no family history of food allergies. Infants and children with food allergies almost always outgrow the allergies by the time they are two to three years old. This is especially true for allergies to milk and eggs and is less true for allergies to peanuts and fish. New allergies can develop at any age; however, the incidence of food allergies decreases with age. Although approximately 20 percent of people experience food allergies at some point in their lives, only about 1 percent to 5 percent of allergies persist into adulthood.

There are two types of food allergies: the immediate or obvious type and the delayed type. Only 5 percent of diagnosed food allergies are the immediate type where a person experiences an allergic reaction within minutes of eating a food. For example, the individual allergic to shrimp will develop allergic symptoms, such as hives, asthma, or a migraine headache, within approximately 30 minutes of eating the shellfish.

The delayed type of food allergy is more common, less obvious, more chronic, and very difficult to detect and correct. Adverse reactions to a food might take up to five days to appear and can occur in unrelated tissues such as the respiratory tract in the form of bronchitis, asthma, or inflammation of the sinuses (sinusitis).

Symptoms blamed on food allergy are extensive and diverse, although actual documented symptoms of food allergies are restricted to the respiratory tract, the digestive tract, and the skin. Any gastrointestinal disorder can result from an allergic reaction to a food, including faulty absorption of food, diarrhea, vomiting, swelling and tenderness of the mouth and throat, or rectal bleeding. Classic skin complaints include burning and itching of the skin, rash, hives, or small bruises (hemorrhages) below the skin. Some forms of dermatitis also are attributed to food allergies. Headaches, blood in the urine, inflammation and reddening of the whites of the eye (conjunctivitis), and joint pain also can occur as a result of food allergy. In all of the above allergic reactions, symptoms can be mild to severe; the most severe symptoms are anaphylactic reactions, which can cause severe itching and hives, perspiration, constriction of the throat, breathing difficulties, lowered blood pressure, shock, and in rare cases, respiratory failure and death. The frequency and severity of other disorders, such as rheumatoid arthritis, bed-wetting, and migraine headaches, have been associated with food allergies; however, evidence supporting these claims are not conclusive.

The diagnosis of food allergies is complicated and the result of a single test does not determine a conclusive diagnosis of the condition. Diagnosis is based on the accumulation of evidence based on a thorough history of the individual's symptoms, foods thought to aggravate, previous medical and emotional history, and a medical exam to identify any possible underlying disorders that might explain or contribute to the allergic-like symptoms.

Several popular tests for food allergies have been developed, but their accuracy and usefulness are questionable. Cytotoxic testing takes a suspected food component, mixes it with a sample of the person's blood, and records changes in the white blood cells (immune response). Sublingual testing takes a drop of the suspected food component, places it under the individual's tongue, and records signs of an allergic reaction. In the provocative and neutralization testing, extracts of the suspected food are injected under the skin and allergic symptoms are recorded. None of these tests produce reliable results. The radioallergosorbent extract test (RAST) and the skin test are the most reliable diagnostic tests for food allergy and are performed by a physician or physician's assistant.

Nutrition and Allergies

FOODS. The most common causes of food allergies are eggs, milk, and wheat. It is a specific protein in wheat—called gluten—that triggers the allergic response. Although corn is low in gluten, some people also are sensitive to corn. Other common foods include nuts, citrus fruits, fish, shellfish, chocolate, and tomato-based products (Table 31). Some fiber or laxative preparations, especially those that contain psyllium, might cause an allergic reaction in some individuals.

Table 31
FOOD INTOLERANCES AND THEIR SYMPTOMS

Food Or Food Ingredient	Symptoms
Chocolate, aged cheese, red wine, brewer's (nutritional) yeast, canned fish	Migraine headaches
Fermented cheese, fermented foods (sauerkraut), pork sausage, canned tuna, sardines	Migraine headaches, skin rash or itching
Shellfish, strawberries, tomatoes, peanuts, alcohol, pineapple	Itching, eczema
Milk	Bloating, flatulence, diarrhea, abdominal pain
Legumes, berries, apples	Diarrhea, abdominal pain, flatulence
Monosodium glutamate (MSG)	Asthma, dizziness, headaches, sleep problems
Metabisulfites	Asthma, itching, fluid retention, congestion of the nose
Food additives and colorings	Asthma, itching, headaches, gastrointestinal disorders, behavioral problems

ADDITIVES. No evidence exists that food additives are responsible for widespread food allergies, but a few additives, such as sulfiting agents, tartrazine or FD&C yellow dye #5, monosodium glutamate

(MSG), the preservatives called benzoates, and yellow azo food dyes do produce symptoms in some people.

The most effective treatment for most food allergies is to avoid the offending food. Alternative foods, such as soy-based formulas instead of cow's milk for infants, can be found in some cases. Waiting until at least four months old to introduce any solid foods might prevent some food allergies. Simple foods used in uncomplicated recipes are easy to avoid, but foods that are common ingredients in a variety of items are more difficult to identify and substitute or avoid. For example, wheat flour is found in a variety of processed foods and recipes, including cakes, bread, pies, gravies, soups, and salad dressings. A person must learn to read food labels and become familiar with the normal composition of standard foods such as mayonnaise, catsup, and peanut butter.

The degree of strictness in avoiding a food will depend on individual sensitivity to the food; some individuals with food allergies suffer extreme allergic reactions to trace amounts of the offending food, while others can consume average amounts if the food is eaten with other foods. In most cases, the offending food can be reintroduced six months to several years after removal from the diet with no allergic symptoms. In other cases, the way in which a food is prepared can alter the reaction. For example, the person might tolerate the food cooked, but cannot eat it raw.

Cross-reactions are possible with foods from the same grouping; if a person is allergic to peanuts, it is possible that other legumes also will be poorly tolerated. Other related foods that might produce cross-reactions include shrimp and crab or cow's milk and goat's milk. Cross-reactions also have been reported between some foods and pollen; for example, melons or bananas and ragweed pollen, celery and mugwort pollen, and carrot, apple, or hazelnut and birch pollen.

The elimination-challenge test is useful when food allergies are suspected, but the offending foods have not been identified. The person is placed on a restricted, simple diet that excludes all foods suspected to cause allergies. After several days, one food at a time is introduced back into the diet and signs of allergy are recorded. The final diet is based on all foods that do not produce allergic symptoms. The elimination-challenge test can take several weeks to complete and should be conducted with the supervision of a registered dietitian (R.D.) or physician (M.D.). Reintroduction of a food can cause immediate or delayed allergic reactions that should be monitored closely by a skilled professional. Self-diagnoses are often wrong and can result in unnecessary avoidance of nutritious foods.

Limited evidence is available for the use of vitamins, minerals, or other nutrients in the treatment of allergies. Vitamin C might reduce some of the nasal congestion associated with the allergic reaction. Pantothenic acid might reduce the allergic drainage and nasal stuffiness associated with allergies. Vitamin B12 shows limited effectiveness in allergic asthma, hives, and allergic dermatitis. Fish oils reduce the symptoms of inflammatory disease, but it is unclear whether they are effective in the treatment of allergies.

ALZHEIMER'S DISEASE

Overview

Alzheimer's disease is characterized by a slow, progressive, irreversible loss of memory. Basic body functions, such as the ability to eat and bladder control, are lost as the disease progresses. Alzheimer's disease usually affects older people, but cases also are reported in young and middle-aged people. It is the cause of dementia and slow death in thousands of Americans each year.

Nutrition and Alzheimer's Disease

Poor nutrition is related to Alzheimer's disease, but it is unclear whether it is a cause or an effect. Early damage to brain cells located in the region of appetite control might explain changes in food intake. A poor diet resulting in low vitamin-mineral intake might predispose an individual to Alzheimer's. Once the disease has reached advanced stages, the patient loses interest in or the ability to choose or consume nutritious foods and the resultant malnutrition can increase the symptoms or speed the progression of the disease. Long-term rejection of food, either by pushing food out of the mouth by tongue movements, rejecting foods, or loss of memory of how to eat results in protein-calorie malnutrition and wasting of the body and nervous system. Long-term use of many medications further depletes the body of vitamins and minerals. (See Chapter 6.)

ALUMINUM. Dietary intake and abnormal accumulation of aluminum in the brain are associated with a variety of brain and nervous system disorders. In addition, aluminum deposits in the brain cells that are most affected in Alzheimer's disease. This association does not prove that aluminum causes Alzheimer's; however, there is a strong relationship between the toxic mineral and this degenerative brain disease.

The intake of aluminum has increased since the development of aluminum cookware, utensils, and foil. The mineral dissolves from aluminum pots into the food or beverage. For example, coffee brewed in aluminum pots contains more aluminum than does coffee brewed in glass pots; the longer the brewing time or the newer the pot, the greater the amount of aluminum in the beverage. Other sources of aluminum are medications and sundries, such as aluminum-containing antacids and antiperspirant deodorants. The safest way to continue using aluminum-containing products is to choose those that include aluminum phosphate instead of aluminum chloride, which is more readily absorbed.

If aluminum intake is a contributor to Alzheimer's disease, prevention would include avoidance of all aluminum-containing substances and the treatment would include medications that bind to the mineral, reduce its absorption, and increase its excretion. Adequate intake of iron or calcium competes with aluminum and decreases its absorption, while fluoride increases the body's elimination of aluminum. Studies on animals report that excessive vitamin D intake might promote the accumulation of aluminum in the muscles, heart, and brain.

VITAMIN B1. Vitamin B1 is essential for the synthesis and release of acetylcholine, a neurotransmitter involved in memory, and metabolism of the vitamin might be altered in the brains of Alzheimer patients. A study conducted at the Medical College of Georgia found that high doses of vitamin B1 (three to eight grams daily) slightly improved dementia symptoms in Alzheimer patients. However, vitamin B1 therapy does not halt the progression of Alzheimer's disease.

VITAMIN B12. More than 70 percent of older persons who are deficient in vitamin B12 also have Alzheimer's disease. Blood levels of the vitamin are significantly lower in Alzheimer patients than in patients suffering from other brain or memory disorders. Scores on cognitive-function tests are lowest in Alzheimer patients with the lowest vitamin B12 blood levels. It is unknown whether the vitamin deficiency causes or results from deterioration of brain tissue. One of the functions of vitamin B12 is to maintain healthy nerve tissue, which might explain how a deficiency of the vitamin might contribute to the progression of Alzheimer's disease.

CHOLINE. Choline and its dietary source lecithin (a fatty substance found in egg yolks, wheat germ and liver, but which can also be taken in supplemental doses) have shown varying effectiveness in the treatment of memory loss and Alzheimer's disease. The attempts to use this vitamin B-like substance are based on the observation that a particular neurotransmitter called acetylcholine, which contains choline and is responsible for the transfer of messages related to memory, is not produced in sufficient amounts in the brains of patients with

Alzheimer's disease. Symptoms, such as slowed speech, shaking, and palsy-like movements, appear when acetylcholine production in the brain is inadequate. Supplementation with choline or purified soya lecithin (containing 90 percent phosphatidylcholine) sometimes has improved brain function in patients with memory loss. In other cases, however, increased intake of choline or lecithin raises blood levels of choline, but has no affect on acetylcholine levels or brain function.

If choline or lecithin are effective in the treatment of memory loss, they are probably useful only in the beginning or mild stages and are then only useful in prolonging the onset of more advanced stages of the disease.

OTHER VITAMINS AND MINERALS. Patients with dementia compared to patients without memory loss consume less vitamin C, vitamin E, and niacin and have lower levels of folic acid in their blood. The relationship between these nutrients and the initiation or progression of Alzheimer's disease is unknown. One study found supplementation with iron, vitamin B6 and the vitamin-like substance ubiquinone (also called co-enzyme Q) slowed the progression of Alzheimer's disease; however, further research is needed to confirm this finding.

Low blood levels of the antioxidant nutrients vitamin A, beta carotene, and vitamin E might indicate increased free-radical activity in Alzheimer's disease. Preliminary research suggests that long-term mild overdoses of vitamin A might contribute to the development of Alzheimer's disease; however, this theory is purely speculative and awaits scientific testing.

Dietary Recommendations

Limited information is available on dietary recommendations for the prevention or treatment of Alzheimer's disease. Until more is known, the best dietary strategy is to consume a low-fat, high-fiber, nutrient-dense diet, adequate in all vitamins and minerals and low in sugars and refined and convenience foods. The diet should contain a variety of fruits, vegetables, whole grain breads and cereals, cooked dried beans and peas, low-fat or nonfat milk products, and extra-lean meats, chicken, and fish. A multiple vitamin-mineral supplement that contains at least 100 percent of the RDA for all nutrients, especially vitamin B12; a calcium-magnesium supplement; regular exercise; effective stress management; and avoidance of aluminum cookware, aluminum-containing medications and sundries, alcohol, and tobacco might be important for the prevention and treatment of Alzheimer's disease.

ANEMIA

Overview

Anemia is a reduction in the number or size of red blood cells or in the amount of hemoglobin within the cells. Red blood cells carry oxygen from the lungs to the tissues and transport carbon dioxide from the tissues back to the lungs to be exhaled. Any condition that reduces the oxygen-carrying capacity of the red blood cells reduces the oxygen supply to the tissues, including the internal organs, the muscles, and the brain.

Symptoms of anemia include lethargy, weakness, poor concentration, or being out of breath after minor physical effort. A pale complexion is sometimes observed in the anemic person. Increased susceptibility to colds and infection might be an early warning of anemia. A desire to eat non-food items, such as chalk, ice, or dirt (a condition called pica), also might indicate anemia. In the later stages of anemia, the fingernails become thin and flat, the tongue becomes smooth and waxy, and stomach disorders are possible.

Anemia can result from severe blood loss from excessive bleeding or chronic low-grade blood loss from a bleeding ulcer or repeated blood donations. Anemia also can be nutritional in origin and can result from insufficient dietary iron, vitamin B12, folic acid, vitamin B6, vitamin C, vitamin E, or copper. The deficiency can result from poor dietary intake, impaired absorption, or faulty use of the nutrient within the body.

Nutrition and Anemia

VITAMIN E. Vitamin E might be beneficial in the prevention and treatment of certain forms of anemia. Patients with kidney disease who are on dialysis often suffer from anemia. The cause of this anemia is unknown; however, the type of anemia resembles the "hemolytic" or fragile-cell anemia characteristic of a vitamin E deficiency. Supplementation with vitamin E increases the number of red blood cells and reduces the rate of red blood cell destruction in some patients.

VITAMIN B2. Increased intake of vitamin B2 combined with iron supplements is more effective in the treatment of anemia than is iron alone.

VITAMIN B12 AND FOLIC ACID. Poor dietary intake of either vitamin B12 or folic acid results in a form of anemia called macrocytic or megaloblastic anemia. In contrast to the pale, small red blood cells common to iron deficiency anemia, the red blood cells are large, fragile, and limited in number. The results are the same; in both forms of anemia, the oxygen-carrying capacity of the blood is reduced and lethargy, poor concentration, and other symptoms of anemia develop.

IRON. Iron is attached to the protein hemoglobin in red blood cells. It is the iron that binds to oxygen in the lungs and releases oxygen to the tissues. The manufacture of red blood cells decreases when the body does not have an adequate amount of iron. The few red blood cells that are formed are small and pale in color.

Iron deficiency is the most prevalent nutritional deficiency in the United States and occurs most frequently in infants, young children, teenagers, women of childbearing age, pregnant and lactating women, and seniors. As many as 80 percent of exercising women and 20 percent of women in general are iron deficient, which is the marginal iron status that precedes anemia. Daily iron supplements improve iron status, even during intensive athletic training in these women.

Adult males are at low risk for iron deficiency because their daily needs are low and their food intake is high. If iron deficiency is diagnosed in this population it is often an indication of internal bleeding from another condition, such as stomach ulcers or cancer. Postmenopausal women, because they are no longer menstruating, also are at low risk of iron deficiency as long as they consume otherwise nutritious diets.

Anemia is the later stage of iron deficiency. The iron in muscles and other body stores has been depleted for months before the red blood cells are affected. Prior to a reduction in red blood cells, moderate to severe iron deficiency in children and adults can result in irritability, headaches, loss of appetite, clumsiness, lethargy, poor school performance, and hyperactivity. Teenagers show poor attention span and reduced perception that interferes with learning abilities.

Tests are available to identify iron deficiency and iron-deficiency anemia. The routine hemoglobin and hematocrit tests only indicate the final stage of deficiency-anemia. The serum ferritin, transferrin saturation, and total iron binding capacity tests are more sensitive indicators of iron status and provide an indication of pre-anemic or marginal iron status. However, women should have several tests done at different times of the month since iron levels fluctuate throughout the menstrual cycle. (See page 116 for more information on iron and anemia.)

SELENIUM. Selenium deficiency might result in or aggravate the symptoms of anemia. Blood selenium levels are low in anemic animals and selenium supplements correct the anemia. Selenium's role as a component of the antioxidant enzyme glutathione peroxidase, which protects red blood cell membranes from free-radical damage, might be an explanation for the mineral's association with anemia.

OTHER VITAMINS AND MINERALS. Vitamin A, in combination with iron supplements, increases hemoglobin levels in anemic patients. Copper, vitamin C, and vitamin B6 aid in the formation of hemoglobin and red blood cells, so a deficiency of any one of these nutrients could result in anemia.

Copper is required in such minute amounts that normal dietary intake usually provides an ample supply of the mineral; however, long-term, inadequate intake of copper will result in abnormal use of iron and anemia. Copper-deficiency anemia is most common in infants fed cow's milk or copper-deficient infant formula rather than breast milk.

Vitamin C is necessary for optimal absorption and use of iron. One of the symptoms of vitamin C deficiency is anemia related to the vitamin's role in iron metabolism.

Vitamin B6 deficiency results in an anemia that resembles iron-deficiency anemia. The blood levels of iron are adequate, but hemoglobin and red blood cells are not formed in the absence of vitamin B6. Treatment consists of a therapeutic trial dose of 50 to 200mg of vitamin B6 each day. The anemia should respond within a few weeks if vitamin B6 is the cause. This treatment requires physician supervision.

Dietary Recommendations

Iron deficiency and iron-deficiency anemia can be prevented and successfully treated with an increase in dietary iron, dietary factors that improve iron absorption, and/or supplemental iron. A moderate dose iron supplement or adding as little as 3 ounces of extra-lean red meat to the diet is often all it takes to prevent iron deficiency. Symptoms improve within three weeks of initiating an aggressive iron program.

Infants and young children might develop iron deficiency anemia after weaning as a result of a prolonged milk-based diet and by over-consumption of foods low in iron. Poor food choices combined with the normal decline in appetite after the first year of life can result in chronic low iron intake in children under 8 years old.

Excess consumption of iron in supplement form has its drawbacks. Large doses of iron can cause stomach upsets and constipation or diarrhea. Huge doses of 3 to 10 grams of iron can be fatal in children. Iron also competes with other trace minerals, such as zinc and copper, for absorption from the intestine and increased intake of one can cause secondary deficiencies of the other minerals. For example, iron-fortified formulas might produce low blood levels of zinc in infants. This nutrient-nutrient interaction adds support to the argument that the "one nutrient/one disorder" approach to vitamin-mineral fortification or supplementation might be an oversimplification of a much more complex and integrated process of nutrient status. An iron supplement for anemia might be an incomplete therapy that causes secondary deficiencies of other nutrients, unless these nutrients also are increased in the diet.

The best dietary advice to prevent or treat anemia in children, women, seniors, and other high-risk groups is to consume a low-fat, high-fiber, nutrient-dense diet that supplies optimal levels of all vitamins and minerals and is low in sugars and refined and convenience foods. The diet should contain a variety of iron-rich fruits, vegetables, whole grain breads and cereals, cooked dried beans and peas, and extra-lean meats, chicken, and fish. Although red wine contains four to five times as much iron as white wine, the iron is poorly absorbed. A multiple vitamin-mineral supplement that contains at least 100 percent of the RDA for all vitamins and minerals, including copper, iron, selenium, vitamin B2, vitamin B6, vitamin B12, folic acid, vitamin C, and vitamin E; as well as regular exercise, effective stress management, moderate use of alcohol, and avoidance of tobacco are important for the prevention and treatment of anemia.

ARTHRITIS

Overview

Arthritis is inflammation of the joints, which can be long-term (chronic) or short-term (acute). Rheumatoid arthritis and osteoarthritis are the most common forms of arthritis, and the symptoms of rheumatoid arthritis are the most severe.

Rheumatoid arthritis is a chronic, disabling, and crippling disease characterized by inflammation of the lining of the joints. The small joints of the hands and feet are the most common sites for rheumatoid arthritis, but any joint can be affected. The causes of rheumatoid arthritis are unclear and are possibly a combination of a disturbance in the body's immune response, infection, heredity, or an as yet unidentified factor.

Osteoarthritis differs from rheumatoid arthritis in that it is a degeneration of the cartilage rather than inflammation of the lining of a joint. The joints most likely to be affected by this degenerative disease are the joints of the feet and toes, the thumb joint, and the joints of the weight-bearing bones, such as the knees, hips, ankles, and backbone. Osteoarthritis is the most common form of arthritis and is found in most people in their later years. There is no single cause of osteoarthritis and this joint disorder is probably a result of physical stresses experienced throughout life, especially injuries or other diseases of the joints and obesity.

Nutrition and Arthritis

It is common for people with rheumatoid arthritis to be poorly nourished. The inflammatory process of arthritis changes the lining of the intestine and reduces the absorption of some nutrients, while increasing the daily nutrient requirements. Nutritional status is further depleted if the person is on long-term medication therapy that increases nutrient needs or causes peptic ulcers and gastritis, which reduces the desire to eat. Finally, the crippling and pain of rheumatoid arthritis can interfere with the purchase, preparation, and consumption of food.

Poor dietary intake of certain vitamins and minerals as well as weight loss and muscle wastage are associated with rheumatoid arthritis, although it is unclear whether poor nutrition is a cause or a result of the disease. Joint pain and stiffness increase when the patient is malnourished, and deficiencies of folic acid, vitamin C, vitamin D, vitamin B6, vitamin B12, iron, magnesium, selenium, and zinc are found in patients with rheumatoid arthritis. The low levels of vitamin D common in women with rheumatoid arthritis might indicate a disturbance of bone metabolism and account for their increased risk for osteoporosis.

In addition, children with arthritis have abnormal blood levels of certain trace minerals, including iron, zinc, and copper. Enriched and fortified foods, convenience and snack foods, and other foods common in the diets of children are not typically good sources of zinc, copper, and other trace minerals and the poor dietary intake might contribute to the development or severity of rheumatoid arthritis. Low blood levels of copper are probably a result of the disease, however, rather than a cause.

In adults, blood levels are low and symptoms improve with the increased dietary intake of calcium, selenium, zinc, and vitamin E. The antioxidant nutrients, such as selenium and vitamin E, might be effective because of their ability to stop free-radical damage to joint linings, which in turn causes the accumulation of fluids, swelling, and associated pain. The addition of several antioxidant nutrients to the diets of patients with rheumatoid arthritis might be beneficial in the prevention and treatment of this disease. However, medications are the most effective treatment for rheumatoid arthritis, and no dietary therapy is widely accepted.

FISH OILS. Eicosapentaenoic acid (EPA), the fatty acid found in fish oils, might be useful in the treatment of rheumatoid arthritis. People with arthritis who take EPA supplements report improvements in morning stiffness and joint tenderness. Evidence linking fish oils to improvements in rheumatoid arthritis is limited and no dietary recommendations can be made at this time.

FOOD INTOLERANCE. Food intolerances have been blamed for some cases of rheumatoid arthritis. Improvements in pain, number of painful joints, duration of morning stiffness, and grip strength are experienced when foods likely to be poorly tolerated, such as wheat or milk, are eliminated from the diet. These improvements in symptoms are maintained as long as the patient follows the restricted diet and symptoms return when a patient returns to previous eating habits.

Dietary Recommendations

Rheumatoid arthritis is linked to poor nutritional status, while good nutrition counteracts the adverse effects of medication therapy. For example, supplementation with calcium and vitamin D can help prevent the bone loss associated with the use of steroids prescribed in the treatment of rheumatoid arthritis. Increased intake of vitamin C can offset the adverse effects of aspirin on the absorption of vitamin C.

Weight loss and maintenance of a desirable body weight is recommended for patients with either rheumatoid arthritis or osteoarthritis. Symptoms of osteoarthritis often subside with a return to a healthy weight.

Until more is known about diet and rheumatoid arthritis, a low-fat, high-fiber, nutrient-dense diet, adequate in all vitamins and minerals and low in sugars, refined and convenience foods is a healthy and safe preventive measure. The diet should contain a variety of fruits, vegetables, whole grain breads and cereals, cooked dried beans and peas, low-fat or nonfat milk products, and extra-lean meats, chicken, and fish. Some patients report less pain, swollen joints, and morning stiffness and fewer tender joints after changing to a vegetarian diet.

A multiple vitamin-mineral supplement that contains 100 percent of the RDA for the trace minerals as well as regular exercise, effective stress management, and avoidance of alcohol and tobacco are important for the prevention and treatment of arthritis. In addition, the patient with either rheumatoid arthritis or osteoarthritis should lie down at least once during the day to rest the joints and remove the weight from them. Massage and heat therapy also reduce pain.

Although adequate intake of vitamins and minerals is essential to the health of the person with arthritis, overconsumption of nutrients also might be harmful. Large amounts of iron might increase the symptoms of arthritis. Excessive doses of vitamin D cause calcium to be deposited in tissues, such as the kidney and heart. The damage caused by calcification of soft tissue is irreversible.

ASTHMA

Overview

The causes of asthma are not clear. The disorder might be inherited, as several members within a family usually suffer from asthma. In some cases, asthma is a result of food allergies. Psychological and emotional influences also contribute to asthma attacks.

Nutrition and Asthma

VITAMIN B6. Increased intake of vitamin B6 might reduce the symptoms of asthma. Some people who consume 100mg of vitamin B6 daily report a reduction in occurrence, severity, and duration of asthmatic attacks. Asthma patients have lower blood levels of vitamin B6 than do healthy adults and although supplementation might not raise these levels, it does appear to improve symptoms. Supplementation with large doses of vitamins or minerals should be supervised by a physician.

VITAMIN C. Blood levels of vitamin C decrease temporarily during an asthmatic attack, while blood levels of the stress hormone cortisone increase. It is not known whether an increased dietary intake of vitamin C might aid in the prevention of the asthmatic attack.

SELENIUM. Blood levels of selenium are low in patients with asthma and these low levels might worsen the inflammation associated with the disorder.

VEGETARIAN DIET. A strict vegetarian or vegan diet (avoidance of all foods of animal origin) might aid in the treatment of asthma. Improvements in the frequency and severity of asthmatic attacks are reported by people placed on a strict vegetarian diet. In addition, dosages of medications usually prescribed for asthma, such as cortisone, are reduced by 50 percent to 90 percent, and some people are able to discontinue medication on the vegetarian diet.

Dietary Recommendations

Some food allergies produce asthma-like symptoms. (See pages 163–168 for more information on food allergies.) For example, some people are sensitive to the flavor-enhancer monosodium glutamate (MSG), the coloring agent FD&C yellow dye #5, salicylates, or the metabisulfites preservatives and develop asthma-like symptoms whenever these food additives are consumed. The asthma symptoms develop within minutes to hours after the food is ingested, so it is possible to identify the offending food and eliminate it from the diet. Specific dietary recommendations for asthma are not available (Table 32).

Table 32
SALICYLATES IN FOODS

Food Group	Contain Salicylates
Beverage	Tea, root beer, birch beer
Meat	Corned beef, meat processed with vinegar
Milk	None
Vegetable	Cucumbers, green peppers, tomatoes, potatoes
Fruit	Apples, apple cider, apricots, blackberries, boysenberries, cherries, currants, gooseberries, huckleberries, maraschino cherries, grapes, melons, nectarines, peaches, raisins, raspberries, prunes, plums
Cereals and Breads	None
Fat	Salad dressing, mayonnaise, avocado, olives

A low-fat, high-fiber, nutrient-dense diet adequate in all vitamins and minerals and low in sugars and refined convenience foods and any food suspected to cause allergic reactions, is a healthy and safe protective measure. The healthful diet should contain a variety of fruits, vegetables, whole grain breads and cereals, and cooked dried beans and peas, low-fat or nonfat milk products, and extra-lean meats, chicken, and fish should be consumed in moderation. A strict vegetarian diet also can be designed to meet all vitamin and mineral needs. Regular exercise, effective stress management, and avoidance of alcohol and tobacco are important in the prevention and treatment of asthma.

BRUISING

Overview

A bruise is a surface injury to the skin where the small blood vessels that reside below and within the skin are broken. Bruises that develop without an injury can be a sign of numerous disorders, including leukemia, low blood levels of platelets (cell fragments responsible for blood clotting), or nutrient deficiencies.

Nutrition and Bruising

Nutrients necessary for the normal healing of bruises and wounds include protein, vitamin A, vitamin B12 and other B vitamins, vitamin C, vitamin E, folic acid, calcium, copper, and zinc. In addition, chronic use of alcohol or some medications depletes the body of these nutrients and impairs the healing of wounds and bruises. A physician should be consulted if the diet is adequate in nutrients and the bruising persists.

VITAMIN C. The classic symptom of scurvy, the vitamin C deficiency disease, is tiny hemorrhages below the skin called petechial hemorrhages. Vitamin C is necessary for the formation of collagen, the protein portion of connective tissue. This tissue holds the body's cells together, while improper formation causes other tissues to fall apart. Consequently, a vitamin C deficiency causes the blood vessels to become fragile, and blood leaks into the surrounding tissues, causing small bruises.

Dietary Recommendations

The best dietary defense against bruising is a low-fat, high-fiber, nutrient-dense diet adequate in all vitamins and minerals and low in sugars and refined and convenience foods. The diet should contain a variety of fruits, vegetables, whole grain breads and cereals, cooked dried beans and peas, low-fat or nonfat milk products, and extra-lean meats, chicken, and fish. Regular exercise, effective stress management, and a limited consumption of alcohol to little or none, and avoidance of tobacco are important in the prevention and treatment of bruises.

BURNS

Overview

A widespread burn is one of the most severe injuries to the body. Repair of damaged tissues and changes in the nervous system and hormone regulation associated with burns can double normal energy (calorie) requirements. Excessive loss of protein, water-soluble vitamins, and minerals caused by the injured tissue increases the daily need for these nutrients. Simultaneous infection further increases protein and nutrient needs. In addition, burn patients often lose their appetites and the maintenance of good nutritional status is challenging.

Nutrition and Burns

The dietary management of patients with severe burns should be supervised by a dietitian and a physician. It will include the replacement of fluids and electrolytes (e.g., sodium, chloride, potassium, and other nutrients) and adequate intake of calories and nutrients based on ideal body weight, percentage of body burned, and a nutritional assessment. The daily need for all vitamins and minerals also increases during the healing process.

CALCIUM. Blood levels of calcium are low in patients with burns that cover more than 30 percent of their bodies. Loss of calcium is exaggerated when the patient is unable to move or exercise. Calcium supplementation and early initiation of exercise might be necessary to prevent bone loss.

ZINC. Low blood levels of zinc are seen in patients with severe burns. Zinc supplementation is recommended to treat post-burn loss of appetite and impaired wound healing.

Dietary Recommendations

Nutritional support for the patient with severe burns will include increased intake of protein, calories, vitamins, minerals, fluids, and electrolytes. Frequent feedings, use of supplementary feedings in the form of tube feedings or intravenous solutions, and sterile serving containers also might be recommended.

Nutrition for the treatment of minor burns does not vary from dietary recommendations for the healthy adult. A low-fat, high-fiber, nutrient-dense diet should be consumed, adequate in all vitamins and minerals and low in sugars and refined and convenience foods. The diet should contain a variety of fruits, vegetables, whole grain breads and cereals, cooked dried beans and peas, low-fat or nonfat milk products, and extra-lean meats, chicken, and fish. Regular exercise, effective stress management, and avoidance of alcohol and tobacco are important for the healing of burns.

CANCER

Overview

Cancer is a group of diseases characterized by the uncontrolled growth and spread of abnormal cells. The abnormal cells trespass into surrounding tissues, interfere with the tissues' ability to function, and eventually damage or destroy the healthy cells. Cancer cells also can break loose, travel through the blood and lymph, lodge in tissues in other parts of the body, and develop into new cancers. This ability to form secondary cancers is called metastasis (Table 33).

Table 33
THE 7 WARNING SIGNS OF CANCER

C hange in bowel or bladder habits
A sore that does not heal
U nusual bleeding or discharge
T hickening or lump in breast or elsewhere
I ndigestion or difficulty in swallowing
O bvious change in wart or mole
N agging cough or hoarseness

Cancer develops in two stages: an initiation stage where the normal, healthy cell or its genetic code is altered, and a promotion stage where the abnormal cell is encouraged to multiply. Both stages are necessary for cancer to develop. The initiation stage happens quickly and frequently and is caused by a substance called a mutagen or a carcinogen. The promotion stage, where a substance called a promoter is in contact with the abnormal cell, is more lengthy, allowing the slow growth of cancer to go undetected for up to 30 years. Cancer will not develop unless the cell exposed to a mutagen or carcinogen is subsequently in contact with something that will promote its growth. In addition, the strength of the immune system might have an important role in the prevention or development of cancer.

Figure 2

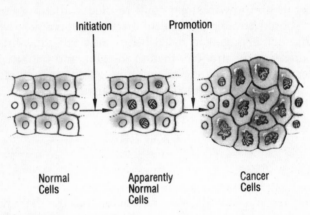

The two stages of cancer.[1]

[1]*Reprinted with permission from Health Media of America, 1578 West Lewis Street, San Diego, CA 92103.*

Nutrition and Cancer

Nutritional excesses and deficiencies are associated with the development of cancer. It is estimated that as much as 70 percent of all cancers are diet-related, which makes diet second only to tobacco as the most influential factor in the development (and prevention) of cancer.

Many substances in food act as mutagens or promoters. For example, the food additives called nitrites, found in processed meats such as bacon and bologna, are converted in the body to nitrosamines, which are potent carcinogens. Alcohol does not initiate cancer, but it promotes the growth of a pre-existing abnormal cell. Other dietary mutagens include aflatoxin (a mold that forms on peanuts), heavy metals such as lead, polychlorinated biphenyl (PCB), and pesticides such as malathione and DDT. Examples of suspected dietary promoters are saccharin, excess dietary fat, and excessive use of coffee or caffeine.

On the other hand, the diet also contains many substances that prevent the development or progression of cancer. A diet low in fat and alcohol, and high in fiber, vitamin A or beta carotene, vitamin C, vitamin E, selenium, and several other nutrients and phytochemicals found in food inhibits the initiation and promotion of several types of cancer.

However, a nutrient that prevents or treats one type of cancer might not necessarily work for another cancer. For example, vitamin A reduces the risk of developing breast cancer, but may have little influence over the course of colon cancer. Vitamin C might help reduce the risk of stomach cancer, but does not appear to provide protection against breast cancer.

BODY WEIGHT. People who maintain a healthy or desirable body weight, as compared to people who are 20 percent or more above their desirable body weight, live longer and are at a lower risk for developing cancers, especially cancers of the prostate, uterus, gallbladder, kidney, cervix, stomach, colon, and breast.

DIETARY FAT. No other dietary change has as profound an effect on lowering the risk for developing cancer than does reducing dietary fat intake. Numerous studies show that a typical American diet that provides more than 30 percent of its calories from fat is linked to and perhaps is a cause of cancer of the ovaries, uterus, colon, and prostate.

Whether or not dietary fat is linked to breast cancer remains controversial. The risk for developing breast cancer is low in countries where people consume a low-fat diet. However, cancer risk increases when these people move to the United States and consume the fatty Westernized diet. Of the two dietary fats associated with the development of cancer (saturated and unsaturated fats), the polyunsaturated fats, found in vegetable oils, salad dressings, and mayonnaise, and saturated fat found in foods of animal origin have the greatest cancer-promoting effects. Monounsaturated fats in olive oil and canola oil appear to have little effect on cancer risk. Oral and esophageal cancer risk rises with increased intake of meat, animal products, and most vegetables oils.

FIBER. A low-fat, high-fiber diet is a person's best safeguard against cancer. People have an 8-fold increase in the risk for certain forms of cancer, such as colon and intestinal cancers, when the diet is low in fiber, as it is in the United States. A high-fiber diet also reduces the risk for developing breast and prostate cancers. The insoluble fibers, such as cellulose in whole wheat products, wheat bran, and some vegetables, appear to be the best protectors against cancer.

VITAMIN A AND BETA CAROTENE. A diet high in vitamin A or beta carotene protects a person against cancer, especially cancers of the mouth, larynx, esophagus (throat), stomach, breast, cervix, bladder, and lungs. In contrast, a person who consumes a diet low in vitamin A or beta carotene is at increased risk for developing cancer. Patients with cancers of the lung, stomach, esophagus, and cervix and their immediate family members have low blood levels of beta carotene.

Free radicals, reactive compounds that damage tissues, initiate cancers and promote tumor growth. Vitamin A and beta carotene are antioxidants that protect the body from free radicals and therefore protect against cancer by inhibiting both the initiation and promotion stages of cancer. Vitamin A plays a stronger role during the promotion stage and beta carotene appears to have more effect during the early initiation stage. Vitamin A and beta carotene work with other antioxidants, such as vitamin E and selenium, to protect cells from free-radical damage. Beta carotene also might aid in the prevention of cancer by:

1. inhibiting the growth of abnormal cells;
2. strengthening the immune response so cancer cells are less likely to grow;
3. fortifying cell membranes so they are less vulnerable to attack or damage;
4. altering cell production so abnormal cells are less likely to develop; and
5. moderating cell communication so that abnormal cell growth is discouraged.

Vitamin A also aids in the prevention of tissue damage caused by radiation. Vitamin A and beta carotene might delay or prevent the transformation of precancerous cells into cancer.

The most common cancers in the United States are cancers of epithelial tissue, the tissue that lines the inside and outside of the body. Skin, mucous membranes, and the tissues that line the lungs, mouth, throat, stomach, colon, prostate, cervix, and uterus are examples of epithelial tissues. Vitamin A aids in the development and maintenance of these tissues. A deficiency of vitamin A produces changes in these tissues that resemble the initial changes in cancer. Tissues low in vitamin A are more prone to develop cancer than are tissues with a high concentration of the vitamin.

Beta carotene is more effective than vitamin A in preventing lung cancer. Lung cancer rates are lower in cigarette smokers who also consume a diet high in fruits and vegetables than in smokers who avoid these foods. The risk for lung cancer rises when the intake of beta carotene is low. Optimal intake of beta carotene also reduces the risk of lung cancer in non-smokers. Both vitamin A and beta carotene help prevent the precancerous changes in the mouth observed in people who chew tobacco. Daily requirements for beta carotene might increase with excessive exposure to sunshine.

People with precancerous conditions also might benefit from adequate vitamin A intake. Benign breast disease is characterized by pain and breast lumps and is associated with a two-fold increase in risk for developing breast cancer. Symptoms of breast pain and lumps are reduced in some individuals when the vitamin A content of the diet is increased. There is no evidence, however, that the vitamin or beta carotene will cure the disorder. High intake of lycopene, a carotenoid found in many of the same foods as beta carotene, might prevent the precancerous condition called cervical intra-epithelial neoplasia (CIN).

Vitamin A or beta carotene also might assist in the treatment of cancer. Vitamin A-rich foods or vitamin A supplements, when taken in conjunction with chemotherapy or radiation therapy, might improve the cancer patient's outcome for recovery and reduce damage to healthy tissue caused by chemotherapy or radiation. A combination of vitamin A and the amino acid arginine might slow the growth of tumors and improve the survival time of the cancer patient.

BEWARE THE ONE-STUDY APPROACH TO NUTRITION

Nutrition made headlines recently when a Finnish study published in the New England Journal of Medicine reported that beta carotene increases a person's risk for developing lung cancer. While the study presented interesting information, it did not deserve the media attention it received.

In the past decade, literally hundreds of research studies have been published showing a potential link between beta carotene and a reduced risk for disease. People who consume too little beta carotene (and vitamin C) are the ones most likely to develop lung cancer, whether they smoke, are passive smokers, or avoid tobacco. People who increase their intake of the carotenoids show elevated levels of these substances in their tissues and a subsequent reduction in cancer risk. The same goes for epidemiological studies that compare smoking and carotenoid intakes across countries; for laboratory studies on rats, mice, and other animals; and in cell culture studies where cells are exposed to carcinogens with and without beta carotene. In clinical trials, beta carotene has proven effective in reversing oral leukoplakia, an established premalignant lesion.

BEWARE THE ONE-STUDY APPROACH TO NUTRITION (CONT.)

Numerous studies have shown that beta carotene affects cell differentiation, immunologic function, and the interaction of cells with growth factors, all mechanisms important for their anticarcinogenic activity. Granted, more research is always useful, but in the case of beta carotene, the research jury has overwhelmingly voted in its favor.

Few of these studies have made the evening news, while the Finnish study made a catchy headline and so was raised to celebrity status. However, while the study presents some interesting findings, it is not as newsworthy as the press would have us believe. First, the study did show that taking a moderate-dose supplement of vitamin E or beta carotene after 36 years of heavy smoking is not likely to undo a lifetime of bad habits. Even then, those subjects with the lowest base-line serum vitamin E and beta carotene levels were the ones most likely to develop lung cancer during the study.

Second, the study lasted for only five to eight years. So, many of the cancers that developed during the study could have been established, but undetected, at baseline. In fact, the researchers admit: "We are aware of no other data at this time...that suggest harmful effects of beta carotene, whereas there are data indicating benefit....In light of the data available, an adverse effect of beta carotene seems unlikely...this finding may well be due to chance."

In a nation addicted to quick fixes, one where the combination of frantic-paced lifestyles and information overload have left many people tolerant of new information only if it is packaged in a sound bite, we must be careful not to allow the media to dictate dietary recommendations by packaging a wealth of scientific research into a too-good-to-be-true magic bullet.

FOLIC ACID. Folic acid's main function in the maintenance of the genetic code of cells and the regulation of normal cell division and growth might explain this B vitamin's link to a reduced risk for developing cancer. A microscopic view of cells shows a folic acid deficiency produces changes in the cell's structure that resemble the beginning of cancer. Preliminary evidence shows folic acid prevents the conversion of a normal cell to a precancerous cell and might convert damaged cells back to normal ones. Folic acid supplementation also might help prevent lung cancer.

Folic acid plays an essential role in the production of another substance, S-adenosylmethionine, that helps block DNA abnormalities that could contribute to cancer growth. A build-up of abnormal DNA fragments occur in patients with benign tumors and colon and rectal cancer. Increased folic acid intake might prevent these initial changes.

VITAMIN B6. Vitamin B6 might have a secondary effect on the prevention of cancer by strengthening the immune system and aiding the body in its efforts to resist cancer. Limited evidence also shows this B vitamin might protect against the initiation of cancer.

VITAMIN C. The risk for developing cancer of the stomach, oral, esophageal, and possibly bladder and breast is reduced when the diet is high in vitamin C-rich foods, while these cancers are more prevalent in people who consume little vitamin C. Limited evidence credits vitamin C with a protective role in lung and cervical cancer. Nitrosamines are potent cancer-causing substances found in cigarette smoke and formed in the stomach from food additives called nitrites. Vitamin C neutralizes these carcinogens and protects the tissues that are in contact with them, such as the stomach, the colon, and the bladder.

Vitamin C might have other anti-cancer actions. Cell membranes and DNA are damaged by reactive compounds called free radicals. Vitamin C, as an antioxidant, scavenges and deactivates free radicals that might initiate and promote cancer growth. The vitamin might strengthen the cells' resistance to invasion by abnormal growth, enhance the immune response, and limit mutations in cells exposed to pesticides.

Vitamin C supplementation also might aid in cancer treatment. Patients who supplement with gram doses of vitamin C prior to radiation therapy can withstand greater doses of radiation with fewer complications than can unsupplemented patients. (See pages 150–153 for information on free radicals.)

VITAMIN D. Vitamin D might prevent or slow the growth of certain forms of cancer, such as cancers of the breast or colon and non-Hodgkin's lymphoma. The likelihood of developing colon cancer is higher in areas where people have limited exposure to sunlight (the necessary factor for the production of vitamin D in the skin) than in areas where the sun shines frequently. In addition, people who consume a diet low in vitamin D are at higher risk for developing colon cancer than are people who consume ample amounts of the vitamin. New studies indicate that vitamin D reduces the number of colon tumors that develop in the presence of a carcinogen. Vitamin D also inhibits the growth of premalignant cells in the lining of the colon, which might prevent and even treat colon cancer.

VITAMIN E. A diet high in vitamin E is linked to a reduced risk for developing cancers of the liver, lung, oral cavity, esophagus, and colon, whereas low blood levels of vitamin E increase the risk for developing cancer. People with lung cancer show depleted vitamin E stores in their tissues when compared to tissues of healthy people.

Although research on vitamin E and breast cancer is controversial, one study found women with low levels of vitamin E in their blood have a five-fold increase in the risk for developing breast cancer when compared to women with normal to high blood levels of vitamin E. Risk for breast cancer is reduced when vitamin E is added to the diet. In addition, tumor formation, growth, and numbers decrease and animals live longer when given vitamin E supplements.

Vitamin E appears to effectively protect cells from cancer initiation and promotion. Vitamin E works with other antioxidants, such as vitamin C and selenium, to prevent free-radical damage to cell membranes or the cell's genetic code that could otherwise lead to the initiation of abnormal cell growth or function. Vitamin E inhibits the growth of pre-existing cancer cells possibly by blocking the synthesis of DNA and protein in the abnormal cells. In contrast, a deficiency of the vitamin results in increased tissue damage by free radicals and nitrites, while adequate intake of the vitamin reduces the formation of nitrosamines from dietary nitrites. (See pages 150–153 for information on antioxidants.)

Another proposed way that vitamin E might protect against cancer is the vitamin's ability to protect the body's genetic code. Cancer often begins as an alteration in the genetic code that regulates the shape, function, and characteristics of each cell. Vitamin E might protect the genetic code from alterations that initiate the growth of abnormal cells and strengthen cell immunity to further resist cancerous changes. In addition, abnormal cells might be converted back to normal cells when a person consumes adequate amounts of vitamin E.

The multifaceted nature of cancer combined with the different forms of vitamin E make the link elusive. Some studies find no association while others show a preventive effect with vitamin E supplementation that depends on the form of vitamin E or intake of other nutrients such as selenium. Vitamin E succinate might be the most potent supplemental form of the vitamin.

VITAMIN K. In laboratory studies, tumor cell growth is curtailed when vitamin K is present. The cancers responsive to vitamin K therapy included breast, ovary, colon, stomach, bladder, liver, and kidney cancers.

IRON. Iron can have either a protective effect or increase the risk of developing cancer. Adequate iron intake probably protects the body from cancer by strengthening the immune system, while a diet low in iron might increase a person's risk for developing cancer. However, excessive iron intake and high tissue stores are associated with an increased risk of cancer. Preliminary research suggests that this increased cancer risk is associated with free iron (most iron is bound to proteins in the blood and other tissues), which generates free radicals. Altered iron absorption or metabolism in cancer-prone individuals also might increase disease risk.

SELENIUM. Increased intake of selenium might reduce the risk for developing cancer. People who live in areas of the country where the selenium content of the soil is high (see page 136) have a low incidence of cancer, especially cancers of the digestive tract, lungs, breast, and lymph system. The incidence of cancer is lower in countries where the people consume a selenium-rich diet than in countries where the selenium content of the diet is poor. A recent study in a region of China where the people consume low-antioxidant diets found that a combined supplement of selenium, vitamin E, and beta carotene reduced the otherwise high risk of stomach and esophageal cancer.

Blood levels of selenium are low in cancer patients with Hodgkin's disease, leukemia, and cancers of the breast, lymph system, stomach and intestine, colon, bladder, and genital tract. People with low blood levels of the mineral have a two-fold greater risk of developing cancer than do people with adequate blood selenium levels.

Selenium might protect an individual from developing cancer by its antioxidant capabilities or its ability to neutralize the toxic effects of certain metals. Selenium works with vitamin E in the protection of cell membranes and the cell's genetic code from free-radical damage that could lead to abnormal cell shape, function, or growth. Selenium also might strengthen the immune response and improve a person's defense against abnormal cell growth. Finally, selenium helps detoxify cadmium and mercury, two minerals that cause cancer.

The form of selenium might be important in the prevention or treatment of cancer. The organic form of the mineral called selenomethionine or selenocysteine might be more potent and less toxic than the inorganic sodium selenite. In addition, garlic grown on selenium-rich soil is more effective at limiting tumor growth than are selenium supplements or regular garlic alone.

CALCIUM. Calcium's protective effect against cancer is limited to the large intestine. The mineral's close dietary association with vitamin D makes it difficult to isolate either nutrient as the one that affects cancer rates. However, it appears calcium binds to cancer-promoting fats in the intestine and reduces their ability to initiate the cancer process.

VANADIUM. The trace mineral vanadium might aid in the prevention of cancer. Limited evidence shows supplementation with vanadium in animals limits the initiation and frequency of tumors.

ZINC. Zinc is related to the prevention of cancer because of its contribution to the formation and regulation of the cells' genetic code, the maintenance of a strong immune system, and the healing of damaged tissues. Patients with cancer have low blood levels of zinc and the progression of the disease is accelerated when zinc levels are low. Zinc supplements also might improve appetite in cancer patients.

OTHER DIETARY FACTORS. The frequent inclusion of cruciferous vegetables (broccoli, Brussels sprouts, kohlrabi, cauliflower, and cabbage) might reduce a person's risk for developing cancer, especially cancers of the stomach, colon, and respiratory tract. The protective effect is caused by substances called indoles in the vegetables. These vegetables have added benefits, as they also provide ample amounts of beta carotene, folic acid, vitamin C, and fiber.

A diet that supplies most of its protein from vegetable sources rather than meats or milk products might reduce the risk for developing cancer, such as prostate, pancreatic, and lymph cancers. Vegetarians are less likely than meat-eaters to develop cancer. People who consume a large part of their food intake as meat, cheese, eggs, and milk have a four-fold increased risk for developing prostate cancer as people who consume primarily vegetable protein from cooked dried beans and peas, whole grain breads and cereals, and tofu.

The omega 3 fatty acids, such as gamma linolenic acid (GLA) found in Evening Primrose Oil and eicosapentaenoic acid (EPA) found in fish oil, might aid in the prevention of cancer and might suppress the growth of tumors. For example, limited evidence from studies on animals shows that the omega 3 fatty acids might limit the growth and spread of breast cancer cells.

Garlic might prevent and treat cancer through its anticarcinogenic properties and stimulation of the immune system. People with the highest intake of garlic have lower risks of developing colon cancer. Garlic might suppress cancer growth by deactivating cancer-causing compounds, inhibiting the growth of tumors, and blocking both the initiation and promotion stages of cancer. However, further studies are needed to identify the most effective dose.

A high intake of sugar and alcohol is associated with an increased risk for some types of cancer, especially cancers of the intestinal tract. These effects are accented when combined with a high-fat, low-fiber diet. Artificial sweeteners, especially saccharin and cyclamates, also are linked to the development of cancer. In contrast, substances in green and black tea might help protect the body against some forms of cancer.

Old or damaged peanuts and peanut butter contain a naturally-occurring contaminant called aflatoxin that is one of the most potent cancer-causing substances known to occur in the food supply. The amount of aflatoxin allowed in commercial peanuts is limited by the

Food and Drug Administration (FDA) to no more than 20ppb (parts per billion). To be safe, avoid the "grind-your-own" peanuts in stores and purchase only well-known brands of peanut butter.

Limited evidence shows that some commonly eaten foods (including commercial mushrooms; chili; sassafras; black pepper; psoralen in celery, parsley, figs, and parsnips; catechol in coffee; gossypol in cotton-seed oil; and certain alkaloids in herbs) might contain cancer-causing substances if eaten in excessively large amounts. However, the amount of these carcinogens in the normal diet is minute and consumption of a wide variety of foods will reduce their impact as well as increase dietary intake of other food substances that protect the body against cancer.

More than 3,000 additives are intentionally added to foods; another 12,000 chemicals migrate unintentionally into the food supply. Intentional additives provide color, texture, taste, consistency, or retard spoilage in processed foods. Unintentional additives, such as vinyl chloride, slip into foods during harvesting, processing, packaging, or storage. Some of these additives might encourage the growth of cancer. For example, butylated hydroxytoluene, better known as BHT, is a preservative used to prolong shelf life that also might promote the formation of tumors. The FDA attempts to regulate the amount of hazardous substances in food and has established guidelines for the ingredients that can be added to foods. Any additive suspected to cause cancer must be removed from the food supply; however, only a portion of the substances added to foods have been adequately tested for their ability to cause cancer.

The method used to cook foods might increase the risk for developing cancer. Frying, barbecuing, or broiling fatty meats and fish at high temperatures can convert the fats and proteins into cancer-causing substances. Benzo(a)pyrenes are formed from fats when meats are cooked over a grill. The amount formed will depend on the temperature of the cooking and the length of time the meat is exposed to the flame. The risk for cancer is reduced when perforated foil is placed over the grill to interfere with the fats contacting the flame or the food is cooked for a short amount of time with no charring of the meat.

Smoked foods, such as ham, sausage, fish, or oysters absorb tar during processing. This tar, like the tar in cigarette smoke, contains several cancer-causing substances that could be harmful to health if consumed in large amounts. Commercially available liquid smoke is less hazardous.

Dietary Recommendations

The anti-cancer diet consists of whole grain breads and cereals, fresh fruits and vegetables, cooked dried beans and peas, and small amounts of nonfat or low-fat milk products, chicken, and fish. Foods are steamed, baked, poached, stewed, or lightly broiled, and fat is limited by avoiding gravies, sauces, creams, and other fats. At least two servings of dark green or orange vegetables should be included in the daily diet to obtain adequate amounts of beta carotene and folic acid. Two or more servings of citrus fruits will provide vitamin C. Frequent inclusion of vegetables from the cabbage family also is recommended. Adequate daily intake of fiber can be obtained from at least six servings of whole grain breads and cereals, four servings of fresh fruit and vegetables, and one serving of cooked dried beans and peas.

Calorie intake should be adequate to maintain a desired body weight. Salt-cured, smoked, and nitrite-containing foods should be avoided or consumed in limited amounts. Contaminated, moldy, or spoiled foods should be avoided, in particular old peanuts that might harbor aflatoxin. A multiple vitamin-mineral preparation that contains all the vitamins and minerals, especially vitamin A, folic acid, selenium (as selenomethionine), and zinc, at a level 100 percent to 300 percent of the RDA and an extra dose of the antioxidants, including vitamin C (250mg daily), vitamin E (200IU to 400IU daily), and beta carotene (15mg daily) will supplement the anti-cancer diet. Excessive doses of vitamins or minerals are discouraged as preliminary evidence suggests that certain nutrients, such as iron and zinc, consumed in large amounts might promote the development of cancer by inhibiting the immune response and increasing the body's susceptibility to infection and disease (Table 34).

Table 34
DIETARY GUIDELINES FOR THE PREVENTION OF CANCER[1]

1. Avoid obesity.
2. Cut down on total fat intake.
3. Eat more high-fiber foods, such as whole grain cereals, fruits, and vegetables.
4. Include foods rich in vitamin A (or beta carotene) and vitamin C in your daily diet.
5. Include cruciferous vegetables in your diet.
6. Eat moderately of salt-cured, smoked, and nitrite-cured foods.
7. Keep alcohol consumption moderate, if you do drink.

[1]Established by the American Cancer Society, Inc., 90 Park Avenue, New York, NY 10016

Regular exercise; effective management of stress; avoidance of all tobacco (cigarettes, pipes, cigars, and chewing tobacco); avoidance of second-hand tobacco smoke; moderate consumption of alcohol; and avoidance of radiation, air and water pollution, and carcinogens at home or on the job are important factors in an anti-cancer lifestyle.

Although the diet and environment contain cancer-causing substances, they also contain cancer-preventing factors. It is impossible to avoid all cancer-causing substances, but it is possible to reduce the body's exposure to them and to increase factors that will aid in the prevention of cancer initiation and promotion.

CARDIOVASCULAR DISEASE (CVD)

Overview

Cardiovascular disease is a general term for any disease of the heart (cardio) and blood vessels (vascular). Diseases in this category include:

Atherosclerosis. Fat-clogged arteries.
Coronary artery disease. Atherosclerosis of the arteries that supply blood, oxygen, and nutrients to the heart.
Heart attack or myocardial infarction. Damage to the heart caused by reduced or blocked blood supply.
Stroke. Damage to brain tissue that results from reduced or blocked blood supply.
Hypertension. High blood pressure.
Congestive heart failure. Poor blood circulation and pooling of blood and fluid in the ankles and feet caused by a weakened heart.

Despite the association between CVD and advancing age, the occurrence of heart disease in the United States is not a natural consequence of aging. Atherosclerosis and other forms of CVD are rare to nonexistent in some countries, even in the elderly. The incidence of CVD increases, however, when these people migrate to the United States and assume the Westernized diet high in fat, salt, sugar, and cholesterol and low in fiber. In many cases, the suffering and death from CVD could be avoided if a person made a few changes in diet, exercise, and other lifestyle habits. The sooner these changes are made, the better; however, it is never too late to begin.

Atherosclerosis is the underlying cause of most heart disease. Several factors are related to the initiation and progression of the atherosclerotic process. These include:

- Elevated blood cholesterol
- Elevated low density lipoprotein-cholesterol (LDL-cholesterol), one of the carriers of cholesterol in the blood
- Reduced high density lipoprotein-cholesterol (HDL-cholesterol), another of the carriers of cholesterol in the blood

- Cigarette smoking
- Hypertension
- A sedentary lifestyle
- Obesity
- Excessive and prolonged stress
- A family history of CVD
- Male gender after 35 years old or female gender after menopause.

The most important indicator of cardiovascular disease is blood cholesterol levels. The risk for developing atherosclerosis increases with increasing levels of blood cholesterol and anything that lowers blood fat levels lowers the risk for developing CVD. The average blood cholesterol level for adults in the United States is approximately 240mg percent and Americans have a 50-50 chance of developing heart disease. The heart disease risk is much lower or nonexistent in countries where the average blood cholesterol level is 150mg percent.

LIPOPROTEINS. How cholesterol is packaged in the blood has an important effect on the risk for developing CVD. Fat-soluble cholesterol cannot float freely in the watery medium of the blood and must be packaged in carriers called lipoproteins. Lipoproteins are ideal for transporting fats because they have a water-soluble exterior that dissolves easily in the blood and a fat-soluble interior that can hold cholesterol and other fats. Different lipoproteins transport fats to different places within the body and some are associated with an increased risk for developing CVD, while others lower a person's risk.

A person's risk for developing CVD is high when a large portion of cholesterol and triglycerides are packaged in LDL-cholesterol and VLDL-cholesterol.

A blood cholesterol below 200mg percent, a ratio of total cholesterol to HDL-cholesterol that is 3.5:1 or lower, and an LDL-cholesterol level below 130mg percent are indicators that a person's risk for CVD is low.

A person's risk for developing CVD is low when a large portion of cholesterol is packaged in HDL-cholesterol.

Blood cholesterol above 200mg percent, LDL-cholesterol above 130mg percent, or a ratio above 4.5:1 indicates a high risk for developing CVD.

Recently, a new lipoprotein, called Lipoprotein(a) or Lp(a) also has been implicated in CVD risk. Lp(a) is a unique, cholesterol-rich lipoprotein found in the blood. Lp(a) resembles LDL-cholesterol. Consequently, Lp(a) often is mistaken for LDL-cholesterol. Both lipoproteins—Lp(a) and LDL-cholesterol—contain the same protein (i.e., apoprotein B-100), however, this protein is slightly modified on Lp(a).

Elevated Lp(a) blood levels are associated with increased risk for CVD and atherosclerosis. Lp(a) levels greater than 30mg/dl increase the risk of CVD two-fold and if LDL-cholesterol also is high, CVD risk is five-fold greater than average. However, no relationship exists between Lp(a) levels and total blood cholesterol levels. In other words, a person can have high Lp(a) concentrations despite low blood cholesterol levels.

Nutrition and Cardiovascular Disease

The incidence of cardiovascular disease escalated in the United States population as the consumption of fat, cholesterol, salt, and sugar increased and the intake of fresh fruits and vegetables and whole grain breads and cereals decreased. In the past ten years, as people have slowly reduced their fat and cholesterol intakes, the rate of cardiovascular disease also has declined. However, fat intake still hovers at 34 percent of total calories (the goal is 25 percent to 30 percent) and heart disease remains this country's number one killer disease.

THE ANTIOXIDANTS. A high intake of foods rich in the antioxidant nutrients—beta carotene, vitamin C, and vitamin E—protects against the development of atherosclerosis, the beginning step in the development of cardiovascular disease. These antioxidants protect the body from oxygen fragments and other free radicals that damage the lining of the blood vessels, alter LDL-cholesterol and increase the clumping of cholesterol along the vessel walls. Individuals with the highest intake of antioxidants have the least amount of free-radical-damaged LDL-cholesterol (called oxidized LDLs), higher levels of HDL-cholesterol (the "good" cholesterol), and the lowest risk of atherosclerosis, stroke, and cardiovascular disease. (See pages 150–153 for more information on antioxidants.)

VITAMIN C. Cholesterol production in the liver and conversion of cholesterol to bile acids for excretion require vitamin C. Supplementation with vitamin C might lower total and LDL-cholesterol, increase HDL-cholesterol, and remove cholesterol from deposits in artery walls. Individuals with a vitamin C-rich diet are less likely to die from a heart attack than those with a low intake of the vitamin. Even a marginal deficiency of vitamin C increases free-radical damage to heart tissue that might initiate CVD, while adequate intake protects the heart, blood vessels, and blood from the harmful reactive compounds. Vitamin C lowers blood pressure and might be an effective way to prevent and treat mild hypertension. Vitamin C also helps maintain levels of prostacyclin, a prostaglandin that discourages the clumping of blood fragments and dilates blood vessels, allowing the blood to flow with less resistance.

VITAMIN E. Vitamin E reduces the risk of CVD. The Nurses Health Study conducted at Harvard Medical School in Boston showed that people who supplement with vitamin E in doses of at least 100IU daily for at least two years have a 40 percent lower risk of developing heart disease than do people who do not supplement. Vitamin E might aid in the prevention of heart disease by strengthening blood vessel walls, protecting LDL-cholesterol from free-radical damage, and preventing the abnormal clumping of blood cell fragments called platelets associated with the development of atherosclerosis. Vitamin E also reduces the symptoms of intermittent claudication, the pain and tension in the legs that results from poor blood flow in patients with heart disease. Vitamin E supplementation improves recovery and prognosis from bypass surgery by reducing free-radical damage associated with the procedure.

Recent studies from the University of Southern California Medical School in Los Angeles and the University of New Mexico in Albuquerque show that vitamin E slows the rate of blood vessel blockage after open-heart surgery or angioplasty and suggests that vitamin E might help reverse the atherosclerotic process. Vitamin E supplementation also reduces free-radical damage following open heart surgery and, thus improves recovery and prognosis in these surgical patients.

Limited evidence links vitamin E with CVD in diabetics. Prostaglandin production is altered in cells damaged by diabetes; whereas vitamin E might restore prostaglandin activity, reducing artery wall damage and CVD risk.

VITAMIN D. Large doses of vitamin D are linked to increased risk for developing premature atherosclerosis and heart disease.

VITAMIN B1. Abnormal heart function and enlargement of the heart result from severe vitamin B1 deficiency; however, no other evidence exists linking this vitamin to heart disease.

NIACIN. Large daily doses of niacin might decrease blood cholesterol and LDL-cholesterol levels, increase HDL-cholesterol levels, and reduce the risk for developing CVD. Cholesterol-lowering medications are more effective when combined with niacin.

VITAMIN B6. Low levels of vitamin B6 might increase the risk of CVD by elevating levels of homocysteine, an amino acid by-product that increases the incidence of heart attack and stroke. Inadequate intake of vitamin B6 also might encourage the formation of atherosclerosis and low levels of vitamin B6 are found in patients who are recovering from a heart attack.

FOLIC ACID. Folic acid might reduce the production of some substances that encourage the formation of atherosclerosis. Low levels of folic acid are associated with increased levels of homocysteine, a significant risk factor for heart attacks. However, information is limited on the effects of folic acid on the prevention or treatment of heart disease.

BIOTIN AND PANTOTHENIC ACID. Blood cholesterol levels increase and cardiovascular problems develop when the body is deficient in either biotin or pantothenic acid. However, deficiencies of these B vitamins are rare to nonexistent in the United States population.

CALCIUM. Adequate intake of calcium from dietary sources or from supplements might aid in lowering blood cholesterol levels and reducing a person's risk for developing CVD. The risk for heart disease might increase, however, when large amounts of calcium are consumed in the presence of a magnesium deficiency.

CHROMIUM. Consumption of a diet low in chromium is associated with elevated blood cholesterol and increased risk of developing CVD. Patients with advanced heart disease have low levels of chromium in their tissues and reduced levels of chromium in the blood might be an indicator of advanced heart disease. In contrast, blood cholesterol levels drop, HDL-cholesterol levels rise, and the risk for developing CVD decreases when chromium is added to the diet.

COPPER. Copper is important in the development and maintenance of healthy arteries and other blood vessels. A deficiency of this trace mineral produces the same type of damage to the blood vessels and heart as does a heart attack. One study showed that dietary intake resembling the copper intake in the American diet produced copper depletion in the heart tissue and heart disease. Low blood levels of copper are associated with high blood cholesterol levels and increased risk for developing CVD. However, some evidence shows that high levels of copper also increase heart attack risk. The ratio of zinc to copper also might be important in the regulation of blood cholesterol.

IRON. Iron deficiency is related to irregular heart beat and abnormal heart function, which disappear when the diet is supplemented with iron. A study from Finland reported that high levels of iron (serum ferritin) are associated with increased heart attack risk in men. However, the study did not investigate whether dietary intake or abnormal iron metabolism is the cause of this proposed association. The men averaged serum ferritin levels of 200ng/ml of blood, while premenopausal women often have serum ferritin values of 20ng/ml or less. Subsequent studies showed no association between dietary iron intake and heart disease risk. At this time, the iron-heart disease link is tenuous at best and, if there is an association, it is only with men, not women, children, or seniors.

MAGNESIUM. Both acute and chronic magnesium deficiencies are associated with increased risk for myocardial infarction and for increased morbidity and mortality following cardiac surgery. Patients with acute myocardial infarction are magnesium deficient and blood magnesium concentrations drop even further during the acute phase of the infarct. Although all of the mechanisms for magnesium's effects on the cardiovascular system are not fully understood, several functions have been identified and place magnesium at the forefront in cardiovascular disease prevention and treatment.

Magnesium competes with calcium. It helps regulate calcium movement across and within cell membranes of cardiac and vascular tissues, and is essential to neuromuscular activity, including muscular contraction of the myocardium and vascular tissues. In essence, magnesium functions as a natural calcium-channel blocker. A deficiency results in increased intracellular calcium activity, which might be responsible for the arterial hypertension that accompanies pre-eclampsia during pregnancy.

The pharmacologic effects of magnesium include its ability to reduce vascular resistance, thus decreasing blood pressure and improving the cardiac index. Blood coagulability also is affected by magnesium administration, including inhibition of platelet aggregation, prolonged clotting time, and the prevention of thrombosis.

Magnesium is strongly associated with the prevention and treatment of hypertension. Magnesium depletion results in hypokalemia, intracellular potassium depletion, and accumulation of sodium inside the cell, a condition resembling digitalis toxicity and associated with the development of hypertension. While magnesium deficiency is associated with cell excitability and ventricular arrhythmias, magnesium supplementation often lowers blood pressure, reduces ventricular ectopic beats (sometimes in patients unresponsive to hypertensive medication), and even is effective in terminating episodes of torsade de pointes (a life-threatening ventricular arrhythmia).

Magnesium also reduces the incidence of arrhythmias in patients with acute myocardial infarction, either because of a direct effect on cardiac conduction and excitability, or because it stabilizes other ions (sodium, calcium, and potassium), maintains cardiovascular hemodynamics, reduces infarct size, and influences myocardial metabolism. Magnesium improves myocardial performance by lowering systemic vascular resistance and reducing blood pressure, thus reducing the load on the left ventricle. In addition, magnesium supplementation reduces the toxic calcium overload in cardiac tissue, induces coronary vasodilation and improves coronary blood supply, and reduces the extent of catecholamine secretion in the myocardium, thus limiting the severity of the infarct.

The current research provides substantial evidence that magnesium exerts a strong myocardial protective effect and enhances the survival of patients recovering from an acute myocardial infarction. Future research is likely to uncover other cardio-protective functions of magnesium.

SELENIUM. The risk for heart disease, atherosclerosis, and death from heart disease increases when blood levels of selenium are low. People who consume diets low in selenium develop heart damage called cardiomyopathy, which might explain the increased risk for heart attack observed in these people. One study found a six- to seven-fold increased incidence of premature heart attacks in patients with low blood levels of selenium. Selenium also might protect against free-radical damage to blood vessel walls that initiates the development of atherosclerosis and heart disease.

ZINC. Zinc supplementation might reduce the risk for developing heart disease by changing lipoprotein concentrations, i.e., decreasing LDL-cholesterol and increasing HDL-cholesterol. However, large doses of zinc, exceeding 50mg a day, lowers the HDL-cholesterol level and thus might increase the risk for developing heart disease. Adequate levels of zinc strengthen the lining of blood vessel walls, preventing damage that might initiate atherosclerosis.

FATS AND CHOLESTEROL. In general, the more fat and cholesterol in the diet, the higher the blood cholesterol levels and the greater the risk for developing CVD. The saturated fats found primarily in beef, pork, and other red meats; fatty dairy products; hydrogenated vegetables, such as shortening and margarine; coconut and palm oils used in snack foods; and eggs, and dietary cholesterol found only in foods of animal origin are the greatest contributors to the development of atherosclerosis and CVD. Bernard Hennig, Ph.D., R.D. at the University of Kentucky in Lexington reports that polyunsaturated fats might contribute to the initiation of atherosclerosis, while reducing these fats and increasing the antioxidants and zinc might help strengthen the blood vessel walls and prevent this initial damage. Monounsaturated fats found in olive oil and avocados do not increase blood cholesterol levels and probably do not increase a person's risk for developing CVD.

FISH OILS. Special fats called omega 3 fatty acids or eicosapentaenoic acid (EPA) and docosahexaenoic acid (DHA) found in fish oils reduce blood cholesterol and LDL-cholesterol, raise HDL-cholesterol, interfere with the abnormal clumping of blood cell fragments associated with CVD, and might reduce a person's risk for developing atherosclerosis.

FIBER. Some forms of fiber, such as pectin in fruits and the fibers in alfalfa, cooked dried beans, oat bran, and guar gum reduce blood cholesterol and LDL-cholesterol. Other fibers, such as wheat bran, have little or no effect on blood cholesterol levels.

Dietary Recommendations

The U.S. Department of Agriculture and U.S. Department of Health and Human Services recently released dietary recommendations in the form of the Food Guide Pyramid. According to the Pyramid, the diet should be based on breads, cereals, rice, pasta, and other grains (6 to 11 servings a day). A person should include at least 3 to 5 servings of vegetables and 2 to 4 servings of fruits in the daily fare. Two to three servings from the low-fat/nonfat milk group, and the extra-lean meat, poultry, fish, dry beans, eggs, and nuts group also should be included. This diet is low in extra fats, oils, and sweets. (See Chapter 7 for more on the Food Guide Pyramid.)

In addition, persons should reduce their consumption of foods high in fats, such as fatty cuts of beef, pork, sausage and luncheon meats, whole-milk products, butter, margarine, oils, salad dressing, mayonnaise, pie crusts, gravies, sauces, and foods cooked in fats and oils. Extra-lean meat intake should be limited to no more than 6 ounces a day and consumption of salt and salted foods, such as processed or convenience foods, snack foods, fast foods, canned soups, soy sauce, and alcohol also should be reduced. One to three cloves of garlic should be added to the daily diet. (Garlic lowers cholesterol by lowering fatty acid and cholesterol levels and helping prevent the clumping of blood fragments associated with the progression of atherosclerosis.)

A diet low in fat, cholesterol, sugar, and salt, and high in fiber will increase vitamin and mineral intake and will aid in the maintenance of a desirable body weight. It also is similar to the diet recommended for the prevention of cancer, hypertension, diabetes, and many other degenerative disorders. In addition, frequent inclusion of omega 3 fatty acid-rich fish, such as salmon and herring, might further protect the heart against disease. A multiple vitamin-mineral supplement that contains the B vitamins, chromium, copper, iron, magnesium, selenium, zinc, and other nutrients; an extra dose of the antioxidant nutrients including vitamin C, vitamin E, and beta carotene; regular aerobic exercise; avoidance of tobacco; moderate intake of alcohol and coffee; effective coping with stress; and prevention of diabetes and hypertension will help in the prevention and treatment of heart and blood vessel diseases.

CARPAL TUNNEL SYNDROME (CTS)

Overview

Carpal tunnel syndrome is a disorder of the hands and wrists. The area (tunnel) that encloses the bones of the wrist (carpus) becomes inflamed and constricts the nerves that are embedded within the area. Carpal tunnel syndrome often occurs in people who have repetitive motion jobs, such as computer operators and assembly line workers.

Nutrition and Carpal Tunnel Syndrome

A vitamin B6 deficiency might encourage the development or aggravate the symptoms of CTS. Patients with CTS are more likely than healthy people to have vitamin B6 deficiencies and often the symptoms of CTS are relieved by vitamin B6 supplementation. In some cases, patients no longer require surgery after vitamin B6 supplementation is initiated.

Vitamin B6 is important in the development and maintenance of healthy nerve tissue. A deficiency can result in inflammation of these tissues similar to that observed in CTS, which might partially explain the vitamin's effectiveness in CTS. People with CTS might either consume inadequate amounts of vitamin B6 or have unusually high requirements for the vitamin.

Dietary Recommendations

Dietary recommendations for the prevention or treatment of carpal tunnel syndrome are limited. Consuming a diet high in fiber, vitamins, and minerals and low in fat, sugar, refined and convenience foods, and fast foods is wise. The diet should contain a variety of fruits, vegetables, whole grain breads and cereals, cooked dried beans and peas, low-fat or nonfat milk products, and extra-lean meats, chicken, and fish. A multiple vitamin-mineral supplement that contains vitamin B6 as well as regular exercise, effective stress management, avoidance of alcohol and tobacco, and moderate exposure to sunshine are important for optimal health and might be useful in the prevention and treatment of CTS. Vitamin B6 intake should not exceed 100mg a day without physician supervision, since large doses of this nutrient can cause nerve damage.

THE COMMON COLD

Overview

The common cold is the most widespread infectious disease. It is caused by a virus that is easily spread from one person to another and is resistant to the body's natural defense system.

Nutrition and the Common Cold

All nutrients related to the strengthening of the immune system are important in the prevention of the common cold or any other infection. (See pages 153–157 for more information on nutrition and the immune system.) In particular, vitamin C and zinc might aid in the prevention and treatment of the common cold.

VITAMIN C. Some studies show that vitamin C does not reduce the frequency or duration, but might reduce the severity of a cold. Other studies show that vitamin C is effective in preventing the common cold or shortening its duration, but has no effect on the severity of symptoms. In some cases, people report fewer colds when they take either a vitamin C tablet or a placebo they think is vitamin C, suggesting that a belief in the vitamin is as important as the vitamin itself.

There might be some truth to the vitamin C-common cold connection despite the contradictory evidence. Adequate vitamin C intake might stimulate the immune system in older adults or other people with poorly functioning immune systems. The vitamin strengthens the immune system by increasing the production or activity of white blood cells, which are responsible for destroying foreign invaders such as viruses and bacteria. There is a reduction in white blood cell formation and impaired wound healing when vitamin C is deficient in the diet, and the body's resistance to infection and disease improves when vitamin C intake is increased.

Athletes who train heavily and participate in an endurance event often have lowered resistance and suffer from infections after the event; however, vitamin C supplements taken prior to the event help prevent colds in this high-risk group. Vitamin C appears to be more effective for women than men in reducing the symptoms of the common cold.

ZINC. Zinc might alter the duration of the common cold by inhibiting the growth of bacteria and by stimulating the immune system. People who consume diets low in zinc are more susceptible than well-nourished people to infection and show signs of immune system impairment. The addition of zinc to the diet increases the amount and activity of white blood cells.

People diagnosed with poorly functioning immune systems have low levels of zinc in their blood; when they increase their intake of zinc their immune system is strengthened and they are more resistant to infection. This evidence shows that reduced amounts of zinc in the blood might contribute to a malfunctioning immune system.

Zinc also has a direct effect on slowing the growth of microorganisms, such as the viruses responsible for the common cold. Certain viruses do not survive in an environment rich in zinc. This effect is the basis for zinc lozenges as a common anticold treatment. The use of zinc lozenges was promoted after one study showed that people with cold symptoms who were treated with zinc gluconate lozenges experienced a reduction in symptoms, such as sore throat and fever, as compared to people who were not treated with the lozenges. The results of this one study have not been supported by further research.

Zinc is an excellent example of how the "some is good, more is better" myth is incorrect. Although optimal intake of zinc appears to stimulate the immune system and protect the body against colds and infections, excess intake of zinc might suppress the immune system and possibly increase a person's risk for infection. In addition, zinc intake in excess of 150 to 200mg in the presence of low to moderate copper intake can reduce the absorption and use of copper and contribute to a secondary copper deficiency.

Dietary Recommendations

A low-fat, high-fiber, nutrient-dense diet should be consumed, optimal in all vitamins and minerals and low in sugars and refined and convenience foods. The diet should contain a variety of fruits, vegetables, whole grain breads and cereals, cooked dried beans and peas, low-fat or nonfat milk products, and extra-lean meats, chicken, and fish. A multiple vitamin-mineral supplement and a vitamin C supplement, as well as regular exercise, effective stress management, avoidance of alcohol and tobacco, and outdoor activity are important for optimal health and the prevention of the common cold.

In addition, several glasses of fluids, such as fruit juice, water, herb teas, or bottled mineral water, several servings of fresh fruits and vegetables, moderate exercise such as a 15-minute walk, and extra sleep and relaxation each day are important for the treatment of and speedy recovery from the common cold.

CYSTIC FIBROSIS

Overview

Cystic fibrosis is the most common genetic disease that causes death in the United States and is the most common cause of lung disease in children. The primary symptoms of cystic fibrosis are chronic lung disease, abnormal functioning of the pancreas that results in poor digestion of food and gastrointestinal discomfort, and very high concentrations of salt in the sweat.

The pancreas produces many important enzymes necessary for normal digestion and absorption of foods. In cystic fibrosis, the pancreas does not function properly and these digestion enzymes are in short supply or lacking. People with mild forms of cystic fibrosis might not experience this poor absorption and subsequent malnutrition. The pancreas also produces the hormone insulin that regulates blood sugar, and it is common for people with cystic fibrosis to have high blood sugar levels and the symptoms of diabetes.

Nutrition and Cystic Fibrosis

The maintenance of optimal nutritional status is very important for people with cystic fibrosis. Adequate intake of all vitamins, minerals, protein, calories, and fiber improves height and weight, allows the formation of normal fat deposits that protect internal organs from damage, and encourages the normal development of puberty and growth. Optimal nutrition also improves the resistance to lung infections common in this disease. It is very important that the planning and monitoring of a nutritious diet for the person with cystic fibrosis be supervised by a physician and dietitian (Table 35).

Table 35
GENERAL DIETARY GUIDELINES FOR THE CYSTIC FIBROSIS PATIENT

Nutrient	Dietary Guidelines
Calories	Adequate intake of calories to maintain ideal body weight and promote growth.
Protein	Two to four times the RDA for age. 12 percent to 15 percent of total calorie intake.
Carbohydrate	Most easily digested of three calorie-containing nutrients (protein, fat, and carbohydrate)
Fat	Fat often poorly absorbed. Intake varies according to tolerance.
Fat-soluble vitamins	Two to three times the RDA for age. Provided in water-soluble form.
Water-soluble vitamins	Intake equal to the RDA. Antibiotic therapy requires increased intake of vitamin B2 (riboflavin).
Minerals	Intake equal to the RDA.
Pancreatic enzymes	Given at meals. Dosage and timing considered to prevent diarrhea and avoid constipation.

People with cystic fibrosis either have a good appetite, absorb and use nutrients well, and show normal growth and development; have a good appetite, do not absorb or use nutrients well, and show signs of malnutrition and stunted growth; or have a poor appetite, eat poorly, and do not gain weight or develop normally.

VITAMINS AND MINERALS. The lack of fat-digesting enzymes increases the likelihood that the fat-soluble vitamins will not be absorbed and blood levels of vitamins A, D, E, and K are often low in the blood and tissues of people with cystic fibrosis. Deficiencies of the fat-soluble vitamins are found even when people receive supplements. It is possible that some of the manifestations of cystic fibrosis are a result of vitamin A deficiency. Not only vitamin A, but its protein carrier in the blood and zinc, necessary in the transportation of vitamin A, are low in the body.

Limited information is available on the water-soluble vitamins and cystic fibrosis. Vitamin B12 deficiency has been identified in patients, as has a vitamin B2 deficiency.

Information on mineral status in cystic fibrosis also is limited. Blood levels of copper are elevated in advanced stages of the disease and some evidence exists that blood levels of zinc and iron are low. Some people with cystic fibrosis have low blood levels of selenium and vitamin E that implies a link between the body's antioxidant system and the development or progression of the disease. Children with cystic fibrosis show improved growth and reduced numbers of lung infections when the diet is adequately supplemented with vitamins, minerals, and other nutrients.

PROTEIN, CARBOHYDRATE, AND FAT. Patients with cystic fibrosis might not digest protein well and artificial diets or modified protein diets are often used. Most carbohydrates, such as breads, cereals, noodles, and rice, are well tolerated, but milk sugar (lactose) might need to be eliminated from the diet. Fat is poorly absorbed in cystic fibrosis patients with abnormal pancreatic function. Much of the dietary fat is excreted, resulting in diarrhea. A low-fat diet, or the use of special fats that do not require the presence of enzymes for digestion and absorption can be used. Essential fatty acids, such as linoleic acid, are likely to be deficient as a result of poor dietary intake or absorption.

Dietary Recommendations

Every nutrient is a concern for patients with cystic fibrosis, but the degree of dietary control will vary with each person. Calories might have to be increased to 50 percent to 100 percent more than the normal requirement for age, and protein intake may need to be doubled. Fat intake should be low (at least 30 percent, but not lower than 20 percent of calories) or divided in small doses throughout the day; administration of pancreatic enzymes with meals is usually necessary. New foods should be introduced into the diet one at a time to assess the person's tolerance.

The low intake or poor absorption of food justifies a multiple vitamin-mineral that supplies all the vitamins and minerals in amounts equal to or slightly greater than 100 percent of the RDA. A supplement that supplies vitamins A, D, E, and K in a water-soluble form is usually recommended. Vitamin B12 and vitamin B2 might be required in amounts exceeding the normal requirements.

DERMATITIS

Overview

Dermatitis is a general term for inflammation of the skin. Usually dermatitis results from chafing of the skin, allergies, long-term medications, or nervous irritability. Symptoms of dermatitis include rash, itching, burning, dryness, blemishes, or other skin disorders, and treatment or cure will depend on the cause of the skin irritation.

Nutrition and Dermatitis

Poor dietary habits, combined with deficiencies of several vitamins, are related to skin disorders and dermatitis. The skin is a primary site for nutrient deficiency symptoms, as skin cells are produced, die, and are replaced by new cells every few days. The short lifespan of skin cells allows deficiencies of nutrients to develop quickly.

VITAMIN A. Changes in skin texture result from vitamin A deficiency. The skin becomes bumpy, scaly, and rough, resembling "goose flesh" or "alligator skin." The skin on the forearms and thighs is the first to be affected, but in advanced stages the entire body is involved.

VITAMIN B2. A deficiency of vitamin B2 results in soreness and burning of the mouth and lips and dermatitis characterized by simultaneous dryness and greasy scales.

NIACIN. Early symptoms of niacin deficiency include skin eruptions and dermatitis. The dermatitis of pellagra is a scaly, dark pigmentation that develops on areas of the skin exposed to sunlight, heat, or mild irritation.

VITAMIN B6. Dermatitis is one symptom of vitamin B6 deficiency. The deficiency can develop from either poor dietary intake or long-term use of medications that interfere with vitamin B6 absorption or use, such as antituberculosis medications or oral contraceptives.

VITAMIN B12. A deficiency of vitamin B12 causes reduced cell and tissue repair and results in dermatitis, changes in the lips and tongue, nerve damage, anemia, and intestinal upsets.

BIOTIN. A deficiency of biotin results in dermatitis, progressive hair loss and hair color loss, and other hair and skin disorders.

PANTOTHENIC ACID. Although a deficiency of pantothenic acid is rare, it has been induced in the laboratory and symptoms include dermatitis, burning sensations, and numbness and tingling in the hands and feet.

VITAMIN C. The primary symptoms of vitamin C deficiency result from the vitamin's function in the formation and maintenance of collagen. Small pinpoint hemorrhages under the skin, poor wound healing, the breakdown of old scars, dry and scaly skin, and swollen and bleeding gums are symptoms of inadequate vitamin C intake.

ESSENTIAL FATTY ACIDS. A deficiency of linoleic acid, a fatty acid found in nuts, wheat germ, and vegetable oils, produces a type of dermatitis characterized by red, dry, scaly skin that resembles eczema or dermatitis. The blotchy areas appear first on the face, clustered near the oil-secreting glands, and then in the folds of the nose and lips, the forehead, the eyes, and the cheeks. Dry, rough areas also appear on the forearms, thighs, and buttocks. Fish oils also show promise as an effective therapy in the treatment of psoriasis and other skin disorders.

Dietary Recommendations

The first line of dietary defense against dermatitis is a low-fat, high-fiber, nutrient-dense diet, which is optimal in all vitamins and minerals and low in sugars and refined and convenience foods. The diet should contain a variety of fruits, vegetables, whole grain breads and cereals, cooked dried beans and peas, low-fat or nonfat milk products, and extra-lean meat, chicken, and fish. A tablespoon of safflower oil in salad dressing to supply linoleic acid, and frequent servings of fish should be included in the diet. During times when the diet is inadequate, a multiple vitamin-mineral supplement should supply at least 100 percent of the RDA for all vitamins, including vitamin A, vitamin B2, niacin, vitamin B6, vitamin B12, biotin, pantothenic acid, and vitamin C. In addition, regular exercise; effective stress management; avoidance of alcohol and tobacco; avoidance of cold, wind, harsh soaps, and detergents; frequent use of moisturizers, superfatted bath bars, and a humidifier; and showering after swimming in chlorinated waters are important for the prevention and treatment of dermatitis and dry skin.

DIABETES MELLITUS

Overview

Diabetes is characterized by a reduced ability to use and metabolize dietary carbohydrates, elevated blood sugar levels (hyperglycemia), and an abnormal amount of sugar in the urine. The two general types of diabetes are Type I, also called insulin dependent (IDDM) or juvenile-onset diabetes and Type II, also called noninsulin dependent (NIDDM) or adult-onset diabetes (Table 36).

IDDM usually begins in childhood. It begins suddenly, severe symptoms develop soon after onset, and control of the disorder requires insulin. NIDDM begins in the adult years, the progression of the disease is slow, and symptoms are mild in the beginning. Although genetics contribute to a person's risk for developing NIDDM, lifestyle factors such as being overweight, consuming a poor diet, and lack of exercise are important contributors to the development of this type of diabetes (Table 36).

Table 36
DIFFERENCES BETWEEN TYPE I AND TYPE II DIABETES

Characteristics	Type I	Type II
Age at onset	Under age 40	Over age 40
Percent of all diabetics	10 percent	90 percent
Inherited	Sometimes	Common
Appearance of symptoms	Sudden/severe	Slow
Obesity	Uncommon	Common
Beta cells of pancreas	Reduced	Normal or reduced.
Insulin secretion	Reduced	Normal or reduced.
Insulin receptors on cells	Normal	Reduced or normal
Remission	Rare	Common with weight reduction, diet, exercise.

Individuals with IDDM usually have reduced numbers of active beta cells in the pancreas, the cells responsible for the production and secretion of insulin. The person with IDDM must inject insulin and balance the entry of insulin into the blood with food intake to maintain normal use of sugar. In contrast, individuals with NIDDM can have reduced beta cells in the pancreas or, more often, show adequate production and secretion of insulin, but the cells of the body are insensitive to the hormone. The insensitivity is often related to obesity. Consequently, excess sugar does not flow into the cells and blood sugar (glucose) levels remain high. Oral hypoglycemic medications or injected insulin are sometimes used to overcome the insensitivity, although insulin insensitivity often is reversible with weight loss.

Nutrition and Diabetes

The goals of a diet program for the treatment of diabetes include improvement of overall health by achieving and maintaining optimal nutritional status and a desirable body weight, stabilization of blood sugar levels within the normal range, and prevention or delay of the development of cardiovascular disease, kidney disease, and eye or nerve disorders. The most important aspect of the diet is the control of carbohydrate, protein, fat, and calories; however, vitamin and mineral intakes also contribute to the prevention and treatment of the disease.

VITAMIN B6. This B vitamin functions in carbohydrate metabolism and a deficiency causes symptoms such as low blood sugar, low glycogen stores in the liver, abnormal glucose tolerance, low blood and pancreatic insulin levels, degeneration of the beta cells in the pancreas that manufacture and secrete insulin, and an altered insulin response to sugar. Insulin sensitivity improves when vitamin B6 intake increases in people who are deficient in the vitamin.

VITAMIN C. Adequate intake of vitamin C might help regulate blood sugar levels and aid in the prevention of diabetes. Diabetics have low blood levels of vitamin C and tissue storage of the vitamin might be impaired with the disease. In diabetic patients with low vitamin C intake, supplements might strengthen fragile blood vessels and lower cholesterol levels, reducing the risk of diabetes-related heart disease. The higher turnover of vitamin C characteristic of diabetes might indicate an increased need for the vitamin, and some researchers suggest raising the recommended vitamin C intake for diabetics to 100mg daily. Caution must be used when diabetics supplement with vitamin C, since large supplemental vitamin C might interfere with the urinary test for glucose.

VITAMIN E. Poor dietary intake of vitamin E might alter blood sugar levels. In contrast, increased intake of the fat-soluble vitamin might help lower blood sugar levels and improve insulin action and insulin responsiveness in diabetics. Blood levels of vitamin E are low in diabetics and people at risk for developing diabetes, which suggests that vitamin E metabolism is altered as a result of the disease. Diabetes might increase free-radical activity and result in an increased need for the antioxidant vitamins, including vitamin E. Limited evidence shows that a diet high in vitamin E decreases platelet clumping and slows the progression of atherosclerosis, a common complication of diabetes. (See pages 150–153 for more information on antioxidants.)

CHROMIUM. Chromium functions in the prevention of NIDDM. Insufficient chromium intake impairs glucose tolerance and increases insulin levels. In contrast, chromium supplementation improves glucose tolerance, increases cell sensitivity to insulin, and reduces circulating insulin levels, while reducing the amount of insulin required to maintain optimal blood glucose levels. Since keeping insulin at low levels is important in the prevention of secondary signs of diabetes, chromium also aids in the prevention of diabetes-related arterial plaque formation and atherosclerosis. Patients with hypoglycemia, hyperglycemia, and NIDDM who are chromium deficient show improvement in symptoms within weeks when supplemented with chromium.

Of the 15 studies that assessed the effects of chromium supplementation on glucose tolerance, only three showed no benefits, while 12 showed positive results, including improved or normalized glucose tolerance and maintained glucose levels with lowered insulin output. The degree of improvement in response to chromium supplementation depends on the degree of impairment, i.e., severe glucose intolerance benefits the most from chromium supplementation. However, patients who already are well nourished in chromium show no additional benefits when chromium supplements are added to the diet.

Elevated blood glucose levels might increase chromium requirements. Plasma chromium levels are elevated with increased urinary excretion of the mineral when plasma glucose levels are high in healthy men. The extent of chromium loss is a function of insulin secretion in response to dietary simple sugars; those sugars that elicit a large insulin output also trigger the greatest urinary loss of chromium. This association between elevated insulin levels and chromium excretion implies that conditions where insulin is chronically or acutely elevated also increase the risk of chromium deficiency and increased chromium requirements.

In addition, poor glucose tolerance and diabetes might alter chromium metabolism. This is reflected in diabetics who lose the ability to convert inorganic chromium to a more useable form and must depend on preformed, biologically active, forms of chromium in foods. Supplementing with inorganic chromium (i.e., chromic chloride) might be ineffective for these people. While most people respond favorably to supplemental doses of 200mcg, diabetics might require either greater amounts or chromium supplied only in biologically active forms, such as brewer's yeast.

In short, response to chromium supplementation is best in the prevention, rather than the treatment of diabetes, especially when consumed in a biologically active form in amounts approaching 200mcg/day for weeks or months and in patients who are marginally or overtly deficient in chromium.

MAGNESIUM. Magnesium functions in the release of insulin and plays a role in transporting sugar into the cells. Blood and tissue levels of magnesium are low and urinary excretion of the mineral is high in diabetics. Children with IDDM have lower levels of magnesium than nondiabetic children. The severity of the disease also appears to be related to magnesium status, i.e., diabetics of all ages with the poorest blood sugar control are at the greatest risk for magnesium deficiencies. Optimal magnesium intake might reduce the risk of complications common in diabetes, such as hypertension, heart disease, and retina damage in the eye.

OTHER MINERALS. Altered calcium metabolism in diabetes might impair insulin secretion and aggravate glucose intolerance. An overload of calcium in body tissues also might provide the link between diabetes and its complications, such as heart disease, cataracts, and premature aging.

Adequate intake of zinc is essential for optimal insulin activity, while zinc deficiency impairs insulin sensitivity. Some studies report that blood zinc levels are lower in diabetics than in healthy controls, which might complicate abnormal blood sugar regulation. Finally, zinc supplementation might reduce pregnancy complications and speed healing of leg ulcers in diabetics.

Limited (and inconclusive) evidence shows that

- a manganese deficiency might impair transport of sugar into cells,
- a copper deficiency might alter blood sugar tolerance,
- a selenium deficiency might reduce insulin secretion, and
- excessive iron levels might impair blood sugar control.

Dietary Recommendations

The primary goal in the dietary management of diabetes, both IDDM and NIDDM, is control of blood sugar levels within a narrow range at least 80 percent of the time. A person with diabetes should work closely with a physician and dietitian to establish a diet and exercise program that balances blood sugar and food intake with exercise, body weight, and medication use.

BODY WEIGHT. More than three out of four diabetics are overweight and, in many cases, blood sugar stabilizes or returns to normal with a reduction in body weight.

COMPLEX CARBOHYDRATES. A diet higher in complex carbohydrates, such as whole grain breads and cereals, vegetables, cooked dried beans and peas, potatoes, and other unrefined starches, than in protein and fat is beneficial in the control of diabetes. The American

Diabetes Association recommends the following percentages based on total calories:

> 50 percent to 60 percent carbohydrates
> 15 percent to 20 percent protein
> 25 percent to 30 percent fat

FIBER. Fiber slows the rise in blood sugar after a meal, aids in the maintenance of normal blood sugar levels, and reduces the amount of sugar excreted in the urine. Oat bran and the fiber in cooked dried beans and peas is especially effective in the control of blood sugar levels, but consumption of all fibers, including the fiber in whole grain breads and cereals, vegetables, and fruits, is encouraged.

VITAMINS AND MINERALS. Consumption of a nutritious diet that derives most of its calories from whole grain breads and cereals, fresh fruits and vegetables, and cooked dried beans and peas with small amounts of extra-lean meats, chicken, fish, and nonfat or low-fat milk products will provide adequate amounts of most vitamins and minerals. If the calorie intake is below 2,000 calories or the diet is not optimal, a multiple supplement that contains all the vitamins and minerals in amounts approaching 100 percent of the RDA should provide adequate intake of these nutrients.

REGULAR EXERCISE. Exercise improves how the body uses insulin and aids in the regulation of blood sugar levels. Aerobic exercise, such as brisk walking, swimming, jogging, or stationary or outdoor bicycling, performed three to four times a week, for 20 minutes or more will have an overall lowering effect on blood sugar. A diabetic's exercise program should be developed with the help of a physician and trained exercise physiologist. Exercise also might help prevent the development of NIDDM, especially in individuals at an increased risk for the disease, such as those who are overweight, have high blood pressure, or have a family history of diabetes.

ECZEMA

Overview

Eczema, also called atopic eczema, eczematous dermatitis, or atopic dermatitis, is a general term for any chronic skin inflammation or irritation. Eczema develops from allergic reactions to pollens, cosmetics, dust, or other environmental factors or is a result of dry air, chemical irritants, or excessive exposure to sunlight. The symptoms of this skin disorder are often increased by anxiety, lack of sleep, or other stresses.

Nutrition and Eczema

Numerous nutrient deficiencies will produce eczema-like symptoms, and increased dietary intake of these nutrients will help if the skin disorder is a result of a vitamin or mineral deficiency.

VITAMIN A. Chronic low intake of vitamin A will produce some of the symptoms of eczema including dry, scaly, and rough skin. The most common locations for vitamin A-induced skin disorders are the shoulders, neck, back, forearms, thighs, and abdomen.

THE B VITAMINS. A deficiency of vitamin B2 results in dermatitis or eczema-like symptoms, including dryness, scaling, or itching of the skin. Symptoms of niacin deficiency include skin eruptions, such as darkened skin that is scaly and dry. Eczema-like symptoms also develop during a deficiency of vitamin B6, vitamin B12, folic acid, biotin, and pantothenic acid.

Other Nutrients: Deficiencies of either vitamin C or the essential fatty acid linoleic acid produce skin disorders, including eczema.

Dietary Recommendations

The first line of defense in the prevention and treatment of eczema is a low-fat, high-fiber, nutrient-dense diet that is optimal in all vitamins and minerals and low in sugars and refined and convenience foods. The diet should contain a variety of fruits, vegetables, whole grain breads and cereals, cooked dried beans and peas, low-fat or nonfat milk products, and extra-lean meats, chicken, and fish. A multiple vitamin-mineral supplement that contains adequate amounts of the B vitamins, vitamin C, and vitamin A should be considered if the diet is not optimal. Regular exercise, effective stress management, avoidance of alcohol and tobacco, and moderate exposure to sunshine also are important for the prevention and treatment of eczema.

When food allergies are the cause of eczema, appropriate steps should be taken to eliminate the offending foods. Foods most often associated with allergies include wheat, corn, milk, eggs, chocolate, oranges, nuts, strawberries, and shellfish. For example, one study showed that when people who suffered from eczema and who had been treated with emollients, topical steroids, and oral antihistamines were placed on a nutritious diet that excluded milk and egg products and used soy-based milk as a substitute, their symptoms improved, including a reduction in itching and redness. The management of food allergies should be planned with the help of a physician or dietitian. (See pages 163–168 for additional information on food allergies.)

EMOTIONAL DISORDERS

Overview

Until recently, the brain was thought to be impermeable to the effects of nutrition. Although other organs such as the liver and the heart show profound changes as a result of poor dietary intake of vitamins and minerals, the brain was thought to be protected from fluctuations in nutrient intakes by a series of partitions, called the blood-brain barrier, which separated the brain from the rest of the body. This concept is now recognized as incomplete and inaccurate. Food and nutrient intake have a powerful effect on a person's mood, behavior, and ability to learn, often before overt physical symptoms are apparent.

Nutrition and Emotional Disorders

Vitamin and mineral deficiencies can change the structure and function of the brain and nervous system and affect behavior, memory, mood, and learning. Even the nutrient content of a single meal or marginal deficiencies of a single vitamin or mineral can alter mood and behavior, and disorders once considered irreversible show improvement when vitamin and mineral intake is increased.

Nutrition affects the fundamental units of the brain called the neurons or nerve cells, and the chemicals, called neurotransmitters, secreted by these cells. Neurotransmitters transmit messages from one nerve cell to another or from one nerve cell to its target organ, such as a muscle or a gland that releases hormones. These processes regulate all thoughts, behaviors, physical actions, and the ability to learn. Nutrition can affect the brain in many ways, impair the ability to remember or learn, and cause depression, anxiety, and other mood disorders. The following examples are ways that nutrient intake affects mood, behavior, and thinking processes:

1. Consuming inadequate amounts of protein or the vitamin-like substance called choline limits the production of several neurotransmitters dependent on those building blocks for production, changing mood, eating habits, and other behaviors.

2. Several vitamins and minerals including vitamin B1, vitamin B2, vitamin B6, vitamin B12, folic acid, vitamin C, iron, magnesium, and selenium act as "helpers" during neurotransmitter production. Inadequate intake of these nutrients will limit manufacture and storage of neurotransmitters and result in mood, cognition, and behavior changes.
3. Restriction or overconsumption of fats or carbohydrates can result in under- or overactive neurotransmitters and these imbalances can affect mood, appetite, and other behaviors.
4. Inadequate intake of nutrients, such as protein, zinc, vitamin B6, iodine, folic acid, and vitamin B12 during the early years of life might impair development of the nervous system and alter personality, mental function, and behavior.
5. Foods additives, including monosodium glutamate (MSG), and chemicals, such as tyramine found in aged cheese might block transmission of neurotransmitters, interrupt production or secretion of neurotransmitters, or affect enzymes that regulate neurotransmitter levels in the gap between nerve cells, resulting in profound, but perhaps subtle, mood, behavior, and cognitive changes.

Several vitamins and minerals also affect how a person feels mentally and physically by affecting the production and maintenance of red blood cells. A nutrient deficiency, such as iron or folic acid, that reduces the number of red blood cells, or the capacity of these cells to carry oxygen, would reduce the supply of oxygen to the brain and other tissues and could cause lethargy, mood disorders, learning disabilities, and depression. It should be noted, however, that treatment of these disorders with food or vitamin supplements requires physician supervision.

VITAMIN E. Symptoms of a vitamin E deficiency include nervous system disorders and anemia, characterized by lethargy and depression. People with rare fat malabsorption syndromes, such as cystic fibrosis and celiac disease, are susceptible to nerve damage, poor coordination, and anemia, probably resulting from inadequate absorption of vitamin E. Increased intake of the fat-soluble vitamin improves or eliminates these symptoms.

VITAMIN B1. Vitamin B1 deficiency causes nerve and brain disorders, such as fatigue, loss of appetite, mental confusion, tingling of the hands and feet, numbness, memory loss, emotional instability, reduced attention span, irritability, confusion, increased aggressiveness, and depression. Increased intake of the vitamin reverses these symptoms.

VITAMIN B2. A severe deficiency of vitamin B2 causes depression or hysteria and lethargy associated with anemia. Some evidence shows that as many as one in every four patients suffering with depression are marginally nourished in this B vitamin. A vitamin B2 deficiency is often accompanied by deficiencies of other B vitamins also related to nerve and brain function, such as niacin, vitamin B1, and vitamin B6. In one study of depressed elderly patients, supplementation with vitamin B1, B2, and B6 alleviated some symptoms of depression and improved thinking processes.

NIACIN. One of the classic symptoms of niacin deficiency is dementia or depression. Other nerve and brain disorders associated with inadequate niacin intake include disorientation, irritability, insomnia, loss of memory, delirium, and emotional instability. As with vitamin B2 deficiency, these symptoms usually are accompanied by other nutrient deficiencies, such as protein, iron, vitamin B1, or vitamin B6.

Niacin supplements have been used in conjunction with antiepileptic medications, such as phenobarbital and primidone, with some success. Large doses of niacin have been used in the treatment of schizophrenia; however, the results are conflicting and recommendations for niacin's therapeutic effectiveness cannot be made at this time. Some psychiatric disorders have been attributed to abnormal absorption or use of niacin or its dietary building block tryptophan. A few reports show improvement in patients with depression, hyperactivity, and sleep disturbances with increased tryptophan or niacin intakes. In addition, some reports show that niacin supplements improve short-term memory.

VITAMIN B6. Vitamin B6 aids in the formation of several neurotransmitters, the chemicals that regulate brain and nerve function and that are secreted by nerve cells. Inadequate intake of vitamin B6 results in reduced production or activity of these chemicals and can cause depression, insomnia, confusion, irritability, and nervousness. Low blood levels of neurotransmitters are found in suicidal or depressed patients and supplementation with vitamin B6 often helps stabilize mood. The relief from depression seen in many depressed patients treated with vitamin B6 indicates that a deficiency of vitamin B6 is a cause, not an effect of the depression.

Increased vitamin B6 intake might alleviate depression in women using oral contraceptives. In fact, side effects, such as mood swings and depression, associated with estrogen medications and oral contraceptives might result from altered metabolism of vitamin B6 and suppressed production of the neurotransmitter serotonin. Several studies report that depression related to Premenstrual Syndrome (PMS) might be effectively treated with vitamin B6 in doses above the RDA (i.e., 50 to 200mg).

Pregnant and breast-feeding women consume as little as 60 percent of the RDA for vitamin B6. Limited evidence indicates that insufficient vitamin B6 of the mother during pregnancy and breast-feeding might impair development of the central nervous system, learning, and memory of her child. Mood improves and memory loss might be slowed when some elderly patients supplement with vitamin B6.

In doses greater than 150mg taken for long periods of time, vitamin B6 can damage the nerves, resulting in numbness and tingling in the hands and feet, poor coordination, and a stumbling gait in some persons. Consequently, high-dose supplementation should be monitored by a physician.

VITAMIN B12. Vitamin B12 is essential for the formation and maintenance of the insulation around nerve cells, called the myelin sheath, that speeds the conduction of nerve impulses. A long-term deficiency of vitamin B12 results in nerve damage, tingling and numbness, moodiness, confusion, agitation, dimmed vision, delusions, dizziness, and disorientation. Marginal intake of the vitamin is associated with an increased risk for developing depression, memory loss, and paranoia, while some cases of mental illness in anemic elderly have been linked to an underlying vitamin B12 deficiency. Supplementation with vitamin B12 in these individuals improves mood and memory function.

Vitamin B12 also is important in the formation of all body cells, and a deficiency results in poor formation of red blood cells and the characteristic lethargy, depression, and fatigue associated with anemia. Anemia can be treated, but the nerve damage that results from long-term vitamin B12 deficiency is permanent.

FOLIC ACID. Folic acid is important in the formation of all types of cells and is essential for the growth and development of the nervous system. Irritability, weakness, apathy, hostility, depression, paranoid behavior, and anemia are some of the symptoms of folic acid deficiency and are responsive to an increased intake of the vitamin.

Inadequate folic acid intake decreases the amount of the neurotransmitter serotonin in the brain, resulting in increased risk for depression. A study of healthy people found that individuals with the highest blood levels of folic acid reported the best moods, and individuals with "low-normal" levels were at greatest risk for depression. Folic acid supplements might improve mood in depressed people, especially in patients on long-term use of drugs, such as anticonvulsants, antituberculosis drugs, alcohol, or oral contraceptives that can interfere with folic acid metabolism.

Limited evidence shows that folic acid supplementation in conjunction with a special diet might be useful in the treatment of violent outbursts, seizures, bouts of amnesia, and sleep disorders in children unresponsive to anticonvulsant medication therapy.

BIOTIN AND PANTOTHENIC ACID. Although a deficiency of either biotin or pantothenic acid is very rare, when it does occur, symptoms include numbness in the hands and feet, nausea, lethargy, lack of coordination, staggering gait, restlessness, irritability, and depression. These symptoms disappear when these B vitamins are added back to the diet.

CALCIUM AND MAGNESIUM. Calcium and magnesium are important in the regulation of nerve impulses. The nerves become overly sensitive in the rare occurrence when blood calcium levels drop below normal. Both of these minerals also aid in the formation of certain neurotransmitters. It is unclear how or if a calcium deficiency would alter mood or behavior, but it is known that depression, confusion, personality changes, lack of coordination, and weakness result from poor intake of magnesium.

IRON. The classic symptom of poor iron intake is anemia, characterized by lethargy, depression, poor concentration, irritability, decreased attention span, apathy, and personality changes. Iron-deficiency anemia or marginal iron intake during infancy results in impaired motor and mental development and infants that seem more unhappy, tense, and withdrawn; increasing infant iron intake to adequate levels can correct the developmental delays and mood alterations.

An iron deficiency affects the ability to understand or learn new information. Iron-deficient children do not perform as well in school, do poorly on intelligence tests, show impaired attention span, and have a more limited capacity to remember information than do well-nourished children. Iron deficiency, even in the absence of anemia, also can affect job performance, mood, and memory in adults.

OTHER VITAMINS AND MINERALS. Other nutrients related to nerve and brain function include vitamin C, chromium, copper, selenium, and zinc. A deficiency of any of these nutrients might produce nervous system disorders, such as depression, poor coordination, numbness, and learning disabilities. For example, selenium supplements given to individuals with low selenium intake improves depression and anxiety. Inadequate vitamin C intake is associated with depression, whereas increasing vitamin C intake improves mood, scores on intelligence tests, and decreases nervousness. Limited evidence suggests that vitamin C supplements might benefit some schizophrenic patients.

CHOLINE AND LECITHIN. Choline is incorporated into the neurotransmitter acetylcholine, which aids in the regulation of memory and other brain and nerve processes. Levels of this neurotransmitter are low in the brains of people with Alzheimer's disease and Huntington's disease and one theory for the development of these disorders blames these low levels as the cause of the related memory loss.

Blood choline levels increase when the choline content of a meal is increased. The rise in blood choline stimulates an increase in brain levels of choline and more acetylcholine is produced. However, choline or lecithin supplementation does not always improve memory, especially in advanced stages of memory loss or in people with degeneration of nerve cells such as Alzheimer's patients.

Dietary Recommendations

Depression, lethargy, and other emotional disorders can result from a variety of factors, including life problems and nervous system disorders that are unrelated to nutrition. In addition, over-consumption of certain metals, such as mercury or lead, affects nerve and brain tissue, causing temporary, and sometimes permanent, damage. However, proper nutrition is safe and potentially helpful in all circumstances.

A low-fat, high-fiber, nutrient-dense diet should be consumed, adequate in all vitamins and minerals and low in sugars and refined and convenience foods. The diet should contain a variety of fruits, vegetables, whole grain breads and cereals, cooked dried beans and peas, low-fat or nonfat milk products, and extra-lean meats, chicken, and fish. Consumption of sugar, highly processed and refined foods, and caffeine from coffee and cola drinks should be limited. Regular meals, including a well-balanced breakfast that includes some complex carbohydrate (such as cereal or whole wheat toast) and some protein (such as milk or cheese), are important for the prevention and treatment of emotional and learning disorders.

Do not ignore cravings! Attempts to rid the cupboards and refrigerator of all sweet temptations or to "will away" an urge to eat is likely to do more harm than good, since you are denying your body the very nutrients it needs to self-regulate the nerve chemicals and hormones that affect mood. Instead, fuel your cravings, but do so in moderation and with planned, nutritious foods.

Avoid large meals. Meals of more than 1,000 calories, especially if they are high in fat, leave most people feeling drowsy. Lighter meals of approximately 500 calories for breakfast and lunch provide ample fuel without dragging you down. In addition, light meals in the evening are more likely to aid in a good night's sleep than are heavy meals that take hours to digest.

Develop a routine that includes several small snacks throughout the day and evening. Include some protein and some carbohydrate at each snack, such as peanuts and raisins, low-fat yogurt and fruit, low-fat cheese melted on an English muffin, or a bowl of cereal with milk. If you want to nibble in the evening, make it a carbohydrate-rich snack, such as fruit, popcorn, toast. Keep the snack light and plan it for approximately one hour before bedtime. Keep on hand a variety of low-fat, nutritious foods to soothe your sweet tooth or food cravings. Plan your snacks so you will not fall prey to impulse eating.

When the diet is not optimal, a multiple supplement should be considered that supplies all the vitamins and minerals in approximately 100 percent to 300 percent of the RDA. Larger doses of vitamin B6 or niacin might be considered, but only with physician monitoring. Exercise might have an anti-depressant, mood-enhancing effect. In addition, effective stress management and avoidance of alcohol, chronic use of medications, and tobacco are important in the prevention and treatment of emotional disorders.

EPILEPSY

Overview

Epilepsy is one of the oldest human diseases and affects approximately 1 percent of the population in the United States. The seizures or attacks vary in severity, duration, and frequency and are basically of two types: generalized epilepsy, also known as grand mal or petite mal seizures, and focal epilepsy. Generalized epilepsy involves all parts of the brain while focal epilepsy involves only a portion of the brain.

Dietary Recommendations

Epilepsy is usually treated with anticonvulsant medications, such as phenytoin (Dilantin), phenobarbital, and primidone. In these cases, the person should consume a low-fat, high-fiber, nutrient-dense diet that is adequate in all vitamins and minerals and low in sugars and refined and convenience foods. The diet should contain a variety of fruits, vegetables, whole grain breads and cereals, cooked dried beans and peas, low-fat or nonfat milk products, and extra-lean meats, chicken, and fish. A multiple vitamin-mineral supplement as well as regular exercise, effective stress management, avoidance of alcohol and tobacco, and moderate exposure to sunshine are important in the treatment of epilepsy.

Nutrition therapy consists primarily of a specialized diet called the "ketogenic diet" and is used for those people who do not tolerate or respond to medication. The diet is very high in fat and low in carbohydrates (starchy foods such as vegetables, grains, breads, and fruits) and must be monitored carefully by a physician and dietitian (Table 37).

Table 37
FOODS TO AVOID ON THE KETOGENIC DIET
USED IN THE TREATMENT OF EPILEPSY

The following foods contain carbohydrates and might be restricted on a ketogenic diet for the treatment of epilepsy:

All breads, bread products, and cereals, unless they are planned in the daily meal plan	Marmalade
Cake	Molasses
Candy	Pastries
Chewing gum	Pies
Cookies	Sherbet
Cough drops/syrup containing sugar	Soft drinks
Fruit flavored drinks	Sugar
Honey	Sweet rolls
Ice cream	Sweetened condensed milk
Jam and jelly	Syrup

Vitamins and minerals most likely to be low in the specialized ketogenic diet are calcium, iron, the B vitamins, vitamin C, and vitamin D. A multiple vitamin-mineral preparation that contains these nutrients in amounts between 100 percent and 300 percent of the RDA should be consumed daily.

Long-term use of anticonvulsant medications can alter vitamin and mineral absorption and use. Vitamin D, vitamin B12, and folic acid are likely to be affected by these medications, and increased intake might be necessary. However, large doses of folic acid can interfere with the action of certain anticonvulsant medications, such as phenytoin, and supplements of this B vitamin should be taken only with the approval of a physician. Limited evidence shows that some patients taking antiepileptic drugs have low levels of vitamin E. Supplementing these patients with vitamin E improves the blood levels of the antioxidant and might reduce the number and frequency of seizures.

EYE DISORDERS

Overview

How well a person sees is often an indicator of the health of the eye. Although the eye works, becomes fatigued, and ages as does every organ, many disorders of the eye, including cataracts and macular degeneration, might be preventable or treatable.

Nutrition and Eye Disorders

Deficiencies of the antioxidants, fish oil, and several vitamins might alter vision and the health of the eye.

THE ANTIOXIDANTS. Recent research suggests that many eye disorders are not an inevitable effect of aging and might be preventable with adequate intake of antioxidants. The lens of the eye filters ultraviolet light, a potent source of highly reactive compounds called free radicals, and is thereby exposed to higher levels of these reactive substances. Free-radical damage to proteins within the lens might form protein "clumps" that scatter light and contribute to cataract progression. A diet rich in antioxidant nutrients protects against the formation and progression of cataracts by counteracting the damaging effects of free radicals. A high intake of antioxidants also reduces the risk of macular degeneration. (See pages 150–153 for more information on free radicals and antioxidants.)

Studies on the effect of vitamin C on light-induced cataracts and of vitamin E and beta carotene on cataracts induced by various agents repeatedly show a protective effect either on the formation or the progression of cataracts. In one study of more than 22,000 physicians, multivitamin supplementation and, in particular, vitamin E and vitamin C supplementation reduced the risk of developing cataracts. Preliminary findings from the nationwide lung cancer prevention study also reported improved visual acuity both with and without glasses when vitamin E and beta carotene supplements were added to the diet.

BETA CAROTENE. The antioxidant beta carotene lessens ultraviolet-light damage to the retina and scavenges free radicals that might damage the eye. Increased intake of beta carotene-rich foods, such as dark green, dark orange, and yellow fruits and vegetables, might delay or prevent the development cataracts and macular degeneration and improve visual acuity.

VITAMIN E. The antioxidant nutrients, including vitamin E, are thought to protect the eyes from "oxidative" or free-radical damage and thus help prevent several eye disorders, including cataract formation. A study from the University of Western Ontario reports that a high intake of vitamin E results in a 50 percent reduction in risk for developing cataracts. Another study from the USDA Human Nutrition Research Center on Aging at Tufts University reports that blood levels of vitamin E and other antioxidants are low in patients with cataracts, while vitamin E supplementation might improve vision with and without glasses.

VITAMIN C. Vitamin C might inhibit the progression and encourage the regression of some forms of cataracts. Some of the highest concentrations of vitamin C are found in various ocular fluids and tissues. In humans, the highest concentration is in the aqueous humor, where vitamin C is concentrated 20-fold with respect to plasma. The retina contains the lowest concentrations of vitamin C in eye tissues. Interestingly, nocturnal animals with limited exposure to UV light have very low concentrations of vitamin C in eye tissue, while diurnal animals have up to 35 times the vitamin C in ocular tissues. This phenomenon suggests that a high vitamin C concentration is an adaptation that protects the eyes against solar radiation.

In most cases, the exact role of vitamin C in ocular tissue is still unclear and it is possible that the most important functions have not been identified yet. Vitamin C helps recycle vitamin E in membranes and also interacts with selenium. The high concentrations of this vitamin in ocular tissue and its well-defined antioxidant properties in other tissues are good arguments that the major function of vitamin C is as a strong protector against oxidative damage, particularly light-induced damage.

For example, vitamin C decreases the membrane damage found in lenses of diabetic rats. The vitamin also functions in lens development and maintenance of transparency during development. Finally, vitamin C also rids the lens of oxygen fragments, thus reducing the probability of oxidative insult. Studies on experimental animals show that vitamin C protects against lens damage induced by radiation. The cornea also is susceptible to damage by radiation and free radicals as a result of exposure to air. The accumulation of vitamin C in these tissues, therefore, could serve to protect them from oxidative damage.

Research supports the link between increased vitamin C intake and reduced risk for developing cataracts. In one study, injections of vitamin C prevented the development of selenite-induced cataracts in rats. Another study on Sprague-Dawley rats (a species of rats that cannot synthesize vitamin C) showed that vitamin C supplementation reduced the incidence of cataracts in animals. Vitamin C levels are low in cataractous tissue and increased levels of oxidized vitamin C are found in human lens with progressive senile cataracts.

In short, cataract formation possibly occurs when the oxidative stress on the lens exceeds the capacity of the antioxidant systems, such as vitamin C, within the eye. Prolonged exposure to oxidative stress, not aging per se, is likely to be a primary cause of cataracts. But, does dietary intake raise vitamin C levels in the eye?

Antioxidant nutrients are found in eye tissue in relation to levels consumed in the diet. A study conducted at USDA Human Nutrition Research Center on Aging at Tufts University reports that supplementation with vitamin C raises ocular concentrations of the vitamin. Subjects scheduled for cataract extraction were given either two grams of vitamin C or a placebo daily for at least two weeks. At the time of operation, samples revealed that vitamin C concentrations in plasma, aqueous, and lens tissues of the supplemented group were significantly higher than the unsupplemented group, even though the unsupplemented group consumed more than twice the RDA (i.e., 120mg) of vitamin C in their daily diets. The results of this study suggest that high dietary intake of vitamin C might not be adequate to prevent cataract formation, while supplementation might increase ocular concentrations in a dose-dependent fashion.

VITAMIN A. Vitamin A is essential to the development and maintenance of normal eye tissue and vision. Vitamin A binds with a special protein in the eye that makes vision possible in dim light. A condition called night blindness or poor dark adaptation is an early sign of poor vitamin A intake. A person with night blindness is unable to see well in dim light, especially when entering darkness from a bright light as in entering a darkened room or driving at night where the eyes must adjust rapidly from bright headlights to darkness.

Vitamin A also is necessary for the development and maintenance of epithelial tissues that line the external and internal surfaces of the body including the eyes. An inadequate supply of this fat-soluble vitamin causes these tissues to shrink, harden, and deteriorate. If the deficiency continues, the changes can include irreversible loss of vision. The first symptoms of vitamin A deficiency in the eye include over-sensitivity to bright light, itching, or burning. The eyes and eye lids become dry and inflamed.

In advanced stages of vitamin A deficiency, the cornea, the clear transparent portion at the front and center of the eyeball, becomes dry, inflamed, and swollen with water. Infection follows, accompanied by cloudiness and blindness.

Severe vitamin A deficiency is rare in the United States. Infants and small children are most susceptible to vitamin A deficiency, but loss of vision from lack of vitamin A can occur in any age group. Increased intake of vitamin A can reverse the damage, unless it has progressed to advanced stages. Vitamin A supplements also benefit individuals with retinitis pigmentosa, a hereditary degenerative disorder of the retina characterized by night blindness and loss of peripheral vision.

VITAMIN B2. Some of the symptoms of a vitamin B2 deficiency are damage to the eye tissue, poor vision, burning and itching of the eyes, and increased blood vessels in the eye. The outer lining of the eye becomes inflamed and ulcers appear on the cornea. Poor dietary intake of this B vitamin must continue for several months before changes in the eyes and vision develop. Increased intake of vitamin B2 and vitamin B2-rich foods, such as milk and low-fat milk products and dark green leafy vegetables, reverses the damage.

Low vitamin B2 intake is associated with cataract formation and blood levels of B2 are low in as many as 80 percent of these patients. A recent study at the National Cancer Institute and National Eye Institute in Bethesda, Maryland reports that supplements of vitamin B2 delay cataract formation in the elderly, a group with an increased risk for cataracts. However, high levels of vitamin B2 in eye tissue can contribute to free-radical formation during metabolism and exposure to light, and potentially damage the eye. The cause of vitamin B2 accumulation in the eyes is unknown, since it does not appear to be related to dietary intake.

VITAMIN B12. A deficiency of vitamin B12 results in poor vision that disappears when intake of the vitamin is increased.

ZINC. High levels of zinc are found in the retinal pigment epithelium (RPE), a colored layer of cells in the retina. The RPE has an increased exposure to free radicals, while zinc acts as an antioxidant to protect the RPE from these reactive compounds that might contribute to the development of macular degeneration. Increased intake of zinc and zinc-rich foods, such as extra-lean meat, poultry, and whole grain breads, might delay or prevent macular degeneration and improve visual keenness. However, supplementation with large doses of zinc can produce serious toxic side effects, including muscle incoordination, dizziness, drowsiness, vomiting, and anemia.

FISH OILS. The omega 3 fatty acids found in fish oils might be essential nutrients for the normal development and maintenance of eyesight. Large amounts of these fats are found in eye tissue and a prolonged deficiency during the early stages of life results in a significant loss of vision that might be permanent.

Dietary Recommendations

For the development and maintenance of healthy eyes and vision, a person should consume a low-fat, high-fiber, nutrient-dense diet that is adequate in all vitamins and minerals and low in sugars and refined and convenience foods. The diet should contain a variety of antioxidant-rich fruits and vegetables, as well as 6–11 servings daily of whole grain breads and cereals. A few servings daily of cooked dried beans and peas, low-fat or nonfat milk products, and extra-lean meats and chicken will help supply optimal amounts of essential vitamins and minerals. Frequent servings of steamed, baked, or broiled fish should be included in the diet. At times when the diet is not optimal, a multiple vitamin-mineral preparation that contains between 100 percent and 300 percent of the RDA of vitamin A, vitamin B2, vitamin B12, and zinc, as well as the other vitamins and minerals, and an extra dose of the antioxidant vitamins C, E, and beta carotene can supplement the diet. Regular exercise, effective stress management, avoidance of tobacco and excessive exposure to sunlight, regular medical check-ups and eye exams, and limiting alcohol use to little or none are also important for the prevention and treatment of eye disorders.

FATIGUE

Overview

Fatigue is a generalized feeling of tiredness or lethargy. There are many causes of fatigue, including poor nutrition, inadequate sleep, stress, overwork, infection, or disease. Fatigue is a common, but vague, symptom of many emotional, mental, and physical disorders.

Intense, disabling fatigue that severely restricts daily activities is one of the main symptoms of Chronic Fatigue Syndrome (CFS), a disorder affecting about 1 percent of Americans, two-thirds of which are young, middle-class women. Other symptoms include, persistent flu-like aches, mild fever, sore throat, swollen lymph nodes, muscle weakness, muscle fatigue (especially after exercise), headaches, joint pain, depression, sleep disturbances, and inability to concentrate. A diagnosis of CFS is usually made when a patient has multiple symptoms persisting for up to six months; however, the cause of this disorder remains unknown.

Researchers have several theories regarding CFS, some suspect the cause to be a viral infection and note that an acute infection is often present before CFS develops. Other researchers report disturbances of the immune system, such as suppression of immune system cells;

while still others note that CFS suffers have some symptoms in common with psychiatric disorders and some patients benefit from anti-depressant drugs.

Nutrition and Fatigue

A marginal deficiency of any nutrient can lead to feelings of fatigue. Inadequate intake of calories or protein produce lethargy and apathy, although this condition is uncommon in the United States except in individuals with anorexia nervosa, some hospitalized patients, and the elderly. A diet low in one or more nutrients might affect energy levels and increase the risk of fatigue by compromising immune function. (See pages 153–157 for more information on immunity.)

THE B VITAMINS. Many of the B vitamins, including vitamin B1, vitamin B2, vitamin B6, pantothenic acid, and niacin are essential for converting food into energy. A marginal deficiency of any of these B's leads to feelings of decreased energy, fatigue, weakness, and sleep disruptions. Inadequate intake of vitamin B2, vitamin B6, vitamin B12, and biotin can result in anemia with its accompanying fatigue, apathy, poor concentration, and exhaustion after mild exertion. Athletes, dieters, pregnant women, and vegetarians are at an increased risk for marginal deficiencies of the B vitamins.

VITAMIN C. One study showed that individuals with the lowest intake of vitamin C, i.e., less than 100mg, report the most symptoms of fatigue; whereas those with a vitamin C intake above 400mg daily felt significantly less fatigue. Increased vitamin C intake might combat fatigue by strengthening immunity and resistance to infection. In addition, the vitamin plays a role in the conversion of tryptophan to serotonin, a neurotransmitter involved in the regulation of sleep, depression, and pain.

IRON. This mineral carries oxygen in the blood to supply all the body's tissues. Inadequate intake of iron-rich foods, such as extra-lean red meats, poultry, fish, legumes, and dark green leafy vegetables, deprives the muscles, organs, and brain of oxygen and results in anemia, fatigue, weakness, poor concentration.

MAGNESIUM. Magnesium plays a role in the conversion of carbohydrates, protein, and fats into energy. A magnesium deficiency can result in muscle weakness, muscle fatigue, lack of coordination, loss of appetite, and depression. Researchers at the University of Southampton in the United Kingdom recently reported that patients suffering from Chronic Fatigue Syndrome have low blood levels of magnesium and supplementation improves their energy levels and mood. Magnesium supplements also might reduce symptoms of anxiety and insomnia.

OTHER VITAMINS AND MINERALS. Deficiencies of vitamin E or folic acid result in anemia and symptoms of fatigue, especially after even minor exertion. Anemia also can result from inadequate cobalt, copper, or selenium in the diet. Sodium deficiency, although very rare, and deficiencies of potassium, chloride, and manganese cause weakness and fatigue. An iodine deficiency can result in goiter and its associated feelings of lethargy. Zinc contributes to the production of energy in the body and helps regulate insulin and blood sugar levels; a deficiency can lead to anemia and sluggishness. Excessive consumption of selenium, cadmium, lead, and aluminum, also can produce symptoms of weakness, lethargy, and fatigue.

Dietary Recommendations

The best protection against diet-induced fatigue is to eat a low-fat, high-fiber, nutrient-dense diet that supplies optimal amounts of protein and calories to maintain a desirable body weight. Diets that severely restrict calories increase the risk of fatigue and should be avoided. Eating a healthy breakfast every morning, eating every four hours, and avoiding high-fat meals are ways to maintain normal blood sugar levels throughout the day.

The diet should provide optimum amounts of vitamins and minerals. If it does not, a multiple preparation containing 100 percent to 300 percent of the RDA for the B vitamins, vitamin C, iron, and magnesium in addition to other nutrients should be considered. Drink six to eight glasses of water daily as even mild dehydration contributes to fatigue. In addition, limit caffeinated beverages, avoid alcohol and sugary foods, and practice effective stress management. Finally, sleeping until rested every night and moderate daily aerobic exercise might improve low energy levels.

FIBROCYSTIC BREAST DISEASE (FBD)

Overview

Fibrocystic breast disease (FBD), the most common breast disorder in premenopausal women, is characterized by tender, painful breasts containing lumps and cysts. More than half of all women have FBD symptoms, perhaps beginning during adolescence with symptoms worsening through the early 40s and 50s. Some studies have linked FBD with breast cancer; although, this link depends on a family history of breast disease, and the type, content, and number of cysts a woman develops. However, breast cancer is found in only one out of every 11 women with FBD.

Nutrition and Fibrocystic Breast Disease

The effect of diet on fibrocystic breast disease is not entirely clear. The risk of developing FBD is associated with increased body weight, high socioeconomic status, and advanced education. Women with these lifestyle factors often consume a high-saturated fat diet, which might be a dietary link to FBD.

CAFFEINE. Years ago, researchers at Ohio State University reported that caffeine, part of the family of chemicals known as methylxanthines, increased the risk of FBD. Many women who eliminated caffeine-containing foods and beverages from their diet, such as coffee, tea, soda pop, and chocolate, claimed the pain and tenderness improved. However, subsequent research has not confirmed the association between FBD and caffeine.

DIETARY FAT. Lowering fat intake might prevent or treat FBD. Although FBD is associated with a high-fat intake, increased intake of saturated fats shows the strongest link. Women who reduce fat intake to 20 percent and reduce saturated fat to less than 7 percent of their total calories report reduced breast pain.

VITAMIN E. Some studies show vitamin E alleviates the symptoms of FBD, while other studies do not find an association. Women given vitamin E supplements have reported less pain, tenderness, and congestion; however, women also claim symptom relief after taking a placebo, an inactive pill thought by the patient to be vitamin E. This indicates a possible psychosomatic aspect to FBD that remains to be investigated.

Dietary Recommendations

Maintaining a desirable body weight might be important in preventing FBD. A high-fiber, nutrient-packed, low-fat diet that supplies no more than 7 percent of calories from saturated fat and that contains ample amounts of fresh fruits and vegetables, whole grain breads and cereals, cooked dried beans and peas, and moderate amounts of low-fat or nonfat milk products, fish and poultry is a woman's best safeguard against FBD. A multiple vitamin-mineral supplement and a vitamin E supplement should be considered if the diet does not meet RDAs. Caffeine-containing foods might be eliminated for four to six months as a trial to improve FBD symptoms. In addition, avoid alcohol, practice effective coping skills, and wear a supportive bra.

GUM AND TOOTH DISORDERS

Overview

A healthy smile is dependent on several factors including strong bones and teeth, adequate blood supply to the developing and mature gums and teeth, healthy gums, and a balance between acid and alkaline in the mouth.

Nutrition and Gum and Tooth Disorders

The cells that line the mouth have a short lifespan and require a constant supply of nutrients for normal repair and replacement. Consequently, symptoms of a vitamin or mineral deficiency often will develop more quickly in the mouth than in other tissues. The hard structures in the mouth, the bones and teeth, are blueprints for dietary intake of calcium and other minerals. Dietary habits and intake of other nutrients, such as starch and sugars, also are determining factors in the maintenance or loss of a healthy smile.

The incidence of tooth decay is strongly influenced by dietary intake during tooth development. Periodontal diseases—diseases of the gums—also have nutritional components.

Tooth decay is the most common long-term disease in the United States. People in primitive cultures living in remote areas of the world far from "civilized" cultures often have little or no problem with tooth decay; however, the incidence of tooth decay increases upon exposure to modernized cultures and dietary habits. Tooth decay is most likely to develop with frequent consumption of sugary foods, especially if the food sticks to the teeth or if the sugary foods are eaten alone. The effects of sugar consumption on tooth decay are most pronounced during infancy and childhood when the teeth are developing. Certain vitamins and minerals, however, can help strengthen the tooth and gum structure and aid in the prevention of tooth decay or periodontal disease.

VITAMIN A. Vitamin A is important in tooth formation and in the proper spacing of teeth. However, no evidence exists that vitamin A functions in the prevention of tooth decay.

VITAMIN D. A major function of vitamin D is in the regulation and use of calcium and phosphorus. The vitamin also aids in the formation and maintenance of normal teeth and bones, including the bones of the jaw. In fact, increased vitamin D intake, even without extra calcium, can help reduce fractures and slow the progression of bone loss.

VITAMIN E. It has been proposed that the mercury in silver amalgam dental fillings leaches out of the tooth and poses a potential health hazard, including increased risk for nerve and brain damage. The amount of mercury lost from dental fillings is extremely small and probably is not a problem to health; however, if this source of mercury is a concern, adequate intake of vitamin E would help protect the body against the toxic effects of this metal.

VITAMIN B2. Early symptoms of vitamin B2 deficiency include burning and soreness of the mouth, lips, and tongue and cracks at the corners of the mouth. The lining of the mouth becomes inflamed in advanced stages of vitamin B2 deficiency. These symptoms are reversed when intake of vitamin B2 or vitamin B2-rich foods is increased.

VITAMIN B12 AND FOLIC ACID. Vitamin B12 and folic acid are essential for the normal repair and replacement of cells. A deficiency of these B vitamins causes cells to form improperly. One of the first areas affected are the cells that line the mouth and tongue, causing soreness and deterioration of these surfaces. These symptoms are reversed with increased intakes of vitamin B12 and folic acid.

VITAMIN C. Vitamin C is required for the normal formation of the connective tissue that holds together the gums and other structures in the mouth. Some of the symptoms of scurvy or vitamin C deficiency are bleeding gums, deterioration of the gums, and loosening of the teeth caused by a deterioration of the connective tissue. Increased intake of vitamin C or vitamin C-rich foods cures the bleeding gums, but some damage caused by long-term vitamin C deficiency might be irreversible.

CALCIUM. Calcium protects against osteoporosis, strengthens the jawbone, and helps prevent tooth loss. In fact, one of the first bones affected by poor calcium intake is the alveolar bone, the portion of the jaw bone where the lower teeth are embedded or where dentures rest. Even excellent dental care, such as regular brushing and flossing, cannot protect against bone loss caused by poor calcium intake. Long-term poor intake of calcium can result in deterioration of the bone, periodontal disease, and problems with ill-fitting dentures.

A study of 329 postmenopausal women showed that tooth loss might be an early sign of osteoporosis. Researchers at the Human Nutrition Research Center on Aging at Tufts University found that women who began wearing dentures because of tooth loss before age 40 had more skeletal bone loss than women who required dentures after age 40 and those who kept most of their teeth. In fact, the more teeth the women had lost, the less bone they had in the spine, wrist, and hip, the areas most susceptible to fractures.

Marginal calcium intake throughout life contributes to periodontal disease. As with any bone, the strength and hardness of the alveolar bone is related to how much calcium a person consumes. When calcium intake is adequate, periodontal disease is less likely to occur. One study reported that alveolar bone loss was reversed when people increased their intake of calcium. When supplementation was stopped, the bone began to deteriorate; bone strength again increased when calcium supplementation was resumed.

Calcium functions in several other ways to prevent or treat dental problems. First, low intake of calcium hinders the production and alters the structure of the connective tissue that holds together the gums (periodontium) and bone. As a result, the bone and tissues dissolve and periodontal disease or poorly fitting dentures are likely to occur. Secondly, calcium is important in the formation of strong, well-developed teeth, because the mineral comprises a large part of both the enamel (the outer layer of the tooth) and the underlying dentin layer.

MAGNESIUM. The balance between magnesium and calcium is important in the formation and maintenance of healthy teeth and bones, such as the jaw and alveolar bones. In addition, a deficiency of magnesium produces swollen and sore gums, which is reversed when magnesium is added to the diet.

PHOSPHORUS. Phosphorus is a major component of the enamel and dentin of teeth. The balance between phosphorus and calcium is essential for the normal formation of bones and teeth. Because much of the calcification of these tissues occurs during the last two months in the uterus and during the first few months of life, it is important that the mother consume adequate amounts of both phosphorus and calcium during these periods. Otherwise, the developing infant will drain the mother's stores of these minerals. However, the typical

American diet contains excessive amounts of phosphorus and too little calcium, so the focus should be on increasing calcium intake, not supplementing or consuming more phosphorus-rich foods.

SULFUR. Sulfur is a component of bones and teeth. A deficiency of this mineral is rare and usually is secondary to a protein deficiency.

COPPER. Copper works with vitamin C in the formation of connective tissue. A deficiency of this trace mineral could result in faulty development of gums, teeth, and the jaw and alveolar bones.

FLUORIDE. Adequate consumption of fluoride during the first 18 years of life could reduce the incidence of tooth decay by more than 50 percent and maintain an increased resistance to decay throughout life. The incidence of tooth decay is high in areas of the United States where the water is not fluoridated and fluoride intake is low.

Fluoride is effective possibly because it discourages plaque accumulation on the tooth surface, discourages the activity of decay-causing bacteria, and encourages calcium deposition while discouraging calcium loss from teeth. The inclusion of fluoride into the calcium structure of teeth makes the teeth more resistant to decay caused by bacterial acids. In addition, fluoride strengthens the bones and reduces calcium loss from the jaw (alveolar) bone, characteristic of osteoporosis.

One milligram of fluoride for every liter of water (1 part fluoride for every million parts water or 1ppm) is considered optimal for the prevention of tooth decay. Excessive intake of fluoride causes mottling and discoloration of teeth.

MANGANESE. Manganese is important in the formation of connective tissue and a deficiency of this trace mineral results in bone deformities, such as a misshapened jaw bone.

ZINC. In animals, a deficiency of zinc, combined with deficiencies of vitamin C and folic acid, results in increased risk for developing periodontal disease. Zinc apparently is important in the formation and maintenance of healthy gum tissue and maintenance of the immune system to prevent infection in humans as well.

Dietary Recommendations

To prevent gum and tooth disorders, consume a low-fat, high-fiber, nutrient-dense diet that supplies an optimal amount of all vitamins and minerals and is low in sugars and refined or sugary convenience foods. Sugary foods that stick to the teeth or frequent consumption of sugary foods, especially if consumed as an only food, are of particular concern. Jams, jellies, desserts, candies, caramels, dried fruit, sugar, heavily sugared beverages and soft drinks, and sugared ready-to-eat cereals should be avoided or consumed infrequently.

Consumption of raw and rough foods, such as raw carrot sticks, apples, and green salads, scrape the teeth and help prevent accumulation of plaque and the development of tooth decay. The diet should contain a variety of fruits, vegetables, whole grain breads and cereals, cooked dried beans and peas, and extra-lean meats, chicken, and fish. At least two to three servings of low-fat or nonfat milk products should be consumed daily.

Vitamin D-fortified milk is the only reliable source of this vitamin and adults need at least two glasses daily (children and seniors may need as many as four glasses) to meet their vitamin D needs. People who turn to yogurt or cheese for their calcium might not get enough vitamin D, since these milk products are not fortified with the vitamin. (Your body can manufacture vitamin D when your skin is directly exposed to sunlight. However, this process is blocked by sunscreens and dwindles as a person ages, thus making dietary sources increasingly more important.) Consequently, an alternative source of vitamin D, in a daily dose of 200IU to 400IU, might be necessary to ensure normal calcium metabolism.

Nursing bottle syndrome, a condition in infants and small children, is characterized by extensive decay and loss of the upper teeth. This condition can be prevented by not giving the child a bottle at bedtime filled with any beverage that contains sugar, including sugared fruit drinks, orange juice, milk, or other fruit or commercial drinks. Water or a pacifier can be given to the child if necessary.

Regular dental visits, daily brushing and flossing, and consumption of fluoridated water also aid in the prevention of tooth decay.

HAIR PROBLEMS

Overview

Skin and hair are composed of the same protein, called keratin; however, they differ in shape, texture, and function.

Nutrition and Hair Problems

Although baldness and other hair disorders can be natural results of aging or symptoms of disease, in some cases vitamin and mineral deficiencies result in hair loss that can be corrected when the deficiency is treated. For example, inadequate intake of protein results in brittle, sparse, lusterless hair. Severe protein deficiency in children causes the hair to turn orange as a result of alterations in the pigments embedded in the hair shaft. These symptoms of protein deficiency disappear when the diet is improved.

VITAMIN A. Hair loss and dandruff develop as a result of vitamin A deficiency. If poor vitamin A intake is not a cause or if these symptoms do not disappear when vitamin A-rich foods are added to the diet, then other causes of the disorder should be investigated. Vitamin A toxicity also causes hair loss and dryness and itching of the skin.

VITAMIN B6, FOLIC ACID, AND VITAMIN B12. The hair is dependent on a constant supply of blood and oxygen for normal growth and health. Any nutrient that reduces the blood's ability to transport oxygen to the hair will have an effect on the health and appearance of the hair. Vitamin B6, folic acid, and vitamin B12 are essential for the normal formation of red blood cells, the portion of the blood that carries oxygen to the tissues. A deficiency of these B vitamins causes anemia and diminished blood supply to the hair and skin.

BIOTIN. A deficiency of the B vitamin biotin causes hair loss. A deficiency is rare, however, as bacteria in the intestine produce biotin that is absorbed.

VITAMIN C. Hair splits and breaks easily as a result of a vitamin C deficiency. When the hair breaks below the surface of the skin, the developing hair is cramped, coils into an abnormal circular pattern, and forms improperly. As a result, the hair is dry, kinky, and tangles. These symptoms occur only in a severe vitamin C deficiency and are reversible when vitamin C intake is increased.

COPPER. Copper is necessary for the formation of red blood cells and the maintenance of an adequate supply of blood to the hair shaft. In addition, copper functions in the formation and maintenance of hair pigments. A deficiency of this trace mineral is associated with color changes and loss of color from the hair. Excessive intake of the trace mineral molybdenum might interfere with the body's ability to use copper and produce symptoms of copper deficiency, such as hair loss.

IRON. Iron functions in the formation of red blood cells and the maintenance of the oxygen-carrying capacity of the blood. Therefore, this trace mineral is essential to the maintenance of an adequate blood supply to the hair. Iron deficiency is associated with hair loss, which is corrected when iron intake is increased.

ZINC. Symptoms of a zinc deficiency include hair loss and baldness. These symptoms are reversible if caused by a zinc deficiency. Zinc also functions in the maintenance of the oil-secreting glands attached to the hair follicle.

Dietary Recommendations

Most cases of balding result from hereditary influences; however, a good diet is safe and potentially beneficial. To maintain healthy scalp and hair, a person should consume a low-fat, fiber-rich, nutrient-dense diet that is optimal in all vitamins and minerals and low in sugars and refined and convenience foods. The diet should contain a variety of fruits, vegetables, whole grain breads and cereals, cooked dried beans and peas, low-fat or nonfat milk products, and extra-lean meat, chicken, and fish. Several glasses of water each day also are beneficial for healthy hair.

Regular exercise, effective stress management, avoidance of alcohol and tobacco, avoidance of severe cold and wind, and washing with a mild shampoo are helpful. In addition, limited use of medications such as anticoagulants that produce hair loss, stimulation of the scalp, and moderate exposure to sunshine are important for the prevention and treatment of non-inherited hair and scalp disorders.

HEADACHES

Overview

Any pain in the head is called a headache. An intense, throbbing headache often accompanied by nausea, vomiting, or disturbances in sensation or muscle movement is called a migraine headache.

Nutrition and Headaches

Several dietary factors are associated with an increased risk for developing headaches or migraine headaches. In addition, migraine headaches are sometimes caused by sensitivity to specific food components and often are successfully treated by removing the offending food from the diet.

VITAMIN A. Consumption of large doses of vitamin A, between 60,000IU and 341,000IU can cause headaches in adults. Children develop toxicity symptoms such as headaches at even lower doses. Large doses of carotene appear to be harmless.

THE B VITAMINS. Symptoms of marginal and clinical deficiencies of several of the B vitamins, including niacin and folic acid, might induce headaches. Vitamin B6 increases levels of the neurotransmitter serotonin, which is implicated in the development of migraine and tension headaches. Increased intake of vitamin B6 might relieve the pain of these headaches. Limited evidence shows that vitamin B6 supplements alleviate headaches early in pregnancy and in women using postmenopausal estrogen or oral contraceptives. Vitamin B6 supplements taken during the five to ten days prior to the onset of menstruation might prevent headaches associated with Premenstrual Syndrome (PMS).

CHOLINE. Blood levels of choline are low in people with headaches and headache symptoms improve when blood levels of choline increase. Whether the changes in choline status are a cause or a result of the headache is unclear.

COPPER. Altered copper metabolism might be the underlying factor in the association between the intake of some foods, such as chocolate, and migraine headaches. Food factors known to trigger migraine headaches also might affect copper metabolism. Changes in the intake, absorption, or use of copper might increase the incidence of migraine because the mineral is important in the production, use, and breakdown of chemicals in the brain that cause blood vessels to constrict or relax. Migraine headaches apparently occur more often when blood levels of copper are low than when blood levels are normal.

IRON. Headaches are a symptom of a marginal or clinical iron deficiency.

MAGNESIUM. Blood, cell, and salivary levels of this mineral are low in migraine sufferers, suggesting that brain levels of magnesium also might be low, which could contribute to the onset and persistence of headaches.

FISH OILS. The severity and frequency of migraine headaches might be reduced when the omega 3 fatty acids found in fish oils are increased in the diet.

AMINO ACID—TYRAMINE. Tyramine is a compound similar to the amino acid tyrosine and is found naturally in foods. It is estimated that between 20 percent and 25 percent of people who suffer from migraine headaches can be successfully treated by tyramine-free diets. Tyramine-containing foods include aged cheeses, herring, organ meats, peanuts and peanut butter, chocolate, sauerkraut, fermented sausages such as bologna and pepperoni, and alcoholic beverages.

PHENYLETHYLAMINE (PEA). PEA is a compound found in chocolate and might be a cause or an aggravator of migraine headaches. PEA causes the blood vessels in the head to enlarge, which places pressure on the surrounding brain tissue and results in migraine headaches in some people.

FOOD ADDITIVES. Nitrites are found naturally in foods and are preservatives added to bacon, hot dogs, and other sandwich meats. Some individuals who suffer from migraine headaches are sensitive to nitrites and the severity, frequency, and duration of headache symptoms might be reduced if foods that contain these additives are removed from the diet.

Monosodium glutamate (MSG) is a common food additive used in Chinese and other ethnic foods. The "Chinese Restaurant Syndrome" includes headache, flushing, nausea, or vomiting within an hour after consuming food high in MSG. The non-nutritive sweetener aspartame (NutraSweet) also increases the frequency of headaches in some people.

Dietary Recommendations

The tyramine-free diet is effective in many cases of migraine headache. If headaches continue after following this diet, then an elimination diet where foods thought to trigger headaches are removed one by one from the diet can be retried with the supervision of a physician or dietitian. A regular schedule of meals and sleeping hours and a record of headaches should be maintained to detect any hidden relationships between headaches and diet or other lifestyle patterns. Headaches might increase in frequency, duration, or severity during times of anxiety, high stress, or inadequate supportive relationships.

The dietary approach to preventing and treating headaches includes a low-fat, fiber-rich, nutrient-dense diet that is adequate in all vitamins and minerals and low in sugars and refined and convenience foods. The diet should contain a variety of fruits, vegetables, whole grain breads and cereals, cooked dried beans and peas, low-fat or nonfat milk products, and extra-lean meats, chicken, and fish. When the diet is inadequate, a multiple vitamin-mineral supplement might be considered. Regular exercise, effective stress management, and avoidance of alcohol, caffeine, and tobacco also are important in the prevention and treatment of headaches.

HEARING DISORDERS

Overview

Hearing is a complex process that begins with the gathering of sound at the outer ear and ends with the interpretation of sound in the higher centers of thought and reasoning in the brain (see Figure 1 on page 29).

Nutrition and Hearing Disorders

VITAMIN D. Inadequate amounts of vitamin D in the body might be associated with ear abnormalities and hearing loss in some people. A lack of vitamin D produces calcium loss from the bones and might cause the fragile bone of the inner ear, the cochlea, to become porous and unable to transmit messages to the nerves that lead to the brain. The association between vitamin D and hearing loss is supported by findings that people with other vitamin D-related disorders often have hearing loss. Deafness caused by changes in the cochlea might respond to vitamin D supplementation. It is unknown whether or not calcium is important in this form of hearing loss.

IODINE. Hearing improves in some people when they increase their consumption of dietary iodine. How iodine affects hearing is unclear; however, iodine therapy appears to be effective only in those few people deficient in the mineral.

Dietary Recommendations

Vitamin D cannot cure all types of hearing loss. Deafness as a result of nerve damage is not affected by vitamin D intake. If deafness is caused by changes in the bony structure of the inner ear and if dietary intake of vitamin D-fortified milk or exposure to sunshine has been minimal over a long period of time, then an increase in the consumption of vitamin D (200IU to 400IU daily) and calcium (800 to

1,200mg daily), and exposure to moderate sunshine might be useful in the treatment of hearing loss.

HERPES SIMPLEX

Overview

The severity, frequency, and duration of the viral infection called herpes varies between individuals and depends on other lifestyle factors such as stress and nutritional status. No cure exists for genital herpes, but the symptoms can be treated by soaking in salt solutions or sitz baths, use of pain-killers or soothing ointments, medication, and possibly an antibiotic cream to prevent secondary infections.

Nutrition and Herpes Simplex

Nutrition functions directly and indirectly by stimulating the immune response to reduce the frequency, severity, and duration of recurrences of herpes infections.

AMINO ACIDS—L-LYSINE. Lysine might reduce the frequency and severity of symptoms of recurrent herpes infections. Doses that exceed one gram of lysine appear to be necessary to obtain satisfactory results. Blood levels of lysine also are related to risk for recurrence; when blood levels of lysine are high, the incidence of recurrent infections is reduced as compared to when blood levels of lysine are low.

The herpes virus thrives in an environment where there are large amounts of the amino acid arginine and low amounts of lysine. If lysine supplementation is an effective treatment for herpes, it is probably because increased intake of lysine upsets the ratio of arginine to lysine and slows viral growth. The evidence in support of lysine for the treatment of herpes infections is limited and controversial and some studies have not found lysine beneficial in the treatment of herpes.

BIOFLAVONOIDS. A few reports state that bioflavonoids might be effective in reducing the severity of symptoms during recurrent herpes infections. More evidence is necessary, however, before dietary recommendations can be made.

VITAMINS AND MINERALS. A person's susceptibility to herpes infection depends on exposure to the virus and the strength of the immune system to fight the infection. All nutrients associated with a well-functioning immune system are important to build the body's defense against infection and reduce the likelihood of recurrence. These nutrients include beta carotene, vitamin E, the B vitamins, vitamin C, iron, copper, selenium, and zinc. (See pages 153–157 for more information on nutrition and immunity.)

Dietary Recommendations

Supplementation with L-lysine combined with limited intake of arginine-rich foods, such as nuts, seeds, and chocolate, might discourage the growth of the herpes virus and reduce the risk for recurrence.

A low-fat, fiber-rich, nutrient-dense diet should be consumed, adequate in all vitamins and minerals and low in sugars and refined and convenience foods. The diet should contain a variety of fruits, vegetables, whole grain breads and cereals, cooked dried beans and peas, low-fat or nonfat milk products, and extra-lean meats, chicken, and fish. A multiple vitamin-mineral supplement that contains between 100 percent and 300 percent of the RDA for all nutrients related to the immune system (see pages 153–157 for more information on nutrition and immunity), as well as regular exercise, effective stress management, adequate sleep, avoidance of alcohol and tobacco, and limited use of caffeine are important for the prevention and treatment of viral infections, such as herpes simplex.

HYPERTENSION

Overview

Blood pressure is the blood's force against the walls of the arteries and heart as the blood is pumped from the heart to the tissues. Two pressures make up blood pressure: systolic blood pressure, or the maximum amount of pressure in the arteries when the heart contracts (heartbeat), and diastolic blood pressure, or the least amount of pressure in the arteries when the heart relaxes between beats.

Hypertension is blood pressure that remains above the normal range and signifies a constant, excessive pulsing of blood against the walls of the arteries and heart. Hypertension is not a disease, but a symptom of an underlying disease. It also is one of the three primary risk factors for the development of heart attack and stroke. The best defense against hypertension is prevention; but one can control existing hypertension with correct diet, lifestyle habits, and medication.

Nutrition and Hypertension

Diet is strongly linked to the prevention and treatment of essential hypertension. For example, body weight is proportional to hypertension risk; as weight increases above the ideal, the risk for hypertension increases. In contrast, weight loss and maintenance of a desirable body weight is often effective in the prevention and treatment of hypertension. The maintenance of a desirable body weight for people with borderline hypertension might eliminate the need for medications, which otherwise have side effects that sometimes increase the risk of heart disease. Even a 10-pound weight loss can reduce blood pressure, whereas blood pressure tends to rise as weight is gained.

A high-fat, low-fiber diet is linked to an increased risk for developing hypertension, while increasing fiber and cutting back on fat might reduce blood pressure. Blood pressure drops when the fat content is reduced from the typical 37 percent to 25 percent of total calories and more polyunsaturated fats from vegetable oils than saturated fats from meat and dairy products are consumed.

Some evidence shows that polyunsaturated fats are changed to the hormone-like prostaglandins that assist the body in blood pressure regulation. It is theorized that if fat was reduced to less than 25 percent, salt intake was restricted, and a desirable body weight was maintained, hypertension might be controlled or eliminated without the need for medication in more than 85 percent of all cases.

Sodium. Excessive salt (sodium chloride) intake is linked to increased risk for developing hypertension. In contrast, as salt intake decreases, so does the risk for developing hypertension. In populations with a high-salt diet, such as in America and Japan, the incidence of hypertension is higher than in populations with a low-salt diet.

Some people are more susceptible than others to salt intake. This sensitivity to salt might be inherited, in which case the consumption of a low-salt diet from childhood would aid in the prevention of this disorder. Some studies show that 40 percent to 50 percent of people with hypertension are salt-sensitive and about 30 percent of the general public is sensitive to salt. However, there is no method for determining who is and who isn't salt-sensitive. As the intake of salt is excessive in the United States and reduction of intake poses no harm, it has been recommended that all Americans reduce their intake of salt.

Sodium does not work alone, but functions in a balance with other minerals, including calcium, chloride, magnesium, and potassium, to regulate blood pressure. Consequently, hypertension is associated with an imbalance in these minerals where sodium (and possibly chloride) are high, while calcium, magnesium, and potassium intakes are low.

POTASSIUM. The ratio of potassium to sodium might be a factor in the development of hypertension. A high intake of sodium-rich foods such as convenience foods, snack foods, and canned soups, coupled with a reduction in intake of potassium-rich foods is associated with a high incidence of hypertension. Low potassium intake encourages sodium retention, which in turn raises blood pressure. In contrast, a diet high in potassium protects against the development of this disorder by lowering systolic and diastolic blood pressures and reducing the need for blood pressure-lowering medications. Potassium also helps regulate calcium levels, which further protects against hypertension.

CHLORIDE. Chloride, the other compound in table salt (sodium chloride), also is linked to hypertension. These electrolytes work together in the regulation of fluid balance and blood pressure. Some evidence shows that dietary intake of sodium without chloride does not increase blood pressure in salt-sensitive people with hypertension and the intake of both sodium and chloride are necessary for the disorder to develop.

CALCIUM. People who consume low amounts of calcium or calcium-rich milk products are more likely to develop high blood pressure than are people who consume at least the RDA or more for calcium. Diastolic blood pressure drops when diets are supplemented daily with 1,000mg of calcium. In animal studies, a high-calcium diet consumed during pregnancy and breast-feeding discourages the development of high blood pressure in the offspring; in contrast, a low-calcium diet increases the risk of high blood pressure in the offspring.

Calcium interacts with sodium, potassium, and magnesium to regulate blood pressure and might be as strongly linked to hypertension as sodium. For example, increased calcium intake might help counteract the hypertensive effects of a high-sodium diet, possibly by increasing urinary excretion of sodium. In contrast, a high-sodium intake increases urinary loss of calcium and elevates hypertension risk.

MAGNESIUM. People with hypertension often have low blood levels of magnesium. In many cases, elevated blood pressure returns to normal with increased intake of magnesium-rich foods or magnesium supplements. Inadequate intake of magnesium can disturb electrolyte balance, especially in the presence of low potassium and/or calcium intake, which increases the risk of developing or aggravating hypertension.

Some anti-hypertension medications affect the amount of magnesium in the body. Diuretic medications, such as the thiazides, lower blood pressure by increasing urinary excretion of fluid and reducing blood volume. They also increase the excretion of magnesium and the risk for magnesium deficiency. Many people with hypertension who take diuretic medications have low blood levels of magnesium and the combination of magnesium and hypertension medication might be more effective in lowering blood pressure than medication alone.

Magnesium also might aid in the regulation of blood pressure by its effect on the blood vessel walls. Magnesium influences how the heart and the blood vessels contract and relax. Artery walls spasm and an irregular heartbeat develops when magnesium intake is low; artery walls relax and the heartbeat returns to normal when blood levels of the mineral are adequate. Constriction or spasms of the blood vessels are linked to hypertension, whereas relaxation of the blood vessels increases the size of the blood vessel, reduces resistance to blood flow, and lowers blood pressure.

VITAMINS. People with hypertension often have low blood levels of vitamin C and consume vitamin C-poor diets. Increasing vitamin C intake might lower the blood pressure of these individuals. Researchers at the USDA Human Nutrition Research Center in Beltsville, Maryland found that vitamin C supplements reduced blood pressure and the researchers concluded that supplementation in conjunction with other therapies might be beneficial for the treatment of hypertension.

Low intakes of vitamin D might increase the risk for hypertension. One study investigated the link between vitamin D and blood pressure in women between the ages of 20 and 80 years old and found that blood pressure increased as vitamin D intake decreased, particularly in the younger women. Vitamin D might affect blood pressure indirectly by altering calcium absorption and metabolism.

FISH OILS. The omega 3 fatty acids found in fish oils might lower blood pressure. Blood pressure drops as much as 24 percent when a person includes frequent servings of fish in the weekly diet or takes fish oil supplements. The blood pressure-lowering effect of fish oils is enhanced when combined with a low-salt diet.

Dietary Recommendations

Maintenance of a desirable body weight is important for the prevention and treatment of essential hypertension. The diet should be low in fat, salt, and sugar and high in fiber, vitamins, and minerals. Salt intake can be reduced by limiting salt use in cooking and at the table, buying low-salt foods, and avoiding highly processed foods that are high in salt. The diet should contain a variety of fruits, vegetables, whole grain breads and cereals, cooked dried beans and peas, low-fat or nonfat milk products, and extra-lean meats, fish, and chicken. Foods should be baked, steamed, and broiled, rather than fried or sauteed. A multiple vitamin-mineral supplement and a calcium and magnesium supplement should be consumed if the diet does not supply at least the RDA for these nutrients.

Regular aerobic exercise, such as walking, jogging, swimming, or jumping rope, is also necessary for weight and blood pressure maintenance. Effective stress management, frequent blood pressure checkups, compliance with medications, moderate use or avoidance of alcohol and caffeine, and avoidance of tobacco are important for the prevention and treatment of hypertension.

INFECTION

Overview

Infection is any invasion of the body by disease-causing microorganisms (germs), such as bacteria or viruses, that results in a reaction of the tissues, inflammation, and a response from the immune system. Many areas of the body are normally inhabited by microorganisms, but disease develops when the body's defense system is faulty or the microorganisms migrate from their natural spot to another area in the body. Other disease-causing microorganisms are transmitted through food, air, contact with other people and the environment, contact with insects and animals that transmit disease, or water. Microorganisms find entry into the body through the skin, nose, mouth, ears, the intestinal or urinary tracts, and other body openings.

In addition to common infections, several diseases are attributed to exposure and susceptibility to specific microorganisms, such as the diseases caused by bacterial infection including scarlet fever, rheumatic fever, meningitis, measles, tuberculosis, whooping cough, and food poisoning. Also included are the diseases caused by viral infections including rabies, mumps, influenza, acquired immunodeficiency syndrome (AIDS), hepatitis, herpes, chickenpox, infectious mononucleosis, and smallpox.

The strength of the immune system is an important factor in the prevention or development and treatment of infection. (See pages 153–157 for more information on the immune system.)

Nutrition and Infection

Nutrition is a major contributor to the functioning of the immune system. All organs and cells of the immune system are affected by a person's nutritional status. General poor nutrition, including inadequate intake of protein and calories, suppresses the immune response and increases the risk for developing infection and disease; however, even single vitamin or mineral deficiencies in the presence of otherwise adequate nutrition can compromise a person's ability to fight infection. On the other hand, optimal intake of all vitamins and minerals and consumption of a diet low in fat and high in fiber enhances the immune response and reduces a person's risk for developing infection.

The vitamins and trace minerals associated with the immune response include vitamin A, beta carotene, vitamin E, the B vitamins, vitamin C, copper, iron, selenium, and zinc. Inadequate intake of any of these nutrients results in reduced activity of the immune system and increased susceptibility to colds and infection. In addition, infection drains essential nutrients from the body and increases the daily requirement in order to fight the infection and repair the damaged tissues. Marginal nutrient deficiencies have a harmful effect on the immune system long before obvious signs of more severe deficiencies and malnutrition develop.

Dietary Recommendations

To maintain a healthy immune system and prevent infections, a low-fat, fiber-rich, nutrient-dense diet should be consumed, optimal in all vitamins and minerals and low in sugars and refined and convenience foods. The diet should contain a variety of fruits, vegetables, whole grain breads and cereals, cooked dried beans and peas, low-fat or nonfat milk products, and extra-lean meats, chicken, and fish. A multiple supplement that supplies between 100 percent and 300 percent of the RDA for all vitamins and minerals should be chosen when the diet is not optimal. Regular exercise, effective stress management, avoidance of alcohol and tobacco, compliance with antibiotic medications, daily consumption of several glasses of water, adequate amounts of sleep, and good sanitation are also important for the prevention and treatment of infection. (For additional information on specific infections see the sections on The Immune System, Acne, AIDS, the Common Cold, Dermatitis, Herpes, and Yeast infection.)

INSOMNIA

Overview

The most common sleep disorder is insomnia. Insomnia can be a result of difficulty falling asleep, difficulty staying asleep during the night, or waking too early in the morning. The relative decrease in the need for sleep that is the normal accompaniment of aging is not included in this category. Insomnia results from numerous disorders such as depression, chronic physical pain, stress, and many medications.

Nutrition and Insomnia

A generally poor diet and inadequate intake of several nutrients can result in disturbed sleep, including insomnia, fatigue, and other sleep disorders. A healthful diet that is optimal in all vitamins and minerals, and avoids or limits intake of caffeinated beverages, alcohol, and food additives is the best start to a good night's rest.

THE B VITAMINS. Deficiencies of niacin and vitamin B6 are related to insomnia; however, supplementation with these nutrients is only effective if a nutrient deficiency is the cause of the sleep disorder. One of the symptoms of a niacin deficiency is insomnia, and increased niacin intake is an effective cure for this form of the disorder. Vitamin B6 is an important contributor to the formation of serotonin, a neurotransmitter that aids in the regulation of sleep. A diet low in vitamin B6 is associated with increased risk for developing insomnia, irritability, and depression, and increased intake of the vitamin reverses these symptoms.

Vitamin B12 supplements improve sleep patterns in chronic insomniacs, while sleep problems resume when the supplements are discontinued. However, individuals with insomnia usually have normal levels of vitamin B12 and a large-dose supplement is required to improve sleep. A physician should supervise any megadose vitamin therapies. Finally, limited evidence shows that increasing folic acid and vitamin B1 intake might improve sleep patterns in some individuals.

MINERALS. Some minerals indirectly affect sleep. For example, calcium and magnesium work together in nerve function and muscle contraction and relaxation. A deficiency of one of these might cause muscle cramps or disturbed nerve function that could disrupt sleep. Low copper intake has been linked to earlier bedtimes, increased time needed to fall asleep, increased length of sleep, and reduced feelings of restedness. Inadequate iron might increase length of sleep, risk of earlier bedtime, and frequency of nighttime awakenings.

AMINO ACIDS—TRYPTOPHAN. The dietary amino acid tryptophan is converted to the neurotransmitter serotonin in the body. Serotonin is one of the chemicals that regulate sleep. Tryptophan supplementation increases serotonin levels, reduces the time required to fall asleep by as much as 50 percent, and can improve the quality and length of sleep. This amino acid is also associated with metabolism of a hormone called melatonin that affects mood and sleep. To elevate blood and brain levels of tryptophan, consume a carbohydrate-rich, low-protein snack (toast and jam) one hour before bedtime.

OTHER DIETARY FACTORS. The caffeine in coffee, tea, many cola drinks, hot cocoa, and chocolate is a stimulant that can result in shakiness, nervousness, irritability, and insomnia. Small amounts of caffeine-containing foods and beverages consumed in the morning probably won't affect sleep in the evening. However, ingesting multiple servings, especially later in the day, or minimal amounts for caffeine-sensitive persons might result in significant sleep disruptions.

Although alcohol produces feelings of drowsiness, this drug actually disturbs normal sleep patterns, resulting in less restful sleep. Sleep disturbances also can be caused by foods containing the flavor-enhancing additive MSG, lactose intolerance or food allergies, eating spicy or gas-forming foods, and large or high-fat dinners that prolong digestion time. Very-low-calorie diets increase the risk of night awakenings and awakening too early, while decreasing the amount of time spent dreaming. Resuming normal eating habits resolves these sleep disturbances.

Dietary Recommendations

Short-term insomnia might be treatable with tryptophan-rich foods, such as milk, cheese, turkey, or bananas. Tryptophan entry into the brain is increased if a meal or snack is high in starchy foods and low in protein. However, tryptophan supplements are not currently available in the U.S. since a late-1980s contaminated supply produced a rare blood disorder. Long-term insomnia should be treated with the help of a physician and may require medication and stress reduction or psychological counseling.

Other dietary approaches include:

1. increase intake of foods rich in calcium, magnesium, copper, and iron,
2. eat larger meals, and spicy or gas-forming foods in the morning or afternoon, instead of at dinner, and
3. avoid strict diets.

Stress reduction techniques, such as regular exercise, establishing an evening routine prior to going to bed, and not taking afternoon naps might aid in the treatment of insomnia. Avoidance of caffeine, tobacco, and other stimulants or drugs also is beneficial.

JET LAG

Overview

Jet lag is a physiological and psychological syndrome experienced by many people when they travel by air across three or more time zones; symptoms are most severe in flights traveling west to east. People do not develop jet lag when traveling north and south. Within the first day at the destination, a person might feel tired, experience poor concentration, have memory lapses, or perform poorly on normal tasks. Later symptoms include increasing weariness, gastrointestinal disturbances such as constipation or diarrhea, insomnia, loss of appetite, headaches, reduced ability to see at night, and limited peripheral vision. The symptoms last from a day to two weeks, depending on individual variation and the number of time zones crossed. In general, it takes the body one day to adjust for each time zone crossed.

Dietary Recommendations

A jet lag diet program has been developed that might aid in the prevention of weariness and related symptoms associated with long-distance air travel. Four days prior to the estimated breakfast time at the destination the meals should be hearty, high in protein at breakfast and lunch, and high in carbohydrates at dinner. Coffee and tea are allowed only between 3 P.M. and 5 P.M. The second day of the program, the meals are light, such as salads, simple soups, fruits and fruit juices, and vegetables. This "fast" day is designed to deplete the body's stores of carbohydrates and help "reset" the internal time clock.

The last two days of the diet the feast and fast cycle is repeated, except on the fourth day people flying westbound drink a caffeinated beverage in the morning, while people flying eastbound drink a caffeinated beverage between 6 P.M. and 11 P.M. The feast-fast cycle is broken at what should be breakfast time at the destination by consuming a high-protein breakfast. The person should eat this meal regardless of when the breakfast hour occurs, even if he/she must get up in the middle of the night or eat at 2 A.M. on the plane.

In addition, sleep and meal times should be shifted one hour each day prior to the trip to prepare the body for the time change. The traveler should begin the trip well rested and not plan activities for the first day after arrival. Fluids should be consumed before and during the flight to replace body water lost due to low humidity in the pressurized airplane cabin.

KIDNEY DISORDERS

Overview

The kidneys and urinary system maintain the chemical balance of all body fluids. They filter out and remove waste products from the blood; maintain the normal ranges of nutrients in the blood by removing and excreting excess amounts of minerals, vitamins, and other compounds; and regulate the normal acid-base (pH) balance of the body. Kidney and urinary disorders include the following:

Acute glomerulonephritis: Temporary inflammation of the portion of the kidneys that filters waste products from the blood.

Chronic glomerulonephritis: Long-term inflammation that sometimes develops from the acute form of the same disorder.

Nephrotic syndrome or nephrosis: A disease characterized by water retention, protein loss in the urine, tissue deterioration, and malnutrition.

Uremia: A toxic condition caused by the accumulation of waste products in the blood that is a symptom of kidney failure.

Acute and chronic kidney failure: The inability of the kidneys to remove waste products characterized by the accumulation of toxic chemicals and acids in the blood.

Kidney stones: Kidney stones are crystals of calcium oxalate, calcium phosphate, uric acid, or a mixture of these or other substances. The urinary concentration of calcium oxalate, and other substances, and the presence (or absence) of factors in the urine that promote or inhibit stone formation, called crystallization, determine whether a stone will develop.

Urinary tract infections: Infections, such as a bladder infection, result from bacteria in the urethra, bladder, or ureters.

Nutrition and Kidney Disorders

Dietary management for all kidney disorders except kidney stones includes consideration for the intake of protein, fluid, salt, potassium, calcium, phosphorus, vitamin D, fluoride, and all vitamins. Dietary control of these kidney disorders must be monitored closely by a physician and a dietitian.

VITAMIN A. Vitamin A is essential for the development and maintenance of the lining of the urinary system.

VITAMIN D. Excessive intake of vitamin D can result in calcium deposits in the kidneys and irreversible kidney damage. Vitamin D, however, also improves zinc status in kidney patients on dialysis.

VITAMIN E. A deficiency of vitamin E produces a form of anemia called hemolytic anemia, where red blood cells are fragile and break easily. This form of anemia is common in patients on dialysis for the treatment of advanced kidney disease, and supplementation with the vitamin might help prevent or correct this secondary disorder.

VITAMIN B6. A vitamin B6 deficiency might increase the risk for developing oxalate-containing kidney stones. Supplementation with the vitamin reduces the amount of oxalate in the urine and reduces a person's risk for developing kidney stones or kidney damage.

VITAMIN C. Some studies report that large doses of vitamin C might encourage the formation of oxalate-containing kidney stones in people prone to stone formation. For example, evidence shows that vitamin C intake should be limited to the RDA in people with kidney disorders because large doses of the vitamin raise blood and urinary levels of oxalic acid, a compound that aggravates kidney disease. However, other studies show no association between vitamin C and kidney stones, even in people prone to stone formation. Consequently, the link between vitamin C and kidney stones remains controversial.

MAGNESIUM. Magnesium inhibits the formation of crystals in the urine, possibly as a result of the ratio of magnesium to calcium in the urine. The magnesium content of the urine of stone formers and stone nonformers is similar; however, stone formers excrete greater amounts of calcium, making their urinary ratio of calcium to magnesium very high. Increased intake of magnesium raises the magnesium concentration in the urine, alters the ratio of calcium to magnesium to resemble the urinary magnesium concentration of stone nonformers, and reduces the formation of kidney stones.

Kidney stones are most common in affluent nations where typical diets are high in protein, refined carbohydrates, fat, alcohol, and phosphorus. These dietary factors also increase the daily need for magnesium.

Dietary Recommendations

For the prevention of kidney disorders, a person should consume a low-fat, high-fiber, nutrient-dense diet, optimal in all vitamins and minerals and low in sugars and refined and convenience foods. The diet should contain a variety of fruits, vegetables, whole grain breads and cereals, cooked dried beans and peas, low-fat or nonfat milk products, and extra-lean meats, chicken, and fish. A multiple vitamin-mineral supplement as well as several glasses of water daily, limited use of bubble baths and hygiene sprays, regular physical examinations that include a urine culture, regular exercise, effective stress management, avoidance of alcohol and tobacco, and daily bathing are important.

Kidney stones are comprised of several different substances including calcium and uric acid. Dietary management of kidney stones should be designed and monitored by a physician and a dietitian and depends on the type of stone. Treatments attempt to reduce these substances in the urine or keep them in solution rather than allowing them to solidify into stones.

The use of acid-ash or alkaline-ash diets in the treatment of kidney stones refers to the products the foods will eventually yield after use in the body. The acids in fruits or milk are used in the body and the remaining products for excretion include alkaline substances such as potassium or calcium. In contrast, the waste products of a diet high in meat are acidic and produce an acid ash, such as uric acid and phosphoric acid, that is excreted by the kidneys.

The most common form of kidney stones are calcium-containing stones that are caused by abnormal absorption of calcium from the intestine, abnormal filtering of calcium from the kidneys, or abnormal activity of hormones that regulate calcium use in the body. A high dietary intake of calcium does not cause kidney stones except in those people who are prone to kidney stone formation. Foods that produce an acid ash, such as meat, starchy foods, cranberries, and prunes, help keep calcium from crystallizing into a stone.

Other techniques for the control of calcium stones include the use of diuretic medications that reduce the amount of calcium in the urine and gel medications that reduce the absorption of calcium from the intestine. A low-calcium diet is often prescribed, but increases the risk for developing osteoporosis and other bone diseases. In contrast, uric acid stones require an increased intake of alkaline ash foods, such as milk, vegetables, and fruits and a reduced intake of meats and other acid ash foods.

Urinary tract infections have been treated with mixed results by drinking large amounts of cranberry juice or consuming large doses of vitamin C to acidify the urine. The best treatment after a diagnosis, based on an analysis and culture of the urine, is the use of prescribed medications such as antibiotics or sulfa drugs combined with increased water intake. Coffee, tea, alcohol, and spicy foods should be avoided during the period of infection.

The treatment of kidney diseases should be designed and monitored by a physician and dietitian, and includes dietary, medication or medical, and lifestyle components.

LIVER DISORDERS

Overview

The liver is the largest and one of the most important organs in the body and has the greatest variety of functions. Most of the nutrients absorbed from the diet are transported directly to the liver for storage, repackaging, or combining with other compounds. Poisons that enter or are produced in the body are detoxified in the liver. Many compounds essential to growth and development are produced in the liver, such as fat, proteins, sugar, cholesterol, and the blood carriers of fat called lipoproteins. The liver serves as a storehouse for nutrients, such as the fat-soluble vitamins, vitamin B12, vitamin C, copper, and iron, and the storage form of energy called glycogen.

The liver also releases substances into the blood when levels are low, such as sugar to maintain blood sugar levels and a special protein called albumin that maintains fluid balance in the blood. The liver packages other compounds for excretion, such as converting cholesterol to bile for excretion into the intestine. The liver converts vitamins to their active forms, such as carotene into vitamin A.

Damage to the liver has profound effects on numerous body processes, including digestion, absorption, storage, and use of vitamins and minerals. In addition, the manufacture of proteins decreases, fat production is altered and results in fat accumulation in the liver, and the manufacture of enzymes necessary for the detoxification of alcohol and other poisons is reduced so that these substances accumulate in the body.

Diseases of the liver include the following:

Hepatitis: Inflammation of the liver caused by a virus, toxin or drug, or blockage of the duct leading from the liver to the gallbladder.

Cirrhosis: A replacement of healthy liver tissue with tough, fibrous tissue resulting in a reduction in liver function,

Jaundice: The symptom of an underlying liver disorder, which is characterized by a yellowish discoloration of the skin and eyes caused by accumulation of bile in the body.

Hemochromatosis: An excessive accumulation of iron in the liver.

Nutrition and Liver Disorders

Liver disease causes malnutrition for three reasons. It

1. hinders the digestion and absorption of food.
2. affects the utilization of nutrients in the body.
3. reduces food intake because of nausea, loss of appetite, and vomiting.

The manufacture, use, and excretion of protein, carbohydrate, and fat are altered and the absorption and use of numerous vitamins and minerals are reduced when the liver is not functioning correctly.

VITAMIN A. Adequate intake of vitamin A might help prevent the accumulation of tough, fibrous tissue in the liver characteristic of disease. Animals with liver disease show reduced damage to the tissue when the diet is high in vitamin A as compared to when vitamin A intake is poor. Long-term and excessive intake of the fat-soluble vitamin might cause liver enlargement and disease.

VITAMIN E. Vitamin E supplementation that raises liver concentrations of the vitamin might prevent liver damage and cirrhosis according to researchers at the University of Turin in Italy. Rats were supplemented with vitamin E to levels that raised liver vitamin E concentrations. The animals were then exposed to carbon tetrachloride to test whether the pretreatment with vitamin E would protect against both acute and chronic liver damage and cirrhosis. Vitamin E supplementation increased the vitamin content of the liver three-fold and reduced oxidative damage to liver tissue, but had no protective effect on the development of fatty infiltration of the liver. Cirrhosis also was significantly prevented in the vitamin E-supplementation rats. Vitamin E apparently provides considerable protection from carbon tetrachloride-induced liver necrosis and cirrhosis, probably by reducing the spread of lipid oxidation processes and reducing the extent of oxidative liver damage.

In another study, the highest blood levels of vitamin E were in healthy subjects and alcoholics with normal liver enzyme levels. Alcoholics with ethanol intoxication showed a 37 percent lower vitamin E-to-fat ratio than controls. Hemochromatosis patients with high blood iron levels and Wilson's disease patients with high blood copper levels had 34 percent to 37 percent lower vitamin E levels as compared to healthy people. These results show that the reduced free-radical scavenging ability of patients with low vitamin E levels might promote liver disease.

VITAMIN K. Large doses of vitamin K produce jaundice and damage to brain tissue in infants.

BETA CAROTENE. Beta carotene levels are low in patients with liver cirrhosis, while a diet high in beta carotene might reduce liver damage. Cirrhosis of the liver often is associated with increased activity of harmful compounds called free radicals that might increase the risk of liver cancer. As an antioxidant, beta carotene might prevent the formation of potentially harmful free radicals.(See pages 150–153 for an explanation of free radicals and antioxidants.)

NIACIN. Although hypercholesterolemia is effectively treated by niacin, researchers at the Virginia Commonwealth University warn that the sustained-release form of niacin is hepatotoxic and the immediate-release form also might produce negative side effects.

In the sustained-released niacin group, 78 percent of the subjects withdrew before reaching 3,000mg/day supplementation, primarily because of gastrointestinal tract symptoms, fatigue, and increased levels of liver enzymes suggestive of liver dysfunction. Hepatotoxic effects developed only in the sustained-release group, not in the group taking regular niacin. The results of this study show that therapeutic doses of sustained-release niacin should be taken only with physician monitoring.

BIOTIN. Large doses of biotin over long periods of time might cause abnormal enlargement of the liver.

CHOLINE. Liver damage might be a sign of choline deficiency. Fat fragments accumulate in the liver because triglycerides must be packaged as VLDLs (very-low-density lipoproteins) to be transported from the liver, but VLDLs require phosphatidylcholine to function. Consequently, VLDLs cannot be exported during choline deficiencies.

Human subjects show liver enzyme dysfunction and decreased blood cholesterol (derived from VLDL secreted by the liver) within three weeks on a choline-deficient diet. These symptoms are reversed within two to six weeks after lecithin supplementation, which raises blood choline levels.

COPPER. An inherited disorder in the use of copper called Wilson's disease is characterized by excessive accumulation of copper in tissues and results in reduced liver function. Treatment of Wilson's disease includes a diet low in copper and the medication penicillamine that binds to copper and increases its excretion in the intestine.

SELENIUM. One study showed that individuals with and without liver disease have similar intakes of selenium, but those with liver disease have lower liver and blood levels of the mineral.

Nutritional consequences of liver disease might include reduced formation of vitamin D, which contributes to osteoporosis, increased loss of vitamin B6 and possible deficiency, and reduced formation of the protein that transports vitamin A in the blood. Additionally, increased loss and possible deficiencies of folic acid, calcium, magnesium, and zinc might occur.

Dietary Recommendations

The dietary management of all liver disorders should be designed and monitored by a physician and dietitian. Protein, carbohydrates, fat, and calories must be balanced, and vitamin and mineral intakes should be optimal to reduce nutritional stress on the liver and provide all the nutrients necessary for repair of the damaged tissue. Vitamins should be consumed in their active forms, especially vitamin A and the B vitamins, as the liver, which is responsible for producing the active forms of vitamins from dietary building blocks, is unable to function normally. Water-soluble forms of vitamins A, D, E, and possibly K might be necessary if the person is unable to absorb fats. In addition, a person should avoid alcohol, environmental and dietary toxins, and substances that stress the body, such as tobacco. Use of medications known to cause liver damage should be monitored closely by a physician.

To prevent liver disease, avoid alcohol, and consume a low-fat, high-fiber, nutrient-dense diet, optimal in all vitamins and minerals and low in sugars and refined and convenience foods. The diet should contain a variety of fruits, vegetables, whole grain breads and cereals, cooked dried beans and peas, low-fat or nonfat milk products, and extra-lean meats, chicken, and fish. A multiple vitamin-mineral supplement as well as regular exercise, effective stress management, avoidance of tobacco, removal of all environmental and dietary toxins, and regular physical examinations are important.

LUNG DISORDERS

Overview

The main function of the lungs is to supply the bloodstream with oxygen and remove unwanted gases, such as carbon dioxide, from the system. Carbon dioxide is removed with each exhalation and oxygen is absorbed into the blood with each inhalation. This exchange of gases is called respiration and is essential to life.

The lungs are exposed to numerous environmental substances that could cause infection, including molds, bacteria, viruses, and pollens. The barriers to infection in the respiratory tract include enzymes that destroy foreign substances, a strong lining (epithelial lining) that forms a physical barrier to contaminants, a mucous coating that covers the lining of the lungs and further prevents invasion by harmful germs and substances, and a layer of minute hair-like structures (cilia) on the lining of the respiratory tract that sweep inhaled debris into the stomach for excretion. In addition, white blood cells and the other factors of the immune system constantly monitor the respiratory tract and prevent establishment of infectious bacteria and other germs. Tobacco smoke, alcohol, and air pollution deteriorate the lining of the lungs and reduce the strength of the immune system, increasing the lungs' susceptibility to disease and infection.

Lung disorders associated with environmental conditions or tobacco use include bronchitis, emphysema, and lung cancer. A healthy immune system combined with an active antioxidant system is important for the prevention and treatment of these lung disorders; however, tobacco use and secondhand smoke are the greatest contributors to these lung diseases. Allergies and asthma, two disorders that involve the respiratory tract, are discussed in detail on pages 163–168 and 177–179.

Nutrition and Lung Disorders

Vitamins and minerals function to maintain healthy lung tissue by strengthening the immune system and increasing the body's resistance to infection, maintaining the lining of the lungs, and deactivating highly reactive compounds called free radicals that cause lung damage and possibly cancer. Other dietary factors, especially a high-fat intake, also can increase the risk of lung cancer.

VITAMIN A AND BETA CAROTENE. Vitamin A and beta carotene are necessary for the development and maintenance of healthy epithelial tissue and mucous membranes, such as the lining of the lungs, bronchi, and other respiratory tissues. Epithelial tissue forms a barrier to bacteria and other foreign substances and directly aids in the prevention of infection and disease.

Beta carotene also strengthens the immune system and provides resistance to infection. Low-birth-weight newborns sometimes are born with low blood and liver levels of vitamin A, which can impair the growth of lung epithelial tissue and increase the risk of lung diseases such as bronchopulmonary dysplasia. Physician-monitored vitamin A supplementation increases blood and tissue levels of vitamin A, promotes healing and growth in the lung, and lowers the risk of lung disease in these newborns.

An adequate intake of foods high in beta carotene reduces a person's risk for developing lung cancer. Preliminary results from one study indicate that supplementation with beta carotene and vitamin E might reduce lung cancer risk by 23 percent in high-risk individuals. In contrast, people who smoke or who develop cancer have lower tissue levels of vitamin A and beta carotene than do healthy people. Vitamin A or beta carotene might reduce cancer risk by strengthening the epithelial lining of the lungs, functioning as antioxidants to defend the tissues against free-radical damage, and discouraging the formation of abnormal cells.

One study published in the New England Journal of Medicine contradicts these findings. This Finnish study reported that supplementation with beta carotene in smokers did not reduce lung cancer risk and, in fact, slightly increased the risk of lung cancer. However, the subjects of the study had smoked for an average of 36 years prior to beginning a moderate-dose beta carotene program. Since the study lasted less than eight years, undetected precancerous lesions could have existed before the study began. Overall, the results of this one study are not strong enough to diminish the overwhelming evidence in favor of a protective role of beta carotene against the development of lung cancer.

VITAMIN D. If vitamin D is important to the maintenance of healthy lung tissue, it is because this fat-soluble vitamin aids in the regulation of the immune system and improves the lungs' resistance to infection.

VITAMIN E. As an antioxidant, vitamin E protects the membranes in the lungs from damage by free radicals found in air pollution and tobacco smoke and aids in the prevention of tumor growth that develops from free-radical destruction of tissue. People with lung cancer, compared to healthy people, show low levels of vitamin E in their tissues. One study showed that a combined supplement of vitamin E and beta carotene lowered lung cancer risk in smokers by 25 percent. (See pages 150–153 for more information on antioxidants and free radicals.)

THE B VITAMINS. Adequate intake of vitamin B6 is necessary for optimal functioning of the immune system; however, large doses of this B vitamin do not provide added benefits. Vitamin B12 is important in the formation and maintenance of white blood cells, necessary components of the immune system and essential to the body's resistance to infection and disease. A deficiency of the B vitamin pantothenic acid might increase the risk for developing respiratory tract infections. Adequate intake of folic acid might help prevent precancerous changes and abnormal cell growth in lung tissue.

VITAMIN C. Adequate intake of vitamin C might increase a person's resistance to colds and other infections. Optimal dietary intake of vitamin C reduces the severity and duration of the common cold, while poor dietary intake increases a person's risk for developing respiratory infections. Vitamin C used in conjunction with the medication indomethacin might improve the symptoms, such as easier breathing, of bronchoconstriction (constriction of the bronchial tubes or air passages in the lungs).

A study conducted at the Environmental Protection Agency in Washington, D.C. and the Harvard School of Public Health in Boston reports that vitamin C might help maintain pulmonary function. Recent studies have linked high vitamin C intake with decreased progression of chronic respiratory symptoms, possibly because the vitamin's antioxidant capabilities help counter oxidant injury that accelerates the loss of lung function.

COPPER. Inadequate copper intake, especially during the formative years when the respiratory tract is developing, might be linked to later development of lung damage similar to emphysema. Copper deficiency is associated with reduced resistance to disease and increased likelihood of developing colds and infection.

IRON. Iron contributes to a healthy immune system and increases a person's resistance to colds, infection, and disease.

MAGNESIUM. One of the symptoms of magnesium toxicity is difficulty breathing. However, magnesium can improve asthma symptoms, such as wheezing, narrowed airway, and constricted bronchial tubes. Magnesium supplements reduce the recurrence of apnea, extended pauses in breathing that frequently occur during sleep and that might play a role in sudden infant death syndrome (SIDS).

MANGANESE. Manganese functions as an antioxidant to protect lung tissue from damage by free radicals in air pollution and tobacco smoke.

SELENIUM. A deficiency of the antioxidant selenium is associated with increased risk for developing lung cancer. Researchers at the University of Limburg in The Netherlands report that people with the highest selenium levels had half the rate of lung cancer compared to those with low selenium levels. Limited evidence shows that selenium also is important in the maintenance of the immune system and the body's resistance to infection.

ZINC. Zinc stimulates the immune response and aids in the prevention of colds and infection. In addition, zinc appears to have a direct effect on slowing the growth of infectious organisms, especially viruses that invade the lungs and increase risk for developing colds or lung infections. Excessive intake of zinc reduces resistance to infection.

Dietary Recommendations

There is no specific diet that will prevent all types of lung disorders, although the dietary guidelines for the prevention of cancer also apply to lung cancer. In general, a low-fat, fiber-rich, nutrient-dense diet should be consumed, optimal in all vitamins and minerals and low in sugars and refined and convenience foods. The diet should contain a variety of fruits, vegetables, whole grain breads and cereals, cooked dried beans and peas, low-fat or nonfat milk products, and extra-lean meats, chicken, and fish.

A multiple supplement that provides between 100 percent and 300 percent of the RDA for all vitamins and minerals, especially vitamin A and the antioxidant nutrients, as well as regular exercise, effective stress management, avoidance of alcohol, and limited exposure to air pollution and other toxic environmental gases are important considerations. Avoidance of tobacco and secondhand smoke is one of the most important contributors to the prevention and treatment of lung and respiratory disorders.

LUPUS ERYTHEMATOSUS

Overview

Lupus erythematosus or lupus is one of a number of autoimmune diseases (auto = self) characterized by a defect in the immune system and an accumulation of white blood cells that attack the body, rather than attacking foreign invaders such as a virus or bacteria.

Nutrition and Lupus Erythematosus

VITAMIN E. Tissue destruction in lupus results from free-radical damage to cell membranes and might be a result of an actual or relative deficiency of the antioxidant vitamin E. Improvement in symptoms, including reduced inflammation of the skin and sensitivity to sunlight, are reported when people with lupus consume between 800IU and 2,000IU of natural vitamin E (d-alpha tocopheryl acetate or d-alpha tocopheryl succinate) daily. Doses of 300IU or below appear to have no effect on the treatment of lupus. Supplemental iron and estrogen therapy reduce vitamin E's effectiveness. Vitamin E should not be taken in large doses for the treatment of lupus without the supervision of a physician.

VITAMIN A. Vitamin A supplementation might improve the immune response and resistance to colds and infection in patients with lupus.

Dietary Recommendations

Although no specific dietary recommendations have been established, a person should consume a low-fat, high-fiber, nutrient-dense diet that is optimal in all vitamins and minerals and low in sugars and refined and convenience foods. The diet should contain a variety of fruits, vegetables, whole grain breads and cereals, cooked dried beans and peas, low-fat or nonfat milk products, and extra-lean meats, chicken, and fish.

A multiple vitamin-mineral supplement and a vitamin E supplement, as well as regular exercise, effective stress management, avoidance of alcohol and tobacco, and frequent monitoring of the disease by a physician are important in the treatment of lupus.

OSTEOMALACIA

Overview

Osteomalacia, or adult rickets, is a bone disorder characterized by softening and deformities of the bones of the legs and arms, spine, thorax, and pelvis and is caused by inadequate intake of calcium or vitamin D. The condition results from the loss of minerals from the bones, called demineralization. Rickets is the childhood form of osteomalacia. It is characterized by severely bowed legs or knock knees, malformed rib cage called pigeon breast, delayed growth, delayed eruption of and malformed teeth, and in infants, an enlarged head.

Osteomalacia is most common in women after multiple pregnancies and chronic calcium and vitamin D deficiency or in women who avoid sunlight or are heavily clothed (thus, reducing sun exposure to the skin). Elderly people living alone are at risk for developing osteomalacia because of poor diet, inadequate exposure to sunlight, limited ability to produce vitamin D, and limited intake of vitamin D-rich foods.

Osteomalacia is often confused with osteoporosis, but there are distinct differences between these two bone disorders. In osteomalacia, people complain of chronic pain and muscle weakness, whereas pain is usually associated only with bone fractures, while muscle weakness is uncommon in osteoporosis. Bone fractures are uncommon, but deformities of the bones are very common in osteomalacia; the opposite is true in osteoporosis. Finally, people with osteomalacia respond quickly to vitamin D therapy, while the vitamin produces little response in people with osteoporosis (Table 38).

Table 38
SYMPTOMS AND DIAGNOSIS OF OSTEOPOROSIS AND OSTEOMALACIA

Symptoms	Osteoporosis	Osteomalacia
Skeletal pain	Periodic, usually associated with a fracture	Chronic, major complaint
Muscle weakness	Uncommon	Usually present, often produces disability or unusual gait
Fractures	Common	Uncommon
Skeletal deformity	Occurs with fractures	Common

Table 38 (cont.)
SYMPTOMS AND DIAGNOSIS OF OSTEOPOROSIS AND OSTEOMALACIA

Symptoms	Osteoporosis	Osteomalacia
Loss of bone density	Occurs in most bones	Infrequent or only in spine
Blood levels of calcium/phosphorus	Normal	Low
Blood levels of alkaline phosphatase	Normal	High
Urinary excretion of calcium	Normal or high	Low
Response to vitamin D therapy	Moderate to small	Dramatic

Nutrition and Osteomalacia

A poor diet that contains marginal amounts of calcium and vitamin D over long periods of time is usually the cause of osteomalacia. In some cases, poor absorption or use of these two nutrients increases the daily requirement above the recommended dietary allowances. Osteomalacia is rare in people who are physically active, spend time in the sunlight, and eat a low-fat, nutrient-packed diet. One dietary survey found that older adults consume daily only 88IU of vitamin D, or less than half the RDA. Those who supplemented their diet had higher blood levels of vitamin D and a reduced rate of bone loss than did those who did not take a vitamin D supplement.

Dietary Recommendations

To prevent or treat osteomalacia, a person should consume a low-fat, high-fiber, nutrient-dense diet that is optimal in all vitamins and minerals and low in sugars and refined and convenience foods. The diet should contain a variety of fruits, vegetables, whole grain breads and cereals, cooked dried beans and peas, and/or extra-lean meats, chicken, and fish. At least two to four servings of calcium- and vitamin D-rich milk products, especially low-fat or nonfat milk, should be included in the daily fare.

A multiple vitamin-mineral supplement that contains vitamin D and a calcium supplement might be necessary if several servings daily of vitamin D-fortified milk is not consumed. Regular exercise, effective stress management, avoidance of alcohol and tobacco, and moderate exposure to sunshine are important for the prevention and treatment of osteomalacia.

OSTEOPOROSIS

Overview

Osteoporosis is a degenerative bone disease characterized by long-term loss of calcium from the bones, especially the bones of the jaw, spine, pelvis, and the long bones of legs. The bones gradually become porous, brittle, and break easily. The humped posture common in people with osteoporosis is called dowager's hump and also results from changes in the spine as the bones deteriorate and compress. The brittle bones in the legs, pelvis, or arms are susceptible to fracture and seemingly harmless movements, such as coughing, walking down stairs, or receiving a strong hug, can cause them to break. In some cases, the first sign of osteoporosis is a bone fracture. Loss of bone tissue in the jaw causes problems with teeth and dentures and can result in limited food intake and malnutrition (see Table 38).

Nutrition and Osteoporosis

For every man who develops osteoporosis, eight women develop the bone disease. Women are at particular risk for developing osteoporosis because of their lifestyle and dietary habits as well as their small body size relative to men. Women are more likely than men to follow calorie-restricted weight loss diets that contain inadequate amounts of nutrients, especially calcium and vitamin D.

A diet of less than 1,600 calories, the average calorie intake of women in the United States, is likely to be low in several vitamins and minerals associated with the development and maintenance of bone density. For example, loss of bone density in women is associated with typical calcium intakes, which are two-thirds of the RDA of 800mg/day. Frequent consumption of diet soft drinks that contain phosphoric acid and avoidance of milk products that contain calcium and vitamin D upsets the ratio of calcium to phosphorus intake and contributes to calcium loss from bones. High intakes of caffeinated beverages, such as coffee and cola drinks, increase the loss of calcium in the urine and might contribute to bone loss. Regular exercise that places pressure on the bones, such as walking, jogging, or jumping rope, increases bone density and discourages bone loss; whereas inactivity results in calcium loss from bones and an increased risk for developing osteoporosis. Finally, women's bones, in general, are smaller than men's bones and less calcium loss is required before signs of osteoporosis develop.

VITAMIN D. Vitamin D is essential to the absorption of dietary calcium from the intestine and deposition of calcium into bone. A long-term deficiency of this fat-soluble vitamin is associated with calcium loss, bone deterioration, and increased risk of osteoporosis. In contrast, a diet high in both vitamin D and calcium is especially effective in reducing bone loss and risk of fractures. Vitamin D also might treat osteoporosis by reducing bone loss and fractures in osteoporotic women.

Blood levels of vitamin D are low in people with osteoporosis, suggesting a reduced production of the vitamin. The ability to manufacture vitamin D in the skin when exposed to sunlight might be reduced as a person ages and the need to depend on dietary sources of the vitamin is even more important than in previous years. Bone loss might increase during the winter months, since exposure to sunlight is reduced as people spend more time indoors; however, a year-round diet high in vitamin D or vitamin D supplements can prevent this seasonal bone loss. New research has found a gene linking vitamin D receptors with a hereditary risk of osteoporosis, suggesting that in the future a vitamin D metabolism test will assess a person's risk for developing osteoporosis.

VITAMIN B6. Vitamin B6 might aid in the healing of bones after a fracture. A deficiency of this B vitamin results in reduced bone density and width.

CALCIUM. Osteoporosis might be a preventable disease, if adequate calcium (combined with vitamin D) intake is maintained throughout life. Calcium intake is important during childhood and adolescence to develop strong, dense bones. Calcium intake during the middle years, when calcium loss from bones exceeds calcium gain, is important to slow the rate of bone loss. Calcium intake during and after menopause is essential to prevent the development of rapid bone loss associated with the advanced stages of osteoporosis.

The adult Recommended Dietary Allowance (RDA) for calcium of 800mg/day might not be adequate to prevent osteoporosis and it is recommended that premenopausal women consume at least 1,000mg daily. Postmenopausal women who are not on hormone therapy require up to 1,500 to 1,700mg of calcium daily. Hormone therapy aids in the prevention of bone loss in postmenopausal women and 1,000 to 1,500mg of calcium combined with hormone replacement therapy (HRT) helps prevent osteoporosis.

Adequate calcium intake might help regenerate bone tissue in people with osteoporosis. Restoration and maintenance of bone tissue is observed in people who consume, over several years, a high-calcium diet plus 750mg of calcium/day from calcium supplements and 375IU of vitamin D/day.

COPPER. A long-term copper deficiency results in reduced bone formation and bone deformities, possibly from the trace mineral's effect on the protein webbing that forms the matrix for calcium and other minerals in bone tissue. Women with low blood levels of copper have reduced bone mineral density compared to women with normal copper levels. Calcium loss from the bones also is associated with a copper deficiency. A diet high in copper enhances calcium's ability to delay and even reverse bone loss.

FLUORIDE. People who live in areas of the country where the water contains fluoride have a lower incidence of osteoporosis than people who do not consume a regular source of fluoride. Fluoride increases bone mass and reduces the risk of new fractures in women with osteoporosis. However, other studies show that fluoride consumption at the level of 80mg of sodium fluoride each day might increase the risk for hairline fractures in the bones of postmenopausal women with osteoporosis. Consequently, the use of fluoride in the prevention and treatment of osteoporosis remains controversial.

MAGNESIUM. Magnesium is important in the development and maintenance of strong bones. Pregnant animals who consume a magnesium-deficient diet give birth to offspring with bone deformities. The magnesium content of osteoporotic bone is altered from that of healthy bones. Bone formation also depends on the ratio of calcium and magnesium and a deficiency of either mineral could result in reduced deposition of calcium into bones and poor formation of bones. How a magnesium deficiency affects bone loss and the effectiveness of magnesium supplementation in the prevention and treatment of osteoporosis is unclear.

MANGANESE. A long-term deficiency of manganese is associated with calcium loss from bone, possibly because of the trace mineral's role in skeletal growth and maintenance. Osteoporotic women have lower blood levels of manganese than do healthy women.

Dietary Recommendations

Calcium intake should meet or exceed the RDAs throughout life. At least three servings a day of calcium-rich milk products, such as non-fat or low-fat milk, low-fat cheese, or low-fat yogurt, plus a variety of nutrient-dense foods, such as dark green leafy vegetables, cooked dried beans and peas, and whole grain breads and cereals, should be consumed daily to supply the 1,000 to 1,500mg of calcium recommended to prevent osteoporosis (Table 39).

Fortified nonfat or low-fat milk is the only reliable source of vitamin D; one quart provides 400IU, the RDA for children and adolescents. Two cups provides 200IU, the RDA for adults. The current RDA might not be adequate for seniors who have a reduced ability to absorb and manufacture vitamin D from sunlight. The previous RDA of 400IU might be a better goal for people in the second half of life. People who do not drink two to four glasses of milk a day should consider taking a supplement of vitamin D.

A calcium supplement should be used if calorie restriction or aversion to milk products prevents adequate consumption of calcium from the diet. A balanced multiple vitamin-mineral supplement provides adequate amounts of most nutrients, including vitamin D, but many preparations do not supply enough magnesium and calcium. Separate mineral preparations might be required to meet the daily need for these nutrients if the diet is poor.

Table 39
HOW TO INCREASE CALCIUM IN THE DIET

- Add nonfat milk powder to casseroles, soups, meatloaf, cheese sauces, or milkshakes.
- Add nonfat milk powder to recipes for french toast, muffins, dips, puddings, pie fillings, homemade breads, mashed potatoes, creamy salad dressings, or creamed soups.
- Cook rice, hot cereals, or other grains in milk.
- Use nonfat or low-fat yogurt as a partial substitute for sour cream in recipes.
- Combine nonfat or low-fat milk with nonfat milk powder in recipes.
- Use low-fat cheeses with fruit and crackers for snacks.
- Increase the daily consumption of calcium-rich foods of plant origin (broccoli, dark green leafy vegetables, or soy products).

In addition, regular weight-bearing exercise throughout life, avoidance of alcohol and tobacco, effective coping skills for stress, limited intake of caffeine-containing beverages, and moderate but not excessive intake of protein are important in the prevention and treatment of osteoporosis.

PREMENSTRUAL SYNDROME (PMS)

Overview

Premenstrual Syndrome (PMS) is a variety of physical and psychological changes that develop before the beginning of menstruation.

More than 150 symptoms, including mood disturbances, water retention, breast soreness, and changes in eating patterns, are attributed
to this disorder.

The causes of PMS are unclear; however, the disorder probably
results from a complex interaction between hormones, chemicals
called neurotransmitters that regulate nerve function, stress, and
dietary factors. Several lifestyle factors, such as a sedentary lifestyle,
a diet high in sugar and fat, consumption of alcohol and caffeine,
and stress might increase the severity of PMS symptoms.

Nutrition and Premenstrual Syndrome

Generally poor dietary intake is associated with an increased risk for
developing symptoms of PMS. Women with PMS tend to have poor
dietary habits; they consume more refined sugars and starch and
consequently less B vitamins and trace minerals, such as iron, manganese, and zinc, than do women who are symptom-free. A multiple
vitamin-mineral supplement sometimes is all it takes to relieve some
PMS symptoms.

The cravings for sweets characteristic of PMS might result from
fluctuations in blood sugar and insulin levels common during menstruation; however, changing hormone levels also might contribute to
the cravings. For example, as estrogen and progesterone rise in the
premenstrual woman, levels of the neurotransmitter serotonin drop.
Snacking on carbohydrates elevates serotonin levels and sometimes
improves mood. However, sweet snacks, such as candy or desserts
may temporarily raise serotonin levels, but aggravate PMS symptoms
in the long run. Instead, women with PMS should choose complex
carbohydrates, such as potatoes, whole grain breads, or crackers to
sooth their cravings and improve their mood.

Although women with PMS consume more calories, they have a
lower intake of many vitamins and minerals, several of which might
be linked to PMS symptoms. For example, vitamin A, vitamin B6,
magnesium, and zinc show promise in reducing some symptoms of
PMS. Dietary treatment of PMS has not produced consistent results,
however, and many times, regardless of the nutrient, both the group
on the supplement and the group on a placebo (a pill that contains
no active ingredient) report improvements in symptoms. This suggests that psychological factors also might affect the development
and treatment of PMS.

VITAMIN B6. A vitamin B6 deficiency might be a contributing factor in
the development of PMS. Vitamin B6 is a necessary nutrient in the
manufacture of certain chemicals called neurotransmitters that regu-

late nerve function. These neurotransmitters, in particular serotonin and dopamine, direct mood, water balance, memory, and sleep.

It has been speculated, but not proven, that the fluctuations in the female hormones progesterone and estrogen prior to the onset of menstruation cause a temporary deficiency of vitamin B6. This deficiency reduces the manufacture and activity of the neurotransmitters and results in some of the symptoms of PMS. In support of this theory, symptoms such as headaches, water retention, bloating, depression, fatigue, and irritability are reduced when vitamin B6 is increased in the diets of some PMS patients.

Limited evidence shows that consumption of 50mg of vitamin B6 throughout the month and increased doses prior to menstruation cause estrogen levels in the blood to drop, progesterone levels to rise, and symptoms of PMS to vanish. Symptoms responsive to vitamin B6 supplementation include depression, irritability, tension, breast tenderness, water retention, bloating, headaches, and acne.

Vitamin B6 supplements also might reduce mastalgia (breast pain) in PMS sufferers. Vitamin B6 also aids in the regulation of magnesium levels in the blood and a deficiency of the vitamin might alter magnesium status and result in temporary symptoms of deficiency that resemble PMS symptoms. The evidence linking a deficiency of vitamin B6 with PMS is preliminary and limited and some studies have found no association between the vitamin and the disorder.

Caution should be used when consuming large doses of vitamin B6. A study of women taking vitamin B6 supplements for PMS found that many women developed adverse side effects, including hand or foot numbness and tingling, shooting pains, and poor coordination.

VITAMIN E. A deficiency of vitamin E might affect the production of the hormone-like substance prostaglandin, which in turn has a possible link to PMS. Breast tenderness, bloating, and weight gain during PMS might be reduced with vitamin E supplementation; however, the evidence is limited and inconclusive.

MAGNESIUM. Magnesium intake and blood levels are low in women with PMS. Some of the symptoms of magnesium deficiency are similar to PMS, such as muscle cramps, changes in appetite, nausea, and mood swings. Headache, dizziness, and craving for sweets sometimes respond to an increased dietary intake of magnesium. Whether this change in blood levels of magnesium is a result of a magnesium deficiency, changes in hormones, or an as yet unidentified factor is unclear.

OTHER MINERALS. Iron levels are low in some women with PMS who suffer from depression, mood swings, and breast pain; whether or not increasing iron intake would improve these symptoms is unclear. A study at the USDA Grand Forks Human Nutrition Research Center in North Dakota reports that increasing calcium intake to 1,300 to 1,600mg (the equivalent of four to five servings of milk or other calcium-rich foods) reduced PMS symptoms, such as mood and concentration problems, pain and water retention.

Dietary Recommendations

No specific dietary recommendations have been established. In general, women should consume a low-fat, fiber-rich, nutrient-dense diet that is optimal in all vitamins and minerals and low in sugars and refined and convenience foods. The daily diet should contain a variety of fruits, vegetables, whole grain breads and cereals, cooked dried beans and peas, low-fat or nonfat milk products, extra-lean meats, chicken, and fish, several glasses of water, and one to two tablespoons of safflower oil, which contains the fatty acid called linoleic acid that might help regulate prostaglandins and reduce PMS symptoms. Caffeine should be avoided by people who experience anxiety and breast tenderness. Salt and salty foods should be limited for people who experience fluid retention.

A multiple vitamin-mineral supplement that contains vitamin B6 as well as other vitamins and minerals, eating several small meals and snacks throughout the day, combining some protein and carbohydrate at each meal and snack, regular exercise, effective stress management, avoidance of alcohol and tobacco, and an adequate amount of sleep are important in the prevention and treatment of PMS.

PSORIASIS

Overview

Psoriasis is an inflammatory skin disorder characterized by dry, red skin patches covered with silvery white scales. Small spots of bleeding appear under the sores. Psoriasis can be a chronic or sporadic condition.

Nutrition and Psoriasis

Psoriasis might result in marginal nutrient deficiencies, particularly of protein, folic acid, and iron, since these nutrients are depleted during increased skin cell growth. Increasing dietary intake of these nutrients will not treat the disease, but will prevent secondary disorders, such as anemia. On the other hand, limited research shows a possible link between high-protein intake and the development of psoriasis; a very low-fat, moderately low-protein diet is effective in reducing symptoms in some people. The diet is difficult to follow, however, and long-term compliance is poor; psoriatic symptoms reappear upon return of normal eating habits.

Dr. Kempner's Rice Diet, developed in the 1940s and used as a therapeutic diet for patients with certain degenerative diseases, also might be effective in the treatment of psoriasis. People with psoriasis who are unresponsive to medication or ointments report improvement in symptoms when they consume the Rice Diet.

VITAMIN D. Vitamin D plays a role in skin cell metabolism and growth, skin inflammation, and might be helpful in the treatment of psoriasis. A few studies show that individuals with psoriasis have low levels of vitamin D and vitamin D supplements or a vitamin D lotion applied directly to the skin improves symptoms in some patients. While a high intake of vitamin D can alter metabolism of calcium, vitamin D analogues such as calcipotriol significantly reduce the adverse affects on calcium without decreasing the effectiveness of psoriasis treatment.

ZINC. Zinc losses through the skin might be higher in people with psoriasis than in healthy people. Zinc is necessary for the absorption of linoleic acid, a nutrient suspected to cause or worsen the symptoms of psoriasis when deficient in the diet. A zinc deficiency might increase the likelihood of a linoleic acid deficiency and subsequent outbreaks of psoriasis.

LINOLEIC ACID. Inadequate dietary intake or poor absorption of the essential fatty acid called linoleic acid, found in safflower oil, nuts, and seeds, might contribute to the outbreak and severity of psoriasis. Increased intake of this nutrient might improve symptoms.

FISH OILS. Fish oils have been used with some success in the treatment of psoriasis. The signs and symptoms of psoriasis improve when patients with active outbreaks of psoriasis are placed on a daily supplement of fish oil for several months.

Dietary Recommendations

Kempner's Rice Diet consists of 10 ounces of dry rice cooked, small amounts of sugar, and fresh or preserved fruit, supplemented with a multiple vitamin-mineral preparation. Use of this diet should be monitored by a physician or dietitian as the diet is extremely imbalanced, lacks adequate amounts of numerous nutrients, such as protein, vitamin A, vitamin C, the B vitamins, and trace minerals, and cannot be expected to sustain life for long periods of time.

No specific diet has been developed to prevent or treat psoriasis. In general, a low-fat, high-fiber, nutrient-dense diet should be consumed, optimal in all vitamins and minerals and low in sugars, refined and convenience foods, and fats, especially saturated fats. The diet should contain a variety of fruits, vegetables, whole grain breads and cereals, cooked dried beans and peas, low-fat or nonfat milk products, frequent servings of water, one to two tablespoons of safflower oil, and extra-lean meats, chicken, and fish.

A multiple vitamin-mineral supplement that contains vitamin D and zinc, as well as regular exercise; effective stress management; avoidance of alcohol, caffeine, and tobacco; and compliance with prescribed medications or ointments might be important for the prevention and treatment of psoriasis.

SICKLE CELL ANEMIA

Sickle cell anemia is an inherited disorder characterized by crescent-shaped rather than the normal kidney-shaped red blood cells. The abnormal cells block the flow of blood to tissues and cause severe pain, growth retardation, liver damage, hepatitis, jaundice, gallstones, and kidney failure.

The treatment for sickle cell anemia centers around reducing the symptoms of pain. The excess accumulation of iron characteristic of this disorder requires a reduction in iron intake and avoidance of iron-rich foods for some people; however, some sickle cell patients are already iron-deficient and should not reduce iron further without physician approval. The diet should be high in folic acid, zinc, vitamin B2, and possibly vitamin E. Improvements in growth rate, pain, and frequency of infections are noted when children with sickle cell anemia are given a multiple vitamin-mineral preparation that contains zinc, iron, folic acid, and vitamin E. Blood levels of vitamin C are low in people with sickle cell anemia and supplementation with the vitamin might protect red blood cells from free-radical damage and prolong red blood cell lifespan.

SKIN DISORDERS

Overview

Skin is the barrier between the body and the environment. One of the main functions of the skin is to physically prevent microorganisms and other foreign substances from entering the body. Other skin functions include temperature regulation, vitamin D production, preventing water loss, removal of some waste products, and sensation. Disorders that affect the skin include acne, cancer, dermatitis, eczema, psoriasis, and sunburn. (Many of these disorders are discussed in more detail in other sections of Chapter 5.)

Nutrition and Skin Disorders

Many vitamins and minerals help maintain healthy skin by maintaining a strong circulation that supplies nutrients and oxygen to the skin and removes waste products. Other nutrients contribute to cell growth and maintenance and deactivate free-radical compounds that damage the skin and possibly cause cancer. The skin is frequently exposed to sunlight, and the potentially harmful UV rays. The longer rays, UVA rays, penetrate deeply, affecting cells and causing skin changes associated with aging. The shorter rays, UVB rays, are only absorbed by the outer layers of the skin, where they might cause precancerous and cancerous cell changes. Exposure to sunlight, with its damaging UV rays, is a significant risk factor for skin cancer. Several vitamins and minerals help protect the skin against the damaging effects of UV light.

VITAMIN A AND BETA CAROTENE. Individuals with skin cancer have lower levels of beta carotene and vitamin A compared to cancer-free persons, and evidence shows that increased intake of these nutrients might help protect against the development of skin cancer. A long-term deficiency of vitamin A can cause xeroderma, a condition characterized by dry, scaly skin and the formation of small hard bumps.

VITAMIN D. This fat-soluble vitamin might help treat psoriasis, a skin disorder causing dry, red patches of skin that are covered by scales. (See the section on Psoriasis, pages 271–273.)

VITAMIN E. Vitamin E is an antioxidant that might protect skin cells from free radicals formed during and following UV exposure. A study from the University of Arizona reported that high-dose vitamin E supplements prevent UV-induced skin cancer in animals. Other research on animals indicates that applying vitamin E directly to the skin, before or up to eight hours after sun exposure, might act as a "sunscreen" to prevent skin damage, tumor formation, and immune suppression caused by UV radiation. The vitamin E lotion also reduces symptoms of inflammation, redness, and tenderness common in sunburn.

VITAMIN C. Vitamin C might prevent and repair UV-induced skin damage by counteracting the harmful effects of free radicals, helping to produce collagen and maintain connective tissue, and reducing inflammation. UV rays might deplete the skin of vitamin C and increase vitamin C requirements to compensate for the loss caused by frequent or prolonged sun exposure. Increased vitamin C intake (with diet or supplements) or topical application of vitamin C in lotions helps protect the skin from sun damage. Using vitamin C with a sunscreen appears to provide more skin protection than either alone.

SELENIUM. Selenium might help protect against skin cancer. Skin cancer patients have lower tissue levels of selenium than do individuals without skin cancer. Studies on animals indicate that selenium taken orally or applied to the skin reduces sunburn, inflammation, pigmentation changes, free-radical damage, and skin cancer in animals exposed to UV rays. (See pages 150–153 for more information on free radicals and antioxidants.)

Dietary Recommendations

There is no specific diet that will prevent all types of skin disorders. In general, a person should consume a low-fat, high-fiber, nutrient-dense diet that is optimal in all vitamins and minerals and low in sugars and refined and convenience foods. The diet should contain a variety of antioxidant-rich fruits and vegetables, whole grain breads and cereals, cooked dried beans and peas, low-fat or nonfat milk products, and extra-lean meats, chicken, and fish.

A multiple supplement that contains between 100 percent and 300 percent of the RDA for all vitamins and minerals, plus an extra dose of the antioxidants—vitamin C, vitamin E, and beta carotene—might be necessary if dietary intake is not optimal. Regular exercise, effective stress management, avoidance of alcohol and tobacco, and limiting frequency or duration of sun exposure and liberal sunscreen use are important in preventing and treating skin disorders.

STRESS

Overview

Stress is the body's response to any demand, such as hunger, a telephone ringing, an unexpected tap on the shoulder, a death in the family, divorce, or a car accident. Stress cannot be avoided and positive stress can encourage a person to strive and achieve goals. Harmful stress is called distress and can cause anxiety, nutrient deficiencies, and emotional or physical disease. Diseases related to stress include atherosclerosis and heart disease, high blood pressure, obesity, peptic ulcer, and asthma. In many cases, these diseases are preventable when effective coping skills and guidelines for a low-fat, nutrient-rich diet are followed.

Nutrition and Stress

Stress and nutrition are related. First, a nutrient deficiency is a stress in itself. Second, how well stress is handled is related to how well the body is nourished. Stress and its widespread effects on body chemistry and functions can interfere with digestion and reduce nutrient absorption and retention. A well-nourished individual is better equipped to cope with stress than is a poorly-nourished individual. Even a diet that contains marginal amounts of one or more nutrients can produce a deficiency when the compounding burden of stress is present. Third, adequate intake of vitamins and minerals is important in preventing the loss of nutrient stores within the body. A tension-filled day increases losses of several nutrients in the urine, and blood levels of many vitamins and minerals are also low during times of stress.

Finally, vitamins and minerals are important contributors to the immune response, the system that defends the body against infection and disease. The body's response to stress includes release of several hormones that suppress the immune response and increase the body's susceptibility to infection. Adequate intake of the vitamins and minerals, such as vitamin A, the B vitamins, vitamin C, and the trace minerals, that maintain a strong defense system stimulates the formation and activity of antibodies, white blood cells, and other aspects of the immune system. Body stores of these nutrients are less likely to be depleted and the immune system is less likely to be jeopardized if nutrient intake is adequate prior to and during times of stress.

Diet appears to make a difference in the body's ability to handle stress. People who consume a diet low in refined carbohydrates, sugar, and caffeine and high in whole grain breads and cereals and other nutritious foods showed greater improvement in their ability to cope with stress as compared to individuals who consume their normal diets with sugar or caffeine.

VITAMIN E. This antioxidant vitamin helps protect the body from the physical stress of free-radical damage that can result in disease and possibly cancer.

THE B VITAMINS. The B complex vitamins are needed for the maintenance of the nervous system. Diets high in sugars and other refined carbohydrates require B vitamins to adequately process these foods for energy. These foods do not supply ample amounts of these nutrients, however, and can cause a relative deficiency. A low intake of the B vitamins or the relative deficiency caused by consuming a nutrient-poor diet can alter nerve function and increase the symptoms of stress, such as depression and irritability.

VITAMIN C. The vitamin C content of stress-related tissues, such as the pituitary and adrenal glands, is reduced during stress. The reduced body stores are a result of either poor dietary intake or increased daily need during times of stress. During physical stress and heart attack, vitamin C levels drop in the blood. Increased intake of vitamin C during times of stress might reduce the harmful effects of the stress hormones, such as adrenaline, and improve the body's ability to cope with the stress response. Optimal vitamin C intake also strengthens the immune system and reduces the risk of infection and disease.

MAGNESIUM. Magnesium stores are depleted and large amounts of the mineral are lost in the urine during times of stress. Some of the symptoms of stress, including stimulation of the nervous system, are reduced when blood levels of this mineral are normal to high but are accentuated in the presence of a magnesium deficiency.

Animals fed a magnesium-deficient diet react violently to previously well-tolerated noise; consuming adequate amounts of magnesium prior to and during the stressful noise reduces the stress reaction. Hospitalized patients who experience physical and emotional stress are often low in magnesium, which might contribute to the stress reaction and interfere with recovery. So-called "type A" people who are overachievers and often experience high levels of stress have lower magnesium levels and higher levels of stress hormones than do more relaxed "type B" people.

ZINC. People in physical stress, such as hospitalized patients, often are deficient in zinc. The zinc deficiency interferes with the body's ability to recuperate from illness and might contribute to chronic leg ulcers, infection, and secondary diseases. The physical stress of strenuous exercise might increase urinary loss and alter blood levels of zinc and other trace minerals, such as chromium, copper, and iron. Whether these changes increase the daily requirement for the trace minerals is unknown.

Dietary Recommendations

No specific dietary recommendations have been established for people during stress. However, it is wise to consume a low-fat, high-fiber, nutrient-dense diet that supplies optimal amounts of all the vitamins and minerals and is low in sugars and refined and convenience foods. The diet should contain an abundance and variety of fruits, vegetables, whole grain breads and cereals, and cooked dried beans and peas, with a few servings of low-fat or nonfat milk products, and extra-lean meats, chicken, and fish. Several glasses of water daily also is important.

A multiple supplement that contains between 100 percent and 300 percent of the RDA for all the vitamins and minerals, plus extra vitamin C, vitamin E, and beta carotene, should be considered. Regular exercise, effective stress management, avoidance of alcohol and tobacco, and avoidance of caffeine-containing beverages, such as coffee and cola drinks, also are important practices prior to and during times of stress.

THYROID DISORDERS

Overview

The most pronounced symptom of thyroid malfunction is enlargement of the thyroid gland or goiter, also called endemic goiter. The thyroid gland enlarges in an attempt to maintain normal function, despite an insufficient supply of iodine necessary for thyroxine production.

Nutrition and Thyroid Disorders

Poor dietary intake of iodine results in goiter in adults and if the diet is low in iodine during pregnancy, the baby will be born with a condition called cretinism. In addition, excessive consumption of foods containing goitrogens, such as cabbage, soybeans, and turnips, reduces the absorption of iodine and increases the risk of developing goiter.

VITAMIN D. Institutionalized elderly men often are marginally deficient in vitamin D and show signs of secondary hyperparathyroidism, despite dietary intakes of up to 610IU (the RDA is 200IU), according to a study conducted at the Medical College of Virginia in Richmond. The results of this study show that vitamin D requirements for the elderly might be considerably higher than current RDA levels to maintain normal parathyroid gland function.

ZINC. Significant changes in how the body uses and stores zinc are present in patients with thyroid disease. It is unknown whether these imbalances are caused by dietary deficiency or result from the disease.

Dietary Recommendations

Daily consumption of iodine-containing foods or iodized salt, especially if a person lives in the goiter belt (the northern states, the states bordering on the Great Lakes, the New England states, and portions of the central-western states, such as Nevada, Colorado, and Arizona) where the iodine in foods and water is low, will prevent goiter and cretinism. People who live in coastal regions obtain iodine from fresh fish and shellfish and produce grown locally.

YEAST INFECTIONS

Overview

Yeast infections are caused by the fungus Candida albicans, which is normally present in harmless amounts in the vagina, mouth, digestive tract, and on the skin. When conditions in the vagina change to favor growth of this yeast fungus, they overgrow other vaginal organisms, causing symptoms such as itching, redness, a thick white discharge, and soreness during intercourse. Factors that alter the vaginal environment and allow the yeast fungus to proliferate include pregnancy, diabetes, frequent douching or using feminine hygiene sprays, taking oral contraceptives or antibiotics, menstruation, and possibly the use of spermicidal creams and jelly for birth control and safe sex.

Nutrition and Yeast Infection

A healthy, strong immune system is essential for reducing the risk of developing a yeast infection. Women experiencing repeated infections have impaired number and activity of monocytes, a specialized cell of the immune system. Optimal intake of several vitamins and minerals can strengthen immunity and protect against yeast infections. In addition, a low-sugar, high-fiber diet that includes lactobacillus acidophilus-containing yogurt might counteract the growth of Candida infection.

VITAMINS AND MINERALS. Vitamin A helps develop and maintain moist, healthy epithelial tissues, such as the lining of the vagina. This vitamin fights infection by stimulating the immune responses. Limited evidence shows that some women with frequent vaginal irritations are deficient in vitamin A; although it is not known if this deficiency is a cause or result of infection.

Some studies find women with recurrent yeast infections to have low dietary or blood levels of vitamin B6, vitamin B2, and biotin. A study by researchers at the University of Pisa, Italy reported that two women with long-term recurrent yeast infections became symptom-free after taking a daily supplement containing vitamin C, vitamin B1, vitamin B2, vitamin B6, niacin, and pantothenic acid.

Other studies note that women with recurrent yeast infections are deficient in magnesium, which might lower resistance to the yeast fungus or reduce the effectiveness of the immune system. Marginal intake of zinc could increase the incidence, frequency, or severity of yeast infections.

FISH OILS. Limited evidence associates yeast infection with fish oils. Eicosapentaenoic acid (EPA), a fatty acid in fish oils, might protect against the growth of the yeast fungus by decreasing inflammation and strengthening immune function.

OTHER DIETARY FACTORS. The vagina contains bacteria that help to keep the vaginal environment in a healthy balance and inhibit uncontrolled growth of Candida albicans. Including yogurt that contains the bacteria Lactobacillus acidophilus in the daily diet might result in as much as a three-fold reduction in yeast infections and lower the numbers of yeast fungus in the vagina. These yogurts with active bacterial cultures also might enhance immune function, thus further protecting against Candida infection.

Too much sugar and too little fiber also might contribute to yeast infections. A diet high in sugar might alter the vaginal environment in favor of yeast growth, while a diet low in sugar might decrease yeast infection risk. A study from the University of Michigan reports that a diet high in insoluble fibers, such as the fiber from whole grains and wheat bran, increase the risk of Candida infection. However, soluble fibers found in fruits, vegetables, oats, and cooked dried beans and peas are not associated with yeast infection.

Garlic and yeast-containing foods also might play a role in the prevention or development of yeast infections. Garlic contains the substance allicin that counteracts the growth of yeasts, including Candida albicans. Increasing garlic intake or garlic supplements that contain allicin might protect against yeast infections. Some women with recurrent yeast infections might be hypersensitive to yeast-containing foods. Reducing the intake of foods that contain baker's and brewer's yeast might reduce the frequency of Candida infection in these women; however, this theory remains controversial.

Dietary Recommendations

No specific dietary recommendations have been established for the prevention of yeast infections. In general, a woman should consume a low-fat, nutrient-dense diet that contains optimal amounts of all vitamins and minerals and limits or eliminates all refined or processed sugars, including table sugar, honey, and corn syrup. The diet should contain a variety of fruits, vegetables, whole grain breads and cereals (but avoid bran cereals and other processed fiber foods), cooked dried beans and peas, low-fat or nonfat milk products (especially daily servings of yogurt that contain the Lactobacillus acidophilus bacteria), and extra-lean meats, chicken and fish.

A multiple supplement that contains between 100 percent and 300 percent of the RDA for all vitamins and minerals related to the immune system (see pages 153–157 for more information on nutrition and immunity), as well as regular exercise, effective stress management, adequate sleep, avoidance of alcohol and tobacco, and limited use of caffeine are important for the prevention and treatment of yeast infection.

Women with recurrent infections might try avoiding foods made with baker's or brewer's yeast for a few months; if symptoms do not improve, the original diet can be reinstated. Wearing cotton fibers that breathe naturally instead of nylon underwear and limiting time in tight-fitting leotards, bathing suits, and synthetic or irritating fabrics also will reduce the risk of developing yeast infections.

CHAPTER 6

How Medications, Alcohol, and Tobacco Affect Vitamin and Mineral Status

OVERVIEW

From the superstitions of primitive cultures to the high technology of today's medical system, medication has had a primary role in the patient's care. Almost two billion prescription drugs are dispensed each year and more than 100,000 different medications are available in the United States.

The widespread use of prescription and nonprescription medications, also called over-the-counter or OTC drugs, coupled with the increasing interest in nutrition and diet, has encouraged research into the interactions between diet and drugs. Drug-nutrient interactions can be as mild as an upset stomach or as severe as paralysis resulting from potassium deficiency. However, studies show that a majority of health-care professionals do not provide adequate counseling on the possible interactions of a prescribed drug and the patient's diet.

Prescription and nonprescription medications can alter vitamin and mineral status in four ways. Medications can:

1. increase or decrease appetite and alter the amount of vitamins and minerals consumed,
2. reduce vitamin and mineral absorption even with adequate intake,
3. alter how a nutrient is used by the body, and
4. increase vitamin and mineral excretion so even if dietary intake and absorption is adequate, the nutrient is not retained in the body.

The result is possible marginal, and sometimes clinical, vitamin and mineral deficiencies.

Changes in Appetite

Some medications increase and other medications decrease appetite and food intake. Examples of appetite-stimulating medications are some antidepressants and certain antihistamines. Many of these drugs stimulate appetite by improving a person's mental status or emotional stability.

Other medications reduce appetite by their effects on the central nervous system; by direct irritant action on the stomach and small intestine causing nausea, discomfort, constipation or diarrhea, and vomiting; or by altering taste. For example, amphetamines act on the central nervous system and reduce the desire to eat.

Some medications reduce appetite by altering the sense of taste and smell, reduce saliva and cause a dry mouth, cause stomach or intestinal irritation, produce nausea and vomiting, or reduce the desire to eat. The reduced desire to eat increases the likelihood of poor food and nutrient intake and vitamin or mineral deficiencies. Medications also reduce food and nutrient intake by altering mood or behavior. In other cases it is not the medication, but the underlying disease or a combination of disease and medication that upsets this balance and causes a loss of appetite.

Reduced Absorption

Medications, vitamins, and minerals are absorbed in the small intestine and can interact to alter the absorption of one another. Some medications bind to a vitamin or mineral in the small intestine and interfere with the nutrient's absorption. For example, mineral oil binds to the fat-soluble vitamins and hinders their entry into the bloodstream. A medication also can alter the shape or function of a vitamin, making it less likely to be absorbed. Other medications increase the speed with which nutrients pass through the small intestine; the reduced contact time vitamins and minerals have with the intestinal wall results in decreased absorption. Some medications physically or chemically block the absorption sites on the wall of the small intestine or alter the absorption sites so the vitamins or minerals cannot pass through.

Finally, medications can interfere with the digestive juices required for normal absorption of vitamins and minerals. Medications that change the acidity or pH of the stomach and small intestine will reduce the absorption of vitamins and minerals dependent on normal acidity for absorption. For example, antacids increase the pH to a more alkaline environment in the small intestine and reduce the absorption of iron and calcium. Other medications inhibit the activity of bile salts, digestive juices necessary for normal digestion of the fat-soluble vitamins. Other medications alter the digestive juices produced by the pancreas.

Altered Functions

Prescription and nonprescription medications alter how the body uses vitamins or minerals in a variety of ways. Certain medications change specific requirements for vitamins and minerals by altering absorption, availability, storage, and use of the nutrient. Some medications are shaped chemically similar to a vitamin, but have no vitamin activity. In the body, these medications are mistaken for the vitamin and block the real vitamin from entering into normal body processes. The vitamin is available but inaccessible, and symptoms of a marginal deficiency develop. Other medications alter the storage sites for vitamins and minerals. For example, oral contraceptives affect the distribution or possibly decrease blood levels of vitamin B12 in the body.

Other medications bind to the biologically active portion of an enzyme where a vitamin normally would attach. The body mistakes the unattached vitamin for an excess of the nutrient and excretes it in the urine, the medication-bound enzyme cannot function, and all body processes depending on the enzyme are stopped. An example of this medication-nutrient interaction is vitamin B6 and oral contraceptives. The effects of this medication-induced vitamin deficiency are subtle and can cause emotional disturbances, altered sleep, irritability, lethargy, and reduced resistance to infection and disease.

Increased Excretion

Diuretics, laxatives, and cathartics are examples of medications that increase the excretion of vitamins and minerals, and if used in excess could result in nutrient deficiencies. Minerals are most susceptible to this form of medication-nutrient interaction.

The absorption, use, and excretion of minerals in the body depend on a delicate balance; a medication that interferes with one mineral will probably upset the status of other minerals. It is common for an individual to take more than one medication at a time, and the combined effects of these medications might result in numerous changes in mineral status.

Medication-nutrient interactions might result in, or increase, a vitamin deficiency. This interaction occurs at a time when optimal nutritional status is important to a person's health and recovery from disease. In addition, these marginal nutrient deficiencies produce subtle symptoms, such as depression or reduced resistance to infection, that proceed unnoticed or are excused as a side-effect of the disease or medication.

Note: Eating patterns and nutrients also can decrease or increase the therapeutic effectiveness of many prescription or nonprescription medications. These nutrient-drug interactions are usually listed with the medication's accompanying literature or are explained by your physician or pharmacist.

WHO IS AT RISK?

A person who is well-nourished, with optimal amounts of vitamin and minerals stored in the body, who has no problems with digestion and absorption of food, who has consumed a nutritious diet prior to and during illness, and who must take a prescription or nonprescription medication for only a short time is at low risk for developing medication-induced nutrient deficiencies.

In contrast, malnutrition and marginal vitamin and mineral deficiencies are most likely to develop in people on long-term medication therapy, especially if they consume a nutrient-poor diet. In particular, the elderly, children, alcoholics, and people who are chronically ill are the most vulnerable to medication-induced nutrient deficiencies. Poor vitamin and mineral status, however, can result from a variety of factors, including poor dietary intake of nutrients prior to the onset of disease and medication therapy. Malnutrition is less likely to develop if the long-term diet contains a variety of fresh and nutritious foods. Everyone should begin preventive and rehabilitative dietary measures and should monitor nutritional status while taking prescription and nonprescription medications.

Seniors

Seniors account for the highest sales of prescription and nonprescription medications, currently averaging almost four medications per person daily with the numbers increasing each year. Many older people are at risk for vitamin and mineral deficiencies, even if they are not taking medications. The added stress of long-term use of one or more medications, coupled with poor dietary habits, chronic disease, and reduced ability to absorb and use vitamins and minerals places this segment of the population at high risk for drug-induced nutrient deficiencies.

In addition, limited income, reduced mobility or access to nutritious foods and food preparation, special diets, reduced appetite, disinterest in food, and oral and dental problems also contribute to poor dietary intake and increase risk for developing vitamin and mineral deficiencies. Finally, living alone, depression, and social isolation can jeopardize nutritional status.

Problem Drinkers

Alcohol is the number one cause of malnutrition in people who are otherwise disease-free. Abuse of alcohol results in loss of appetite and reduced food and nutrient intake, especially the B vitamins, the trace mineral zinc, and protein. Alcohol damages the lining of the small intestine and reduces the absorption of nutrients. Deficiencies of several vitamins and minerals are common in people who abuse alcohol. Vitamin and mineral deficiencies also develop secondary to alcohol-induced disorders, including inflammation of the stomach, intestine, pancreas, or liver; lactose intolerance; and cirrhosis of the liver.

People with Long-Term Illness

Medication-induced vitamin and mineral deficiencies might develop in people with long-term diseases, such as cancer, diabetes, epilepsy, disorders of the gastrointestinal tract, behavioral or emotional disorders, or heart and blood vessel diseases. Nutrient deficiencies are possible because of long-term exposure to medication and the likelihood of multiple-medication therapies.

Dosage also contributes to the potential for nutrient deficiencies; a high-dose medication taken over long periods is more likely to cause vitamin and mineral deficiencies than a low dose over a short time. This dose effect also holds true for nonprescription medications, such as laxatives and aspirin.

Nutrient depletion of tissues, as a result of the disease or the medication, is gradual and often goes undetected until nutrient stores are exhausted. Preventive measures to maintain or replenish nutrient stores are essential, as long-term medication therapy might threaten nutritional health.

People with Increased Needs or Decreased Intakes of Nutrients

People on weight reduction diets or calorie/food restricted diets; children or adolescents who eat sporadically, but have high vitamin and mineral requirements; and pregnant and breastfeeding women are at risk for medication-induced vitamin and mineral deficiencies. People in these groups often are marginally nourished because of restricted food intake, reliance on high calorie-low nutrient foods, or increased need for vitamins and minerals. Poor dietary intake, coupled with long-term use of medications, increase the possibility of malnutrition. A malnourished person, particularly a child, taking medications is especially vulnerable to adverse side effects from medications.

SPECIFIC MEDICATIONS AND OTHER SUBSTANCES: EFFECTS ON VITAMIN AND MINERAL STATUS

Alcohol

Chronic or abusive alcohol consumption predisposes the drinker to malnutrition in several ways. First, alcohol supplies between 10 percent and 20 percent of the calories in the diet of the average person, but provides little or no other nutrients and requires additional vitamins, such as vitamin B1, vitamin B6, biotin, and niacin, for its detoxification in the liver. For example, vitamin E and other antioxidant nutrients are needed to repair the tissue damage from alcohol, and vitamin C, folic acid, vitamin B12, and vitamin B6 are needed to build new tissue. The body functions in a deficit without adequate amounts of these nutrients. Although beer and wine contain some vitamins and minerals, the amounts are minute (i.e., the nutrient content of 1 ounce of bread exceeds the nutrient content of 12 ounces of beer). The calories from alcohol either replace more nutritious foods or are supplied in addition to a day's allotment of calories. Whether it is nutrient deficiencies or obesity, malnutrition can result.

Second, alcohol irritates the stomach, pancreas, and intestine, and inhibits absorption of vitamin C, vitamin B1, vitamin B12, folic acid, the fat-soluble vitamins, calcium, and other nutrients. A cycle might develop where poor absorption of nutrients results in malnutrition, which further limits absorption of vitamins and minerals and encourages the development of alcohol-related diseases, such as liver disease.

Third, alcohol and its by-products can inhibit the body's ability to use vitamins. Many dietary vitamins must be altered by the liver before they are of use in metabolic reactions. In the presence of excess alcohol, vitamins D, B1, B6, and folic acid are not converted to their active forms and deficiency symptoms might develop even if dietary intake is adequate.

Fourth, alcohol sabotages vitamin stores in the body. For example, liver stores of vitamin A are decreased with long-term alcohol intake. Alcoholism also depletes the body's store and blood levels of antioxidant nutrients, such as beta carotene, selenium, and vitamin E. Levels of beta carotene decline as alcohol-induced liver damage increases. Alcoholics have lower levels of selenium, while a selenium deficiency can compound health and nutrition problems by causing liver damage similar to that seen in alcoholism. This effect on antioxidant nutrients might leave the body defenseless against damage from highly reactive substances called free radicals that are linked to the development of cancer and premature aging. The consumption of alcohol might increase the requirement of selenium and other nutrients that counteract free radicals.

Preliminary research indicates that supplementation with these nutrients might halt or retard the damage induced by alcohol. For example, vitamin A supplementation reduces alcohol-induced free-radical damage to the fatty areas of the body, such as the lining of cells. One study found that the impairment in immune function noted with alcohol abuse can be at least partially reversed if the person consumes a low-fat, nutrient-dense diet. (See pages 150–153 for more information on antioxidants and free radicals.)

Fifth, alcohol increases urinary loss of some nutrients, such as magnesium, potassium and zinc, and is associated with reduced tissue levels of several vitamins and minerals. In particular, a zinc deficiency might initiate a cycle where the alcohol-induced zinc deficiency then encourages excessive consumption of alcohol. In studies on animals, excessive alcohol consumption stops when animals are fed a diet high in zinc.

The best treatment for malnutrition caused by abuse of alcohol is to stop drinking and consume a diet rich in vitamins and minerals and low in fat. Supplements cannot protect the body from the toxic effects of alcohol and cannot prevent the formation of scar tissue or fatty infiltration of the liver. However, they might help minimize the long-term nutritional consequences. The vitamins and minerals most likely to be depleted with alcohol abuse are vitamins A, D, B1, B6, B12, and C; folic acid; and the minerals calcium, iron, magnesium, potassium, and zinc.

Antacids

Antacids are sometimes used in excess to minimize the discomfort experienced from the misuse of other dietary substances such as alcohol or coffee, excessive eating, or to curb the stomach pain from high levels of stomach acid secreted during times of stress. Pregnant women experiencing heartburn also may consume unusually high levels of antacids. This overuse of antacids might result in vitamin or mineral deficiencies.

Large doses of magnesium and aluminum hydroxides in antacids interfere with the absorption of phosphorus and calcium and might upset the delicate balance between these minerals. The result is that calcium and phosphorus are not deposited properly into bones and there is an increased risk for bone disorders. The risk of antacid-induced bone disease is higher in older people than in other segments of the population because the ability to absorb calcium decreases with age, and older people often do not consume adequate amounts of calcium-rich foods, such as milk, yogurt, cheese, and dark green leafy vegetables. However, they rely heavily on antacids.

Antacids can affect calcium and bone health. Sodium bicarbonate (baking soda) used to buffer stomach acid might increase the risk for calcium deficiency. This possible effect on calcium and bone status is only a concern if sodium bicarbonate is consumed daily and the diet is low in calcium. Aluminum absorption from antacids might be increased when they are consumed with citrus fruits and juices. Aluminum toxicity is associated with damage to the nervous system and bones.

Mineral and vitamin deficiencies and anemia might develop with overconsumption of antacids. These nonprescription drugs neutralize stomach acid and alter the acidity or pH of the stomach. Nutrients, such as iron, calcium, magnesium, zinc and vitamin B12, are not absorbed well in the more alkaline environment created by antacids. The absorption of folic acid and vitamin A also is reduced with abuse of antacids. Iron, vitamin B12, and folic acid are essential to the formation of red blood cells and reduced dietary intake or excessive or long-term antacid use could result in anemia. Antacids that contain calcium carbonate might reduce the absorption of the trace mineral chromium and contribute to a chromium deficiency. Another medication that inhibits the secretion of stomach acid and is used in the treatment of ulcers or "nervous stomach," cimetidine (Tagamet), also reduces the absorption of vitamin B12.

The potential for vitamin or mineral deficiencies varies depending on when the antacids are taken. Aluminum hydroxide antacids should be taken 1 to 2 hours before a meal or before bed to maximize their buffering action on stomach acid in the treatment of ulcers. A larger quantity of antacids is sometimes required in the treatment of duodenal ulcer than is required in stomach ulcers because the patient with duodenal ulcer usually also has excessive secretion of stomach acid. In this case, the antacid is taken when no food is present in the stomach, so the antacid will not interfere with nutrient absorption and is not likely to produce vitamin or mineral deficiencies. When the same medication is taken with meals, there is a greater likelihood that the absorption of calcium, iron, vitamin B12, and folic acid will be decreased (Table 40). Aluminum hydroxide is particularly effective in neutralizing stomach acid and is often the preferred antacid for the treatment of ulcers; however, it also is most likely to reduce the absorption of phosphorus and other minerals and vitamins. This type of antacid should be consumed between meals if it is taken for long periods of time.

Table 40
THE EFFECTS OF ANTACIDS ON VITAMINS AND MINERALS

Type of Antacid	Nutritional Effects
Aluminum hydroxide	Aluminum toxicity, reduced absorption of calcium, iron, and vitamin B12
Aluminum or Magnesium hydroxide	Phosphate depletion, reduced absorption of calcium, iron, and vitamin B12
Magnesium hydroxide	Magnesium overload
Sodium bicarbonate	Sodium overload, milk-alkali syndrome

Antibiotics

Antibiotics are important in the treatment of infections but might have nutritional side effects. Antibiotics are effective because they interfere with the growth of disease-causing bacteria; however, antibiotics also interfere with bacteria that promote health. Some essential nutrients are produced by bacteria living in the large intestine, and this source of a vitamin or mineral contributes an important proportion of the daily recommended allowance. Antibiotics disturb the normal intestinal bacterial growth and limit or destroy the vitamin-producing bacteria. For example, a deficiency of vitamin K or biotin might result with long-term use of antibiotics. In contrast, optimal vitamin C intake enhances antibiotic activity by weakening the defenses of harmful bacteria, thus reducing the antibiotic dose needed to effectively suppress bacterial growth.

Long-term use of the antibiotic tetracycline, especially in conjunction with a poor diet, has produced deficiencies of vitamin K and might reduce vitamin C stores in the body. Tetracycline interacts with dietary minerals, such as calcium, iron, magnesium, and zinc, and absorption and use of both the medication and the minerals are reduced when these minerals and the medication are consumed at the same meal. Neomycin causes malabsorption of vitamin B12, calcium, iron, and potassium, which is reversed when the medication is discontinued.

Para-aminosalicylic acid (PAS), an antibacterial prescription medication used in the treatment of tuberculosis, alters the absorption of several nutrients, including vitamin B12 and folic acid. In some cases, the reduction in vitamin B12 absorption results in anemia. The malabsorption of vitamin B12 and folic acid is reversible with discontinuation of the medication or with physician-supervised injections of folic acid and vitamin B12.

Antibiotic-induced vitamin and mineral deficiencies are not likely to develop if the diet contains a variety of fresh and nutritious foods prior to and during medication therapy and if the use of antibiotics is temporary.

Anticonvulsants

Anticonvulsant medications are used in the treatment of epileptic seizures and to prevent or treat seizures resulting from head injuries or surgery on the nervous system. Long-term use of the anticonvulsant medications phenytoin (Dilantin), phenobarbital, primidone, or carbamazepine might cause bone disorders, such as rickets in children or osteomalacia in adults. These medications interfere with the manufacture of vitamin D in the body. A person taking anticonvulsants cannot synthesize adequate amounts of this fat-soluble vitamin, even with adequate exposure to sunlight. As vitamin D acts as a hormone in the regulation of calcium absorption and use, a deficiency of this vitamin, even with adequate calcium intake, might cause calcium loss from bones and bone deterioration. The severity of these bone changes increases with long-term treatment and large doses of the medication.

More than 15 percent of people on long-term use of anticonvulsant medications show reduced blood levels of vitamin D and skeletal disease. Because of the high incidence of drug-induced vitamin D deficiency, it is recommended that everyone on long-term anticonvulsant medication therapy take a vitamin D supplement that contains 400IU to 800IU of the vitamin or consume one quart or more of vitamin D-fortified milk each day.

Long-term use of anticonvulsant medications also might cause deficiencies of the vitamins associated with red blood cell formation and maintenance, which would result in anemia. Phenytoin, phenobarbital, and primidone induce a folic acid deficiency and birth defects in infants born of women on anticonvulsant therapy might be a result of the drug's effect on folic acid. Consumption of large doses of folic acid in an attempt to counteract this deficiency might upset vitamin B12 metabolism. Vitamin B12 is usually unaffected by anticonvulsant medications, but the increase in red blood cell production stimulated by increased intake of folic acid increases the demand for vitamin B12. The combined deficiency and altered metabolism of these two vitamins results in reduced production of red blood cells and anemia.

Vitamin K levels might drop on long-term anticonvulsant therapy, resulting in hemorrhage and blood loss. It is important for a physician to monitor folic acid, vitamin B12, and vitamin K status in patients on anticonvulsant therapy and to prescribe supplements of these nutrients where necessary. Supplements of folic acid should not be taken without the supervision of a physician as large doses of this vitamin might interfere with the effectiveness of the anticonvulsant medication and increase the likelihood of convulsions. Long-term use of anticonvulsants also lowers blood and tissue levels of copper and zinc.

Antidepressants

Long-term use of antidepressant medications and tranquilizers might alter nutrient status because these prescription drugs influence the desire to eat, reduce or increase food intake, and increase vitamin or mineral excretion. Some of the side effects of the antianxiety medications meprobamate, lorazepam, oxazepam, alprazolam, chlordiazepoxide (Librium), and diazepam (Valium) include nausea, vomiting, dry mouth, loss of appetite (anorexia), diarrhea, reduced salivation, and stomach upsets. Prozac can alter appetite in some patients, especially underweight depressed patients, and contribute to further weight loss. Any one of these symptoms might interfere with an optimal vitamin and mineral intake.

The tricyclic antidepressants amitriptyline, imipramine, doxepin, amoxapine, protriptyline, or lithium carbonate and the tranquilizer chlorpromazine increase or decrease appetite and might cause weight gain or weight loss. These drugs also might cause nausea, vomiting, diarrhea, flatulence, peculiar taste sensations, sore mouth, and abdominal cramps; all symptoms that could impair optimal food and nutrient intake. In addition, these medications increase urinary excretion of the B vitamins and vitamin C and alter the body's use of magnesium. For example, diazepam might alter magnesium status and increase the urinary excretion of calcium. Urinary loss of calcium during long-term antidepressant therapy coupled with medication-induced loss of calcium from the bones increase risk for developing bone disorders when taking these medications over long periods of time.

Patients on antidepressants also might need to supplement with B vitamins. One study showed patients on lithium therapy have low blood levels of folic acid, and supplementation in moderate doses (approximately 200mcg) reduces behavioral problems in these people. However, more information is necessary before dietary recommendations can be made. Lithium also interferes with copper absorption, which could result in a deficiency of the mineral, and should not be taken with meals rich in copper unless more copper rich foods are introduced into the diet. In one study, patients on the antidepressant phenelzine (Nardil) showed symptoms of vitamin B6 deficiency, including depression and hyperirritability, that responded to vitamin supplementation. Vitamin B6 deficiency also might contribute to the pre-existing depression.

The sedative-hypnotic medication glutethimide (Doriden) increases the daily requirement for vitamin D and might cause loss of calcium from the bones and bone disease if large doses are taken over an extended period of time.

The monoamine oxidase inhibitors (MAOI) are used in the treatment of depression, usually for adult patients unresponsive to other antidepressant medication therapies. Acute hypertension (high blood pressure) might occur in people taking MAOIs when foods high in a non-nutritive substance called tyramine are consumed. Tyramine-containing foods include aged and fermented foods, such as cheese, yogurt, sour cream, tenderized meats, fermented sausages, pickled herring, beer, red wine, yeast, and soy sauce. Alcohol and caffeine should be avoided when taking MAOI medications as these substances could cause headaches and other unusual symptoms. Alcohol also should be avoided with the use of tranquilizers such as valium and xanax, tricyclic antidepressants, and the sedative phenobarbital.

In general, vitamin and mineral deficiencies are unlikely if the diet is adequate in vitamins and minerals prior to and during medication. However, poor diet coupled with long-term or high dosage antidepressant medication therapy might encourage deficiencies.

Arthritis Medications

D-penicillamine (Cuprimine) is used in the treatment of rheumatoid arthritis. Possible side effects resulting from D-penicillamine use that might affect food and nutrient intake include sores and inflammation of the mouth and tongue, loss of appetite, stomach pain, nausea, vomiting, occasional diarrhea, altered taste sensation, ulcer, disorders of the pancreas and liver affecting the release of digestive juices, and inflammation of the large intestine. Loss of appetite might result in weight loss, muscle wastage, and general malnutrition.

D-penicillamine binds to iron, zinc, and other essential dietary minerals. For this reason, this anti-arthritis medication should be taken on an empty stomach, one hour before or two hours after a meal and at least one hour apart from any other medication, food, or beverage other than water. The loss of appetite, hair loss, and skin changes associated with D-penicillamine use might be partially a result of a drug-induced zinc deficiency, as the medication has been shown to reduce absorption of zinc and clinical symptoms of zinc deficiency include these signs. The potential for iron deficiency is also possible, especially in children and in menstruating women. Supplements of iron should be taken in small doses, two hours before or after the medication, as iron interferes with the effectiveness of the medication.

Long-term use of D-penicillamine increases the daily requirement of vitamin B6 and supplementation during periods of medication prevents the development of a vitamin deficiency. It is recommended that patients take a supplement containing 25mg of this B vitamin each day. In Wilson's disease, the supplement must be free of copper, as supplemental copper intake could block the action of the medication. Anyone taking D-penicillamine should consult a physician or pharmacist before taking a daily vitamin and mineral supplement.

Aspirin, Pain-Killers, and Anti-Inflammatory Medications

Moderate to excessive use of aspirin causes bleeding in the stomach or intestines in many people. The loss of blood means a loss of iron, and iron deficiency can result. People with pre-existing stomach disorders, such as ulcer, are especially susceptible to aspirin-induced blood and iron loss. Deficiencies of folic acid, vitamin C, and potassium, and malabsorption of vitamin B12 also have been reported in people on long-term large doses of aspirin.

Vitamin A might help prevent stomach ulcers and bleeding in people on long-term medication with aspirin. Moderate intake of vitamin A within the recommended dietary allowance of 800RE to 1,000RE might be sufficient to prevent stomach disorders induced by low intake of aspirin (325mg/day). However, more information is necessary before dietary recommendations can be made.

Ibuprofen is both a nonprescription medication (Advil and Nuprin) and a prescription medication (Motrin and Rufen) for the treatment of minor pains and aches. The possible side effects associated with ibuprofen that affect food and nutrient intake include stomach irritation, heartburn, vomiting, nausea, cramps, diarrhea, flatulence, and ulcers. However, these side effects are rare.

The anti-inflammatory medication colchicine is used in the treatment of gout because it reduces the inflammation and pain associated with this joint disorder. Colchicine reduces the absorption of vitamin B12, increases the excretion and tissue loss of calcium and potassium, and reduces the absorption of folic acid and iron. Other side effects that influence the intake of food and nutrients include nausea, vomiting, diarrhea, and abdominal pain, especially when large doses are taken.

The anti-inflammatory medication salicylazosulfapyridine (Azulfidine) decreases the absorption of folic acid and the inclusion of several servings each day of folic acid-rich foods might be necessary to counteract the effects of anti-inflammatory medications on folic acid status.

Cyclosporine is an immunosuppressant often given to patients after liver transplant surgery to reduce the risk of organ rejection. Vitamin E might enhance the bioavailability of cyclosporine and reduce the amount of the immunosuppressant needed by up to 72 percent. One study by researchers at the Ochsner Clinic and Alton Ochsner Medical Foundation reports that children with liver transplant grafts taking cyclosporine were able to discontinue use of the immunosuppressant sooner if they were also given water-soluble vitamin E supplements.

Cancer Medications

Chemotherapy is the treatment of a disease with chemicals or medication. The term is most commonly used in reference to cancer.

Although chemotherapy is an effective therapeutic effort, it has numerous side effects, one of which is nutritional consequences.

The effects of chemotherapeutic agents are not limited to the growth or function of cancer cells, but extend to healthy tissues as well. These toxic effects influence dietary intake and vitamin-mineral status. For example, many chemotherapeutic drugs produce sore or dry mouth, inflammation of the mouth and throat, and altered taste sensation. Nausea and vomiting are common for most chemotherapies. Loss of appetite results from this drug-induced damage to tissues of the mouth, throat, and stomach and the variety and quantity of appealing food choices decreases. The medication 5-fluorouracil alters taste sensations, affects appetite, and produces nutrient deficiencies, including vitamin B1. The results of these conditions are malnutrition, tissue wastage, and weight loss.

The lining of the intestine is also harmed by some chemotherapies, and diarrhea, constipation, or reduced absorption of vitamins and minerals might result. The toxic effects on the stomach and intestine are usually short-term and subside within a few days after each chemotherapy treatment; however, in some cases the damage is severe and prolonged. Some chemotherapies, such as the corticosteroids, damage tissues and cause excessive loss of potassium, calcium, and other minerals in the urine. The vitamin and mineral deficiencies that might result from these medications reduce the effectiveness of the immune system to fight disease, and alter mood and behavior, resulting in a greater likelihood of depression and sleep abnormalities, and generally are counterproductive to regaining health.

Some chemotherapeutic medications interfere with the use of vitamins within the cells and tissues. For example, methotrexate alters folic acid metabolism. Cells cannot divide and multiply without an available supply of folic acid and they die. Cancer cells multiply more rapidly than healthy cells and are more dependent on the folic acid levels in the body; therefore, a deficiency of this B vitamin affects them most severely. However, all cells in the body are affected by a folic acid deficiency including red blood cells. People on methotrexate therapy should not self-medicate with folic acid supplements without the prior approval of a physician, as large doses of this vitamin could alter the effectiveness of the medication therapy.

It is difficult, but possible to maintain adequate vitamin and mineral status during chemotherapy and it is vitally important to the outcome of the treatment. Chemotherapy is most effective when a person is adequately nourished. An adequate supply of all nutrients, including vitamins and minerals, lessens the harmful effects of chemotherapy on healthy tissue and enhances the destruction of cancer cells. Optimal supplies of all vitamins and minerals improves the sense of well-being, preserves healthy tissue function, repairs tissue damage caused by the disease and the chemotherapy, and strengthens the body's natural defense system to fight infection and disease.

In contrast, poor nutrition and inadequate intake of vitamins and minerals are harmful to the outcome of the therapy because a malnourished person has a narrow margin of tolerance to chemotherapy as compared to a well-nourished person. Poor dietary intake of vitamins and minerals and the resultant malnutrition can be the most disabling aspect of cancer. Malnutrition reduces the person's quality of life and contributes to an increased risk for continuation of the disease.

The two goals of nutrition therapy during treatment for cancer are to maintain optimal nutritional status or correct pre-existing deficiencies of vitamins, minerals, and other nutrients and to minimize weight loss resulting from the disease or the medication. The guidelines for meeting these goals must be individualized to the person and should be designed and monitored by a physician and registered dietitian (Table 41).

Table 41
NUTRITIONAL GUIDELINES DURING CHEMOTHERAPY

Problem	Diet	Foods To Avoid
Nausea	Choose small, frequent meals. Eat slowly. Chew food well. Eat dry foods (crackers). Drink cold liquids.	Liquids at meals, sweets, and fatty foods.
Acute stomach or intestine toxicity/pain	Drink clear, cold liquids.	Milk products, soups, cereals, sandwiches.
Post-treatment stomach or intestine pain	Choose liquid and soft foods, carbonated beverages, frozen fruit.	Citrus juice, milk, milk products, meat, raw foods.
Dry mouth	Choose high-fluid foods: gravies, sauces, soups, casseroles. Drink beverages with meals. Include citrus fruits.	Dry foods, meat, bread products.
Reduced taste	Choose a regular diet. Season foods. Choose spicy foods and textured foods with aroma.	Bland foods.

Table 41 (cont.)
NUTRITIONAL GUIDELINES DURING CHEMOTHERAPY

No taste	Choose a regular diet of cold foods: milk, milk products. Experiment with different foods and textures.	Red meats, chocolate, coffee.
Diarrhea	Choose liquid or soft foods, high-protein and high-calorie foods.	Raw fruits, vegetables, milk, spicy foods.
Fullness/Bloating	Take meals with no fluids. Eat slowly. Choose easily digested foods and small meals.	Gas-forming foods, fatty foods.
Heartburn	Choose small, frequent meals.	Pureed foods, coffee, tea, spicy foods, fatty foods, alcohol.

Medications for Cardiovascular Disease

Some of the medications used to lower blood cholesterol in the treatment of atherosclerosis and cardiovascular disease (CVD) include cholestyramine, clofibrate, and colestipol. These medications are called cholesterol-lowering agents or sequestrants. Lovastatin and pravachol are medications that reduce cholesterol synthesis in the liver. Their nutritional side effects, if any, are unknown.

The sequestering medications reduce the absorption of the fat-soluble nutrients, such as the fat-soluble vitamins A, D, E, and K, and the essential fatty acid called linoleic acid. The risk for nutrient deficiencies is high because cholesterol-lowering medications are used for chronic diseases that require long-term drug therapy. Gradual depletion of body stores of the fat-soluble vitamins resulting from long-term poor absorption of these dietary nutrients could produce night blindness and increased risk for some forms of cancer in the case of vitamin A, osteomalacia and related bone disorders in the case of vitamin D, and susceptibility to hemorrhage in a vitamin K deficiency. A linoleic acid deficiency produces skin disorders, such as eczema. It is advised that people on long-term medication with sequestering agents take a supplement of vitamins A, D, E, and K in water-soluble form.

The sequestrant cholestyramine (Questran) also interferes with the absorption of vitamin B12, folic acid, and iron, and chronic use of this cholesterol-lowering medication is associated with low blood levels of folic acid and other nutrients. Long-term medication therapy might result in anemia unless supplementation with these vitamins and iron is combined with the medication therapy. Cholestyramine increases the urinary excretion of calcium, increases blood levels of other fats, called triglycerides, and reduces body stores of iron when taken over a long period of time or at high doses. However, a recent study from the University of Minnesota reports that cholestyramine does not interfere with vitamin D absorption or increase the risk of osteomalacia.

Other possible side effects from long-term use of cholesterol-lowering agents include constipation, abdominal pain, bleeding in the stomach or intestine, belching, flatulence, nausea, vomiting, diarrhea, heartburn, loss of appetite, and steatorrhea (loss of excessive amounts of fat and fatty substances in the stool). Clofibrate causes changes in taste sensation and might reduce the desire to eat.

Colestipol is another medication used in the treatment of elevated blood cholesterol and heart disease. Deficiencies of the fat-soluble vitamins A, D, and E and the B vitamin folic acid are possible when this medication is taken over long periods of time. Vitamin K supplementation also is required, but only in the presence of poor blood clotting and episodes of prolonged bleeding. The effectiveness of colestipol might be increased when it is combined with the B vitamin nicotinic acid (niacin).

Medications classified as calcium-channel blockers (slow channel blockers or calcium antagonists) are popular treatments for cardiovascular disease. Nifedipine (Procardia), diltiazem (Cardizem), and verapamil (Calan, Isoptin) are examples of calcium-channel blocking agents. The terms used for these medications falsely suggest a possible danger in taking calcium supplements or eating calcium-rich foods during medication therapy. The assumption is dietary intake of calcium should be reduced, because these drugs reduce heart disease and hypertension by blocking calcium and calcium therefore must be the "bad guy." This assumption is wrong.

A high-calcium diet in conjunction with a reduced intake of sodium (salt) lowers blood pressure and reduces the risk for developing cardiovascular disease. Any dietary advice for people with cardiovascular disease who are on calcium-channel blockers should include a recommendation to maintain adequate calcium intake and blood levels.

Another class of medications used in the treatment of cardiovascular disease and hypertension is the beta blocking agents propranolol, metoprolol, acebutolol, and timolol. Possible side effects that might affect vitamin and mineral intake include stomach pain, flatulence, constipation, nausea, diarrhea, dry mouth, vomiting, loss of appetite, bloating, abdominal cramping, and inflammation of the pancreas or liver. No vitamin or mineral deficiencies have yet been identified with long-term use.

Medications for Hyperactivity

Amphetamines, such as dextroamphetamine (dexedrine), and psychotherapeutic agents, such as methylphenidate (Ritalin) are examples of drugs used in the treatment of hyperactive children. Long-term use of these medications is associated with reduced growth, specifically in suppressed gains in height and weight. This medication-induced effect on growth is possibly a result of the loss of appetite and subsequent food and nutrient intake that often accompanies amphetamine use.

Amphetamines are appetite suppressants, so much so that similar compounds are used in weight loss or diet pills. Evidence shows children on methylphenidate (30mg to 40mg/day) or dextroamphetamine (10mg to 15mg/day) consume less food and gain weight at a much slower rate than do children who discontinue these medications. The growth retardation stops and catch-up growth occurs when children discontinue amphetamine use. Other possible side effects of long-term amphetamine use that might influence food and nutrient intake include nausea and abdominal pain.

Vitamin and mineral deficiencies are possible during growth spurts when the child's nutrient needs are high, but the appetite is low because of amphetamine therapy. Every attempt should be made to encourage a child to eat a variety of fresh and wholesome foods, such as fresh fruits and vegetables, low-fat milk products, whole grain breads and cereals, and extra-lean meats or cooked dried beans and peas and to avoid nutrient-poor foods such as fatty convenience or fast foods, commercial snack foods such as potato chips and corn chips, and sugary foods. A multiple vitamin-mineral preparation containing approximately 100 percent of the RDA for the fat-soluble and water-soluble vitamins, calcium, magnesium, and the trace minerals also is recommended.

Hypertensive Medications

The diuretic medications (water pills) used in the treatment of high blood pressure (hypertension) and congestive heart failure include ethacrynic acid, furosemide, mercurials, spironolactone, thiazides, and triamterene. These diuretics increase the urinary excretion of sodium and chloride (salt) and probably are effective in the treatment of hypertension because of this influence on sodium and fluid balance; however, other nutrients are lost in the urine as well. Many of the diuretics, unless they are called potassium-sparing diuretics, such as amiloride HCL, triamterene, or spironolactone, increase urinary excretion of potassium and can precipitate symptoms of a potassium deficiency, including irregular heartbeat.

An individual should include several servings each day of potassium-rich foods or take a potassium supplement when using these medications. A person might experience bone disorders, paralysis, temporary sterility, muscle weakness, nerve disorders, and kidney damage if severe potassium deficiency is allowed to progress. A physician or pharmacist should be consulted about whether or not a diuretic requires potassium supplementation before self-medicating with the nutrient. Other medications that deplete the body of potassium include:

- L-DOPA
- Salicylates
- Senna (Senokot)
- Phenolphthalein (Ex-Lax, Feen-A-Mint)
- Gentamicin
- Corticosteroids
- Amphotericin B
- Bisacodyl (Dulcolax)

Magnesium is another mineral that can be depleted when diuretics, such as thiazides or furosemide, are used. Magnesium deficiency is observed in people on long-term diuretic therapy for cardiac (heart) failure or hypertension. This diuretic-induced marginal magnesium deficiency might be a result of the loss of appetite experienced by some people on these medications and subsequent poor dietary and nutrient intake and the increased urinary excretion of the mineral.

Magnesium is important for normal heartbeat and the regulation of blood pressure. Artery walls spasm and an irregular heartbeat develops when magnesium intake is low; artery walls relax and the heartbeat returns to normal when blood levels of the mineral are adequate. Constrictions or spasms of blood vessels are linked to hypertension, whereas relaxation of the blood vessels increases the size of the blood vessel, reduces resistance to blood flow, and lowers blood pressure. Magnesium deficiency also is associated with heart failure, atherosclerosis, and destruction of the heart muscle.

People with hypertension, especially those who take diuretic medications, often have low levels of magnesium in their blood. Elevated blood pressure returns to normal in many cases when the intake of magnesium-rich foods is increased or if magnesium supplements are included in the daily diet. Individuals with hypertension treated with beta blockers might enhance the lowering of blood pressure if they are supplemented with magnesium. (See pages 298–300 for information on the beta-blocking agents and calcium channel-blocking medications in the treatment of hypertension.)

Increased loss of other minerals, including calcium, iodine, and zinc, and low blood levels of folic acid are associated with long-term use of diuretics and might result in marginal mineral and vitamin deficiencies unless the dietary intake of these nutrients is adequate. Long-term treatment with furosemide also is associated with a clinical deficiency of vitamin B1, which might further impair heart function. Vitamin B1 supplements should be considered in patients deficient in this B vitamin.

Laxatives

Laxatives interfere with the absorption of nutrients by reducing the amount of time vitamins and mineral are in contact with the intestine. The laxatives phenolphthalein (Alophen, Ex-Lax, Feen-A- Mint), senna (Senokot), and bisacodyl (Dulcolax) alter the intestinal lining so nutrients might not be optimally absorbed. As a result, several vitamins and minerals, including calcium, potassium, and vitamin D, are excreted rather than absorbed and deficiencies could result if laxatives are used frequently or over a long period of time.

Mineral oil is another laxative that binds to the fat-soluble vitamins A, D, E, and K and the essential fatty acid linoleic acid. These nutrients are then lost because mineral oil is not absorbed and the complex of oil and nutrients is excreted. Long-term use of mineral oil could produce deficiencies of these nutrients, and cause conditions such as night blindness and increased risk for developing cancer in the case of vitamin A, bone disorders with vitamin D deficiency, and frequent hemorrhage with vitamin K deficiency.

Oral Contraceptives

Oral contraceptives affect the absorption and use of several nutrients within the body. They increase appetite and encourage weight gain, reduce the absorption of folic acid and other vitamins, and redistribute nutrients within tissues. Some women who take oral contraceptives have high blood levels of vitamin A and copper and low blood levels of vitamin E, vitamin C, vitamin B6, folic acid, vitamin B1, vitamin B2, vitamin B12, iron, and zinc. Limited evidence shows oral contraceptives also might increase the absorption of calcium. These nutritional effects are moderate to mild, vary between individuals, and might be related to other physical disorders or poor dietary intake of nutrients.

Although low blood levels of iron have been reported in users of oral contraceptives, other studies show blood levels of this mineral are increased. The low blood levels of iron in some studies might be a result of poor dietary intake of iron-rich foods rather than a medication-induced nutrient deficiency. Menstrual flow is reduced in women on oral contraceptives, which reduces loss of blood and iron and should help prevent iron deficiency. Previous research reported that vitamin C interfered with the metabolism of estrogen in oral contraceptives; however, a recent study conducted at the Truman Medical Center in Kansas City, Missouri reports that even high doses of vitamin C do not alter the absorption of oral contraceptives.

The effects of oral contraceptives on vitamin B6 status are of particular interest because the behavioral changes, such as depression, irritability, and insomnia, that are common side effects of these medications might be at least partially a result of the medication's effect on vitamin B6 status. Vitamin B6 is an essential component in the body's production of several chemicals responsible for nerve transmission, behavior, and body processes, called neurotransmitters and hormones.

For example, serotonin is a neurotransmitter found in the brain and is responsible for regulating sleep, several emotions, and mood. Low levels of serotonin are associated with depression, irritability, and insomnia. The amount of serotonin available and its activity depends on the dietary intake and availability in the body of the building blocks for this neurotransmitter, tryptophan and vitamin B6. Inadequate intake or reduced availability of either of these nutrients can result in limited production of serotonin and mood and sleep disorders. Medications, such as oral contraceptives, interfere with vitamin B6 metabolism and might suppress the production of serotonin. In some cases, the mood swings and depression accompanying these medications are reduced or eliminated when vitamin B6 intake is increased.

Some people are more sensitive than other people to medication-induced vitamin and mineral deficiencies, which might result in vulnerabilities to other health problems. For example, low levels of folic acid in women taking oral contraceptives are associated with an increased risk of infection by the human papillomavirus, the virus that causes genital warts. Nutrient deficiencies also might be dependent on the particular oral contraceptive used, the length of time it is used, and the nutritional status of the woman prior to and during the use of the medication.

Steroid Medications

The nutritional side effects of using steroid hormones include nausea, vomiting, diarrhea, abdominal pain, loss of appetite, and burning of the tongue. Steroid medications should only be used with the consent of a physician.

Estrogen therapy for the treatment of menopause symptoms might cause abdominal pain, loss of appetite, diarrhea, and nausea in some women. These side effects reduce food and nutrient intake or increase nutrient losses. Salt and fluid retention and weight gain also are possible on estrogen therapy.

Tobacco

Cigarette smoke affects the smoker's and nonsmoker's nutritional status. Low levels of the antioxidant nutrients, such as vitamin C, beta carotene, vitamin E, and zinc in smokers impairs the body's ability to deactivate harmful and reactive compounds called free radicals that can be found in cigarette smoke; this might contribute to cardiovascular disease.

Inhalation of cigarette smoke depletes the tissues of vitamin C and increases the daily need for this water-soluble vitamin. Although the RDA for vitamin C was raised to 100mg for smokers, some evidence shows that smokers might require twice that to maintain vitamin C levels similar to nonsmokers consuming only 60mg of the vitamin. Despite this, smokers are more likely than nonsmokers to eat diets low in vitamin C and other antioxidant nutrients. A recent study at Duke University in North Carolina found that a fine spray of vitamin C, delivered in a cigarette-shaped tube, might help smokers quit the habit. (See pages 150–153 for more information on free radicals and antioxidants.)

Vitamin A and beta carotene levels in lung and mouth tissues exposed to cigarette or cigar smoke or chewing tobacco are low, while tissues that contain adequate amounts of vitamin A are less likely to become cancerous. In addition, vitamin E might reduce the damage to lung tissue from outside air pollution. Limited research indicates that high-dose supplementation with vitamin E reduces damage to lung tissue by indoor air pollution, such as cigarette smoke.

Smokers have lower zinc levels, while zinc supplements might reduce the risk of atherosclerosis in smokers. Women who smoke during pregnancy have low zinc levels in their blood and are more likely than are nonsmokers to give birth to zinc deficient babies. These babies are at an increased risk for birth defects and disease.

Levels of folic acid also are lower in smokers compared to non-smokers, while increasing intake might prevent some of the damage caused by tobacco use. Vitamin B6 metabolism is altered with cigarette smoking and the residual effects might last as long as two years after cessation of smoking.

Nonsmokers are passive smokers. They inhale both the mainstream smoke (the exhaled cigarette smoke from the smoker) and the sidestream smoke (the smoke from the end of the burning cigarette). Sidestream smoke contains greater amounts of dangerous gases than the smoke filtered through the cigarette before entering the smoker's lungs; it contains twice as much tar and nicotine, three times as much benzo(a)pyrene (a cancer-causing substance), three times as much poisonous carbon monoxide, and 73 times as much ammonia. These toxic gases enter the lungs and bloodstream of the smoker and surrounding nonsmokers and remain for hours after the person leaves the smoke-filled room or puts aside the cigarette.

Inhalation of carbon monoxide reduces the oxygen supply to the heart, brain, and other tissues. The nonsmoker or smoker might experience headaches, and the risk for developing lung cancer and heart disease increases in both groups. Nonsmokers, including the children of smokers, also experience a higher incidence of breathing difficulties, bronchitis, pneumonia, eye irritations, and tonsil operations. The smoke also increases the symptoms of asthma and allergies. Stillbirths and deaths in infants up to one year old are more common when the mother smokes.

The best prevention of lung cancer and respiratory disease, such as emphysema and bronchitis, is to not smoke or quit smoking and avoid others' cigarette, pipe, and cigar smoke. In addition, adequate intake of some vitamins might help prevent the harmful effects of others' smoke.

Tuberculosis Medications

Isoniazid (isonicotinic acid hydrazide or INH) kills actively growing tuberculosis bacteria and is used in the long-term treatment of this disease. It is usually recommended that the medication be taken between meals, but isoniazid can be consumed with food to reduce stomach upset. Alcohol should be avoided while taking this antituberculosis medication. Certain foods, such as tuna and tyramine-containing foods, also should be avoided. The medication can produce toxic symptoms in the liver and symptoms of nausea, headache, fatigue, loss of appetite, vomiting, or numbness of the hands and feet should be reported immediately to a physician or pharmacist.

The potential nutritional side effects include a possible vitamin B6 deficiency. Isoniazid binds to the vitamin and the two are excreted, and the medication interferes with normal use of vitamin B6 in the body. Supplementing the diet with 50mg of vitamin B6 each day might be sufficient to prevent the nerve damage observed in patients on isoniazid. However, this vitamin therapy should be followed only with the consent and supervision of a physician, as moderate to large doses of vitamin B6 has reduced the effectiveness of isoniazid in animals with tuberculosis.

Niacin deficiency has been reported in people taking isoniazid. The symptoms disappeared with a combination of niacin and vitamin B6 therapy. However, the niacin deficiency is probably a result of vitamin B6's role in converting the amino acid tryptophan to niacin rather than poor dietary intake of niacin. In addition, patients with tuberculosis often do not feel like eating, so food and nutrient intake might be poor. The poor diet and niacin intake prior to and during medication therapy coupled with the medication-induced effects on vitamin B6 and the manufacture of niacin from tryptophan might encourage a previous marginal vitamin deficiency to develop into a clinical vitamin deficiency.

Weight Control "Diet" Medications

While obesity is considered the number one public health problem in America, it is the only chronic disorder that has not been typically treated with medication. Recently, this is changing as more research accumulates showing the effectiveness of some pharmacological treatments for obesity. Granted, not all "diet pills" work. For instance, a recent study on ephedrine, an appetite suppressant and decongestant, found that women taking this appetite suppressant while on a calorie restricted diet lost no more weight than did calorie-restricted women taking a placebo.

But, other studies are more hopeful. The active ingredient often used in nonprescription weight control medications is phenylpropanolamine (PPA), which is chemically similar to ephedrine. Although research on PPA is controversial, several studies have found that this appetite suppressant enhances weight loss by increasing the amount of calories the body burns during the day. In fact, women taking PPA lose twice as many pounds as women eating the same number of calories, but not taking the medication.

Other studies report side effects from PPA, including elevated blood pressure, heart damage, nervousness, irritability, insomnia, restlessness, headache, dizziness, and serious central nervous system effects, such as seizures, hallucinations, agitation, and stroke. People with a history of heart disease, diabetes, moderate to severe high blood pressure, kidney disease, hyperthyroidism, depression, or glaucoma should not take PPA. In addition, more than 10,000 cases of toxic effects attributed to PPA have been reported to FDA's Poison Control Center. Of course, anything that suppresses appetite also reduces food and nutrient intake, thus increasing a person's risk for vitamin and mineral deficiencies.

Other appetite suppressants, such as phentermine and fenfluramine, might help in losing and maintaining loss of weight, but they can cause side effects, including dry mouth, diarrhea, insomnia, fatigue, and possibly gout. Medications such as naloxone, naltrexone, and nalmefene can reduce daily food intake by a third and are sometimes used to treat obesity and other eating disorders. However, they can cause serious side effects and should not be used without medical supervision.

Orlistat can contribute to weight loss by reducing the amount of fat that the body absorbs from food. However, Orlistat might lower blood levels of vitamin A and vitamin E. Some users of Orlistat report abdominal pain, diarrhea, nausea, vomiting, flatulence, and oily stools; these symptoms reverse when Orlistat use is discontinued.

The only effective "diet" for long-term weight loss and weight maintenance is one that contains a variety of low-calorie, nutrient-dense foods combined with frequent aerobic exercise. This diet and exercise program must be followed for life if weight loss is to be maintained. Appetite-suppressant medications or other medications, such as flenfluramine, that alter appetite-control chemicals in the brain, are only effective for long-term weight maintenance when used in conjunction with a low-fat diet, regular exercise, and behavior modification.

SECTION 3

THE VITAMIN/ MINERAL-RICH DIET

CHAPTER 7

Vitamins, Minerals, and Food

Most people equate nutrition with the "balanced diet." When people ask what they should eat, it is common to hear, "a balanced diet." Nutritionists recommend the balanced diet rather than vitamin-mineral supplements to meet most people's daily nutrient needs. Parents are told their children should eat a balanced diet. Teenagers are scolded about their unbalanced diets, and the family meal planner worries about preparing at least one balanced meal for the family each day. The term balanced diet is used loosely and the vagueness of the term often leaves people confused. What is a balanced diet?

Only a few years ago a Sunday meal of baked ham, candied yams, buttered beans, and gravy was considered a balanced and wholesome meal. Scientific research now states a diet that contains large amounts of fat and cholesterol, as found in baked ham, buttered beans, and gravy, elevates blood cholesterol levels and increases the risk for developing heart disease and cancer. The salt in the processed ham and the salt added during cooking and at the table contributes to the development of hypertension. Although the evidence on sugar, as found in candied yams, is controversial, the extra calories with no additional vitamins and minerals contribute to either obesity or malnutrition, not to mention dental caries. In addition, even marginal deficiencies of vitamin C, vitamin A, magnesium, chromium, zinc, calcium, or other vitamins and minerals have been

311

linked to suppressed immune function and increased risk for infection and disease, osteoporosis, arthritis, depression, and numerous other emotional and physiological disorders. It appears the balanced diet of years past can no longer be considered healthful.

What can a person eat and how much is enough? First, it is important to recognize the benefits of good nutrition. Healthy dietary habits and proper food and meal selections

- improve resistance to colds and infections,
- reduce the risk for developing acute or chronic disease,
- increase resistance to stress and stress-related disorders,
- maintain a feeling of well-being,
- aid in the prevention of premature aging,
- aid in the maintenance of a healthy appearance,
- help maintain each individual's maximum energy level to enjoy life and perform necessary work,
- improve the outcome of pregnancy and the health and well-being of the infant, and
- aid in the regulation of a stable emotional and social life. Nutrition is one of the most important factors in a long and healthy life.

The good news is that the guidelines for good nutrition, a balanced diet, and optimal vitamin and mineral intake are simple and require, in most cases, only moderate changes in current eating habits.

1. Base the day's food intake on the Food Guide Pyramid.
2. Limit the fat in the diet to no more than 30 percent of total calories and limit cholesterol to 300mg/day or less.
3. Increase the fiber in the diet to at least 25grams daily. Limit processed, refined, or commercial convenience foods that are often high in fat, sugar, salt, cholesterol, or highly processed ingredients.
4. Choose a variety of wholesome, minimally processed, nutritious foods every day.
5. Exercise moderation in food selection, portion size, and all other dietary habits in order to obtain a wide variety of nutrients, avoid excessive intake of harmful substances in foods, and maintain a desirable weight.
6. Be patient. Gradually make dietary changes.

The above six guidelines combined with careful selection of fresh and wholesome food and proper food preparation methods will help guarantee consumption of a balanced, vitamin-and-mineral-rich diet that aids in the prevention of disease and premature aging and helps maintain optimal health.

THE FOOD GUIDE PYRAMID

There are numerous ways to design a vitamin- and mineral-rich diet today. The Food Guide Pyramid outlines dietary recommendations recently released by The U.S. Department of Agriculture and U.S. Department of Health and Human Services that replaced the now out-dated Four Food Groups Plan. The Food Guide Pyramid consists of the familiar four food groups; however, they have been rearranged into tiers within the pyramid shape to reflect the importance of grains, fruits, and vegetables as the primary foods in the daily diet (Figure 3).

Figure 3

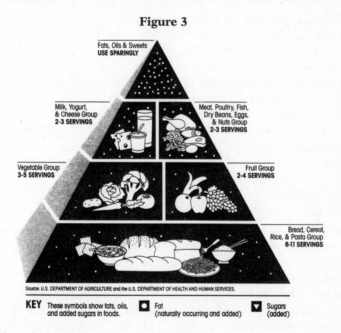

The Food Guide Pyramid.

The base of the Food Guide Pyramid, which should form the foundation of a healthful eating plan, is comprised of grains, cereals, and breads. The Food Guide Pyramid recommends 6 to 11 servings from this group (Table 42). These foods, especially the whole grains such as 100 percent whole wheat bread, oatmeal, and brown rice, are low in calories, fat, cholesterol, sugar, and salt. They are vitamin- and mineral-packed, high-fiber additions to the diet.

Table 42
GUIDELINES FOR PROPER SERVING SIZES

WHOLE GRAIN BREADS AND CEREALS (6–11 SERVINGS/DAY)
1 serving   1 slice of bread; or ½ English muffin, hamburger bun, bagel;
              or ½ cup cooked grain, such as cooked oatmeal, brown rice,
              whole wheat noodles, wheat berries, barley, or millet.

VEGETABLES AND FRUITS (3–5 SERVINGS OF VEGETABLES/DAY,
2–4 SERVINGS OF FRUIT/DAY)
*(at least 1 serving dark green or orange and at least 1 serving citrus or other vit-
amin C-rich selection)*
1 serving   one piece of fruit or vegetable, such as a medium apple,
              orange, carrot, or tomato; or 1 cup raw such as lettuce salad,
              cole slaw, or carrot sticks; or ½ cup cooked, such as spinach,
              broccoli, or lima beans; ¾ cup fruit or vegetable juice.

LOW-FAT MILK PRODUCTS (2–3 SERVINGS/DAY)
1 serving   1 cup (8 ounces) nonfat or low-fat milk/yogurt; or 1½ ounces
              hard, low-fat cheese; or 2 cups low-fat or nonfat cottage
              cheese.

MEAT, POULTRY, FISH, DRY BEANS, EGGS, AND NUTS (2–3 SERVINGS/DAY)
1 serving   3 ounces of lean meat, poultry, or fish; 1 cup cooked legumes,
              such as kidney beans, black beans, split peas, lentils, soy-
              beans, or garbanzo beans; or 2 Tbsp peanut or nut butter

OTHER FOODS
1 serving   1 tbsp safflower, corn, or other vegetable oil (excluding palm
              or coconut oils)

The second tier on the Food Guide Pyramid is split between fruits and vegetables. It recommends 3 to 5 servings of vegetables and 2 to 4 servings of fruit. These foods are good sources of fiber, vitamin C, vitamin A, and folic acid, as well as several trace minerals.

The third tier contains the milk, yogurt, and cheese group. Two to three servings daily will help supply the day's requirements for calcium, magnesium, zinc, vitamin D, protein, and vitamin B2. Low-fat or nonfat selections are your best choices. This tier also contains the meat, poultry, fish, dry beans, eggs, and nuts group. Two to three extra-lean selections from this group each day helps meet the recommendations for protein, iron, zinc, selenium, copper, B vitamins, and phosphorus.

The top level of the Pyramid emphasizes the minor role fats, oils, and sweets, such as oils, salad dressing, mayonnaise, desserts, high-fat snack foods, sugar, and high-sugar desserts, play in a nutrient-packed diet. This group, which also includes cooking preparation methods such as frying and sauteeing, should be used sparingly. A diet based on the Food Guide Pyramid supplies as little as 2,000 calories, while providing 75 percent to 100 percent of the RDA for all vitamins and minerals.

Limit Dietary Fat

The Food Guide Pyramid is not foolproof. Poor choices can be made within each group that can result in a nutritionally-lacking diet. One way to ensure optimal vitamin and mineral intake, while maintaining a desirable weight and low risk for disease is to limit the intake of fats, fatty foods, and fatty methods of food preparation. A beneficial side effect of this dietary change is that as fat (and sugar) intake is reduced, vitamin and mineral intake increases.

Dietary fats come in a variety of forms including visible fats, such as butter, sour cream, cream cheese, margarine, vegetable shortening, vegetable oils, and the visible fat surrounding meat or in chicken skin. Invisible fats are found in pie crust and other desserts, the marbled fat in meats, the hidden fats in fatty fish, doughnuts, croissants, many frozen entrees and other convenience foods, commercial snack foods such as potato chips and corn chips, and gravies and sauces. Limiting fatty foods also includes fatty food-preparation methods, such as frying and sauteing; foods served in cream sauces and gravies; and curtailing the use of salad dressings, mayonnaise, shortening, and other added fats and fatty spreads (Table 43).

Table 43
THE FAT CONTENT OF SELECTED FOODS

FOODS THAT CONTAIN MORE THAN 75 PERCENT FAT CALORIES[1]

Avocado	Luncheon meats (bologna)
Bacon	Nuts
Beef (sirloin, hamburger)	Olives
Coconut	Peanut Butter
Coleslaw	Pork (sausage, spareribs, loin,
Cream	untrimmed ham)
Cream cheese	Seeds (sesame, sunflower)

FOODS THAT CONTAIN 50 PERCENT TO 75 PERCENT FAT CALORIES[2]

Beef (rump, corned)	Fish, fried
Cake, pound	Ice cream
Cheese (blue, cheddar, Swiss)	Lamb (chops, rib)
Chicken, with skin	Pork (Ham loin, shoulder)
Chocolate	Tuna, packed in oil
Creamed soups	Veal
Eggs	

Table 43 (cont.)
THE FAT CONTENT OF SELECTED FOODS

FOODS THAT CONTAIN 30 PERCENT TO 50 PERCENT FAT CALORIES[3]

Beef (lean, flank steak, chuck)	Milk, low-fat (2 percent)
Cake, no icing	Pumpkin pie
Cheese, cottage	Salmon, canned
Chicken, roasted no skin	Soup, bean with pork
Fish, halibut broiled	Turkey, roasted dark skin
Ice milk	Yogurt, low-fat (2 percent)

FOODS THAT CONTAIN 30 PERCENT OR LESS FAT CALORIES

Beans, peas, lentils	Milk, non-fat
Beef (sirloin, lean only)	Pancakes
Bread	Seafood (scallops, shrimp)
Cake, angel food, sponge	Soups, split pea or vegetable
Cereal	Tuna, packed in water
Cheese, cottage uncreamed	Turkey, roasted white meat
Fish, broiled	Vegetables
Fruits	Wheatgerm
Grains	

[1]*More than 8 grams of fat for every 100 calories.*

[2]*Between 5 grams and 8 grams of fat for every 100 calories.*

[3]*Between 3 grams and 5 grams of fat for every 100 calories.*

Limiting fat does not mean reducing the quantity of food intake. In fact, you probably can eat more food if fat intake is reduced. For example, a medium baked potato contains approximately 100 calories and is a rich source of vitamin C, fiber, and several minerals. The addition of butter and sour cream can more than triple the calorie intake without changing the portion size. A 3½-ounce breast of fried chicken contains twice the calories of the same piece baked or broiled. Two tablespoons of dressing contain more calories than two cups of lettuce and assorted salad vegetables. In short, as fat is cut from the diet, a person can eat more vitamin- and mineral-rich food for fewer calories!

Increase Dietary Fiber

A high-fiber diet, based on minimally processed whole grains, fruits, vegetables, and dried beans and peas, is a vitamin and mineral-rich diet. A high-fiber intake also is associated with a reduced risk for colon cancer, cardiovascular disease, diabetes, hypertension, and several intestinal disorders.

A recommendation for the optimal quantity of fiber in the daily diet has not been established, but intakes between 25 grams and 40 grams are associated with a reduced risk for developing chronic diseases. Currently, typical American diets average only 10 grams daily. More than 50 grams of fiber each day is not recommended, as excessive intake (remember the moderation guideline) can cause intestinal upset and might reduce the absorption of certain trace minerals, such as iron and zinc. A fiber-rich diet is easily designed, by including the following foods from the Pyramid Food Guide:

```
6 servings of whole grain breads and cereals........13 grams
4 servings of fresh fruits and vegetables................15–23 grams
1 serving of cooked dried beans and peas.............9 grams
Total.................................................................37–45 grams
```

Choose a Variety of Foods

Variety in the diet is important in guaranteeing adequate intake of the more than 45 essential nutrients, phytochemicals, and possibly as yet unrecognized nutrients, and to avoid excessive consumption of potentially toxic compounds found naturally in some foods or unintentionally added during processing or storing.

For example, eating a variety of foods will increase the amount of phytochemicals in the diet, non-nutritive substances such as indoles, bioflavonoids, and carotenoids found in many vegetables and fruits that might protect against cancer and cardiovascular disease. Many people repeatedly consume the same foods and often choose from less than 50 foods for their weekly diet. In these cases, many highly nutritious foods—low in fat and high in fiber, vitamins, and minerals—are ignored. Individuals should try to include at least three new foods in the diet each week.

Moderation

Good nutrition and choosing a healthful diet is not an "all-or-nothing" decree. It is a process of emphasizing wholesome, minimally processed, low-fat foods and limiting intake of highly processed, refined, and fatty foods. There are no perfect foods and no one food needs to be included in a diet in order for the diet to be nutritious. For example, adding wheat germ or broccoli to a diet otherwise comprised primarily of highly processed, high-fat foods will not make up for the abundance of other poor food choices.

On the other hand, the occasional addition of one fatty or processed food to an otherwise nutritious diet will not reduce the diet's nutritional quality. Bacon and eggs for breakfast every day is not advised because of the high amount of fat, cholesterol, nitrites (cancer-causing substances), and low fiber provided by this meal. However, a breakfast of bacon and eggs once a month is harmless for most people. But, while an occasional poor food choice will not harm an otherwise good diet, repeatedly choosing highly processed and refined foods high in fat, salt, sugar, or cholesterol will jeopardize vitamin and mineral intake, and the risk for developing numerous diseases escalates. The diet should be reviewed according to the daily or weekly food intake, not according to each food.

Moderation also applies to serving size. Remember, each of the foods in the Food Guide Pyramid supplies specific vitamins and minerals necessary for optimal health. Overemphasis of one group to the exclusion or limitation of another group increases a person's risk for developing deficiencies of vitamins or minerals. For example, avoiding low-fat milk products increases the risk for low intake of vitamin D, calcium, and vitamin B2. Consuming insufficient servings of fresh fruits and vegetables results in marginal intake of vitamin C, beta carotene, folic acid, and many trace minerals.

Be Patient

Making dietary changes can be difficult. Success is more likely and discomfort is minimized if changes are made gradually; failure, resentment, frustration, and loss of motivation are more likely if too many difficult changes are undertaken at one time. A person must recognize that lasting change occurs slowly, even if major adjustments in dietary intake are needed.

A nutritious diet is based on a few, simple guidelines. A low-fat, high-fiber diet based on the Food Guide Pyramid, that includes a variety of wholesome foods, that limits consumption of highly refined and processed foods, and that maintains a desirable body weight is most likely to supply the more than 45 essential vitamins, minerals, and nutrients in the proper ratio and combination to maintain optimal health (Table 44). Limiting salt and alcohol and drinking at least six glasses of water each day are also recommended. Fresh foods should be selected and should be prepared to retain the most vitamins and minerals.

Table 44
RATE YOUR DIET

	Usually	Sometimes	Seldom
1. I eat a variety of foods, such as fresh fruits and vegetables, whole grain breads and cereals, lean meats, cooked dried beans and peas, low-fat milk products, and nuts and seeds, and consume at least 2,000 calories worth of these foods every day.	4	1	0
2. I limit the amount of fat in the diet, including meats, oil, butter, cream, desserts, fried foods, salad dressings, mayonnaise, and other fatty foods.	2	1	0
3. I avoid sugar and sugary foods,including soft drinks, candy, desserts, hidden sugars in processed foods, and highly sugared ready-to-eat cereals.	2	1	0
4. I include at least one dark green leafy vegetable, one citrus fruit, and two to three calcium-rich foods in the diet each day.	2	1	0
5. I am not on long-term prescription or non-prescription medications.	2	1	0
6. I avoid quick-weight-loss diets.	2	1	0
7. I avoid tobacco and consume alcohol in moderation or not at all.	2	1	0

Add the circled numbers.
1. A score of 11 to 16 is excellent. It is unlikely you need to take a supplement, unless you want to include an extra dose of the antioxidant nutrients.
2. A score of 7 to 10 is good, but some changes need to be made in eating habits and a multiple vitamin-mineral supplement would improve daily intake.
3. A score of 4 to 6 indicates a health risk. Dietary changes and the inclusion of a multiple vitamin-mineral supplement in the daily nutrient intake should begin immediately.
4. A score less than 4 indicates a high risk to health and nutritional status. Major dietary changes are required that include supplementation. You might benefit from dietary advice from a registered dietitian.

How those foods are consumed, whether it be in three square meals a day or six small meals throughout the day, depends more on an individual's preference and time schedule than on biological needs. Food intake, however, should be evenly dispersed throughout the day so that no more than four to five hours passes between meals and snacks. That means breakfast is an essential meal. In fact, people who eat breakfast are more likely than breakfast skippers to consume a higher intake of vitamins and minerals.

A person also should take time to relax while eating so that the stomach and intestine can function optimally in digesting and absorbing nutrients. It should never be forgotten that food is more than nutrients; it is a source of pleasure, socialization, and enjoyment.

MEAL-PLANNING GUIDELINES

Guidelines for a vitamin- and mineral-rich diet are only as effective as the understanding of how to apply them. Reducing dietary fat and increasing vitamin and mineral intake sounds simple, but often fats are hidden in foods and a diet can remain high in fat or other unwanted substances without the person knowing it. In contrast, preparing vitamin and mineral-rich meals does not have to be time-consuming or complicated. Simple adjustments to favorite recipes and a few additions to the menu might be all that is needed.

Shopping for Nutritious Foods

Most of the foods included in the Food Guide Pyramid plan are found around the periphery of the grocery store. The produce section, the dairy section, the meat section, and the bread section or bakery usually line the side walls and back of the grocery store. The other foods, such as whole grain cereals, noodles, canned and frozen vegetables, and legumes are located on a few aisles, while the greatest percentage of the aisle shelves are devoted to foods that are often highly processed, and convenience foods (Table 45).

Table 45
THE GROCERY LIST FOR VITAMIN- AND MINERAL-RICH FOODS

DAIRY
Nonfat (skim) milk or yogurt (less than 1 percent fat, by weight)
Low-fat milk or yogurt (less than 2 percent fat, by weight)
Buttermilk (less than 2 percent fat, by weight)
Low-fat cheeses
　　Pot cheese
　　Dry curd cottage cheese
　　Low-fat (1 percent fat, by weight) or nonfat cottage cheese

Table 45 (cont.)
THE GROCERY LIST FOR VITAMIN-AND-MINERAL-RICH FOODS

Partially-skimmed mozzarella cheese
Partially-skimmed ricotta cheese
Fat-free cheeses

EGGS
Use only the whites

BREAD
Corn tortillas
Crackers
Rice cakes
Rye crisp
Snack Well's fat-free wheat crackers
Wasa crackers
Whole wheat pita bread
Whole wheat, rye, pumpernickel, multi-grain, or sourdough bread

HOT CEREALS
4-grain and 7-grain hot cereals
Cornmeal
Cracked wheat
Oat bran
Orowheat hot cereal
Rolled oats
Wheatena

COLD CEREALS
Grape-Nuts
NutriGrain, wheat, barley, rye, corn cereals
Puffed wheat, rice, millet, or corn
Shredded Wheat

GRAINS
Barley
Bran
Brown rice
Cornmeal
Couscous
Kasha
Millet
Oat flour
Popcorn (dry pop)
Rye
Rye flour
Tabouli mix, rice pilaf, wheat pilaf, Spanish rice
Triticale
Whole wheat berries

Table 45 (cont.)
THE GROCERY LIST FOR VITAMIN-AND-MINERAL-RICH FOODS

Whole wheat flour, graham, and pastry flour
Wild rice

PASTAS
All pastas, including whole wheat, spinach, buckwheat, rice flour

FRUITS AND VEGETABLES AND JUICES
All fresh fruit
All fresh vegetables (olives and avocados are high in fat)
Fresh and canned 100 percent vegetable or fruit juices
Tomato products: paste, sauce, enchilada sauce, picante sauce, tomato juice, V-8
    juice, whole tomatoes, plum tomatoes, crushed tomatoes, green chili salsa
Raisins, apricots, prunes, and other dried fruits (no added sugar)

OTHER CANNED ITEMS
Apple juice, unsweetened
Artichoke hearts, in water
Bamboo shoots
Beans, rinsed
Beets
Corn
Green chilis
Milk, Evaporated nonfat
Pineapple juice, unsweetened
Pumpkin
Salmon, water-packed
Tuna, water-packed
Water chestnuts

FROZEN VEGETABLES/FRUITS AND THEIR JUICES
All frozen vegetables without sauces
Apple, grapefruit, orange, or pineapple juice, concentrated, unsweetened
Strawberries, blueberries, boysenberries, frozen, unsweetened

BEVERAGES
Caffix
Herb teas
Mineral water
Postum
Seltzer water
Spring water

CONDIMENTS
All spices, herbs, and seasonings (check for added salt)
Dry mustard
Horseradish
Miso
Mustard

Table 45 (cont.)
THE GROCERY LIST FOR VITAMIN-AND-MINERAL-RICH FOODS

Picante sauce
Soy sauce
Tabasco sauce
Tamari
Vinegar
Wines (white, burgundy), sherry, sauternes, dry vermouth, port

LEGUMES
All beans, including soybeans, kidney, black, garbanzo, dried limas, navy,
    white, and mung
Soybean cheese
Tempeh (fermented soybean curd)
Tofu

MISCELLANEOUS STOCK ITEMS
Active dry yeast
Arrowroot
Baking powder
Baking soda
Cornstarch
Fat-free salad dressings
Gelatin, unflavored
Lemon juice (unsweetened)
Lime juice (unsweetened)
Matzo meal
Milk, nonfat dry
Pearl tapioca
Whey powder

READ LABELS. The Nutrition Labeling and Education Act of 1990
(NLEA) created new guidelines for what information is contained on
nutrition labels. Food packages with the new Nutrition Facts label
contain information on calories, calories from fat, total fat, saturated
fat, cholesterol, sodium, total carbohydrate, dietary fiber, sugars, protein, vitamin A, vitamin C, calcium, and iron. Calories and how many
grams of fat are in a product can be easily compared between two
items because serving sizes are now standardized. For example, the
grams of fat in two brands of potato chips are based on the same
amount of chips.

The Nutrition Facts section on a label indicates what percentage
of the daily fat intake (based on a 2,000 calorie diet) is provided by
the product. The grams of sugar can be equated with the number of
teaspoons of sugar in the product (e.g., 4 grams = 1 teaspoon). The

NLEA also regulates the use of label terms such as "reduced," "free," "light," "lite," "more," "fresh," and "lean," which are now defined by the Food and Drug Administration (Figure 4).

The new labels were intended to simplify the process of identifying nutritious foods for the shopper, but in some ways they only add further confusion. First, few people eat or know whether they eat a "2,000 calorie diet." In addition, since no one eats only labeled foods and takes the time to add up Daily Values, providing a % Daily Value for fat, sodium, and other substances in the food is not very useful. Second, the new labels do not provide information on the percentage of calories that come from fat, so the consumer must calculate this information by multiplying the fat grams by 9 and dividing by the total number of calories in a serving. (A short version of this method is to identify foods that have 3 grams of fat or less per 100 calories, which equates to 30 percent fat calories or less.)

THE RDIs. The term Reference Daily Intake (RDI) is the new name for the United States Recommended Daily Allowance (USRDA) that was developed by the Food and Drug Administration (FDA). The USRDAs were condensed lists of nutrient requirements based on the Recommended Dietary Allowances (RDAs). The RDI for any nutrient is identical to the old USRDA. The % Daily Values are equal to % RDI (Table 46).

Table 46
THE REFERENCE DAILY INTAKES (RDIs)

Nutrients	RDI
Vitamin A	5,000IU
Vitamin D	400IU
Vitamin E	30IU
Vitamin B1	1.5mg
Vitamin B2	1.7mg
Vitamin B6	2.0mg
Folic Acid	400mcg
Niacin	20mg
Vitamin B12	6mcg
Biotin	300mcg
Pantothenic Acid	10mg
Vitamin C	60mg
Calcium	1,000mg
Copper	2mg
Iodine	150mg
Iron	18mg
Magnesium	400mg
Phosphorus	1,000mg
Zinc	15mg

Figure 4
THE NEW FOOD LABELS

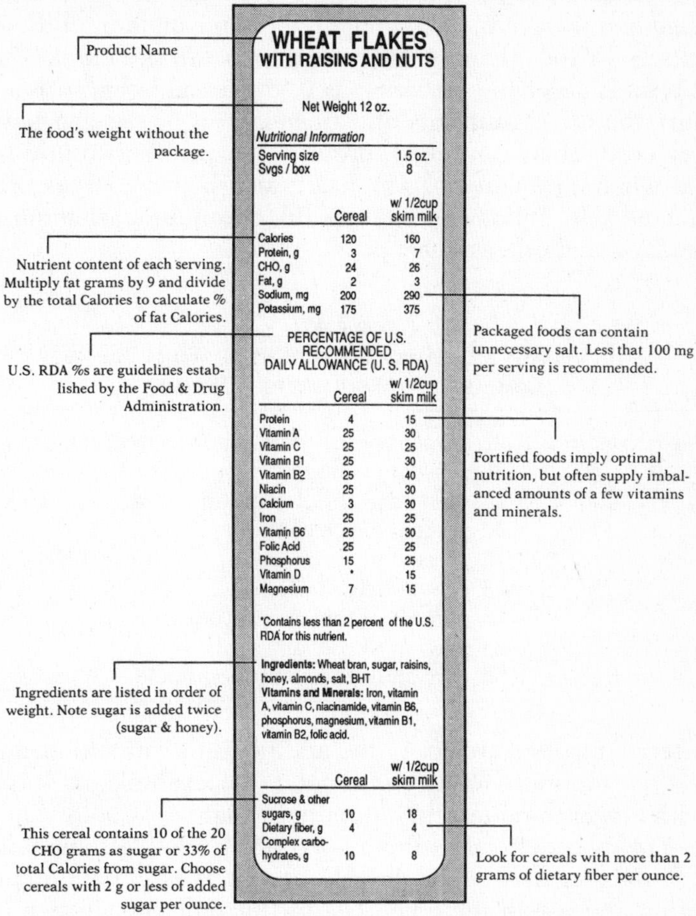

Product Name

WHEAT FLAKES
WITH RAISINS AND NUTS

Net Weight 12 oz.

The food's weight without the package.

Nutritional Information

	Cereal	w/ 1/2cup skim milk
Serving size		1.5 oz.
Svgs / box		8

Nutrient content of each serving. Multiply fat grams by 9 and divide by the total Calories to calculate % of fat Calories.

	Cereal	w/ 1/2cup skim milk
Calories	120	160
Protein, g	3	7
CHO, g	24	26
Fat, g	2	3
Sodium, mg	200	290
Potassium, mg	175	375

Packaged foods can contain unnecessary salt. Less that 100 mg per serving is recommended.

U.S. RDA %s are guidelines established by the Food & Drug Administration.

PERCENTAGE OF U.S. RECOMMENDED DAILY ALLOWANCE (U. S. RDA)

	Cereal	w/ 1/2cup skim milk
Protein	4	15
Vitamin A	25	30
Vitamin C	25	25
Vitamin B1	25	30
Vitamin B2	25	40
Niacin	25	30
Calcium	3	30
Iron	25	25
Vitamin B6	25	30
Folic Acid	25	25
Phosphorus	15	25
Vitamin D	*	15
Magnesium	7	15

*Contains less than 2 percent of the U.S. RDA for this nutrient.

Fortified foods imply optimal nutrition, but often supply imbalanced amounts of a few vitamins and minerals.

Ingredients: Wheat bran, sugar, raisins, honey, almonds, salt, BHT
Vitamins and Minerals: Iron, vitamin A, vitamin C, niacinamide, vitamin B6, phosphorus, magnesium, vitamin B1, vitamin B2, folic acid.

Ingredients are listed in order of weight. Note sugar is added twice (sugar & honey).

	Cereal	w/ 1/2cup skim milk
Sucrose & other sugars, g	10	18
Dietary fiber, g	4	4
Complex carbohydrates, g	10	8

This cereal contains 10 of the 20 CHO grams as sugar or 33% of total Calories from sugar. Choose cereals with 2 g or less of added sugar per ounce.

Look for cereals with more than 2 grams of dietary fiber per ounce.

New headline signals a new label.

More consistent serving sizes in both household and metric measures replace those that used to be set by manufacturers.

Nutrient information emphasizes fat, cholesterol, sodium, and sugar.

Conversion guide helps consumers learn caloric value of the energy-producing nutrients.

New mandatory component helps consumers meet dietary guidelines recommending no more than 30 percent of calories from fat. However, new labels provide no information on percentage of calories that come from fat in the labeled food.

Percent Daily Value shows how a food fits into the overall daily diet. However, this information is not very useful unless a person follows a 2,000-calorie diet and totals all labels every day to meet 100 percent of daily needs.

Reference values help consumers learn good diet basics. They can be adjusted depending on a person's calorie needs.

ENRICHED AND FORTIFIED. The term "enriched" traditionally refers to the addition of three vitamins (vitamin B1, vitamin B2, and niacin) and one mineral (iron) to processed grain. Breads and rice that have been processed and then "enriched" contain the same amount of these four nutrients as did the original whole wheat or brown rice (Table 47).

The term is deceiving, however, as it implies added nutrition when in reality the other nutrients and fiber lost in processing have not been replaced. These "enriched" products are poor substitutes for the original whole grain items, which are also better sources of fiber, pantothenic acid, folic acid, vitamin B6, chromium, selenium, magnesium, zinc, and other nutrients.

TABLE 47
THE VITAMIN AND MINERAL CONTENT OF WHITE BREAD
COMPARED TO WHOLE WHEAT BREAD

White bread contains...	22 percent of the magnesium in whole wheat bread
	38 percent of the zinc
	28 percent of the chromium
	42 percent of the copper
	12 percent of the manganese
	4 percent of the vitamin E
	18 percent of the vitamin B6
	63 percent of the folic acid
	56 percent of the pantothenic acid

The term "fortified" refers to the addition of a vitamin or mineral to levels not naturally found in the food. For example, milk is fortified with larger amounts of vitamin D than is usually found in nature. This is beneficial as there is no other reliable source of vitamin D in the diet, and the fat-soluble vitamin is essential for calcium absorption and use in the body. The fortification of salt with iodine resulted in a marked reduction in the incidence of goiter and cretinism. The FDA is currently considering fortifying breads with folic acid to help prevent birth defects.

Fortification can be misused to sell otherwise nutrient-poor foods. Vitamins and minerals may be added in arbitrary amounts and combinations to breakfast cereals, protein powders, breakfast drinks, fruit-flavored or sugary beverages, granola bars, or even candy bars. Fortification with a few nutrients gives an otherwise poor product the facade of being nutritious. These processed foods are never fortified with all the essential vitamins and minerals in balanced amounts that promote optimal nutrition. The natural product, such as orange juice, is always more nutritious and less expensive than a processed product, such as an orange-flavored, vitamin C-fortified fruit drink.

Fortification also might not be a reliable way to obtain nutrients. A recent study at Boston University that analyzed the vitamin D content of milk across the United States and Canada reported that 80 percent of vitamin D-fortified milk sampled contained either 20 percent more or 20 percent less vitamin D than claimed, 14 percent of the samples contained no vitamin D, and one sample had 914 percent more vitamin D than the label stated.

INGREDIENTS LIST. The ingredients in packaged food must be listed in descending order according to weight. For example, a loaf of bread labeled "whole wheat" that lists enriched wheat flour as its first ingredient is made primarily from white flour. A product will be primarily sweet and nutrient-poor if the first or second ingredient listed is sugar.

Sweeteners come in a variety of names and their total contribution to the product should be considered. For example, if sugar is listed second on the list of ingredients, honey listed fourth, and dextrose or "natural sweeteners" listed sixth, a product should be considered high in sugar.

Food Storage

To maximize the vitamin and mineral content of foods:

- Purchase only the amount of fresh fruits and vegetables that will be eaten within a few days.
- Store refrigerated foods at less than 40°F, frozen foods below 0°F, and canned and dry goods in a cool, dry place. Even small fluctuations in temperature can result in considerable loss of vitamin C in frozen foods.
- Store canned or frozen foods for no more than three to five months, as the vitamin content can decline as much as 75 percent or more with longer storage times.
- Store bulk dried beans and peas, noodles, rice, and flour in dark containers or in the refrigerator to reduce their exposure to ultraviolet light, which destroys vitamin B2.

Food Preparation

The three most important considerations in cooking are the preservation of the vitamin and mineral content of the food, the maintenance of an overall low-fat menu, and the preservation of the taste, texture, color, smell, and appearance of the food.

PRESERVING VITAMINS AND MINERALS. In general, vitamins and minerals are best preserved by cooking in a minimal amount of water, for a minimal amount of time, with a minimal amount of chopping or dicing of the food, and by keeping the cooked food for a minimal amount of time prior to serving and eating (Tables 48 and 49).

Table 48
PRESERVATION OF VITAMINS AND MINERALS DURING FOOD PREPARATION

- Cook food in a minimal amount of water for a short amount of time.
- Cook food to a temperature above 140°F to destroy harmful bacteria.
- Carefully read cooking instructions on packages.
- Use low to moderate heat for cooking meats.
- Thaw frozen meat, poultry, and fish in refrigerator before cooking.
- Cook frozen vegetables without thawing.
- Add shredded or grated cheese at the end of the cooking time.
- Cook eggs and milk mixtures over low heat.
- Use a vegetable peeler to remove only the outer layer of skin on produce.
- Cook produce in covered pan for a short amount of time.
- Cook vegetables just until crisp-tender.
- Peel, cut, chop vegetables just before eating or cooking.
- Prepare salads just before serving.
- Immediately refrigerate or freeze leftovers.
- Use leftover liquids for sauces, soups, stews, or cooking water for cereals, rice, or noodles.
- Save celery leaves, parsley, and other leftover vegetables for soup stock.

Table 49
VITAMIN AND MINERAL LOSSES DURING FOOD HANDLING

The following vitamins or minerals are destroyed when exposed to light, heat, air, cooking water, or changes in pH.

EXPOSURE TO LIGHT
Vitamin B2   Vitamin E
Vitamin A and beta carotene   Vitamin K
Vitamin D

Table 49 (cont.)
VITAMIN AND MINERAL LOSSES DURING FOOD HANDLING

EXPOSURE TO PROLONGED HEAT
Vitamin C   Folic acid
Vitamin B1   Vitamin B12
Pantothenic acid   Vitamin A

EXPOSURE TO AIR
Vitamin C   Vitamin A
Folic acid   Vitamin D
Vitamin B12   Vitamin E
Biotin   Vitamin K

LEACHING INTO COOKING WATER
Vitamin C   Vitamin B6
Vitamin B1   Selenium
Vitamin B2   Potassium
Niacin   Magnesium
Pantothenic acid   Phosphorus

ACID/ALKALINE pH
Vitamin C (alkaline)   Folic acid (alkaline or acid)
Vitamin B1 (alkaline)   Vitamin B12 (alkaline)
Vitamin B2 (alkaline)   Biotin (alkaline)
Pantothenic acid (alkaline or acid)

THE VITAMIN- AND MINERAL-RICH MENU. The lower the fat content of the diet the more foods rich in vitamins, minerals, and fiber can be included in the daily fare and the less risk for developing marginal vitamin or mineral deficiencies, disease, or obesity. The common recommendation is to reduce dietary fat to no more than 30 percent of total calories.

A reduction in dietary fat and cholesterol is accomplished by following a few simple guidelines (Table 50).

1. Emphasize low-fat and nonfat milk products (Table 52).
2. Use only extra-lean meat, chicken without the skin, and fish, and only consume the amount recommended by the Food Guide Pyramid.
3. Limit or avoid cooking with fats (butter, margarine, vegetable oil, or animal fats, such as bacon fat or lard). Limit total daily intake to less than 2 tablespoons.
4. Emphasize whole grain breads and cereals, fresh fruits and vegetables, cooked dried beans and peas, and nuts (Table 53).

Table 50
REDUCING FAT IN THE DIET: MEAT AND GENERAL GUIDELINES

Rather than...	Choose to...
1. using gourmet recipes as is	eliminate egg yolks (use egg substitute or two egg whites for every whole egg), butter, cream, salt, and substitute spices, wine, and other seasonings.
2. making fatty homemade soup	refrigerate stock and skim fat before preparing soup, stews, gravies, or sauces.
3. basting in oil	baste with wine, fat-free liquids, and spices.
4. using mayonnaise	mix imitation or low-calorie mayonnaise with nonfat yogurt. Use for tuna or chicken salad.
5. preparing grilled sandwiches in butter	use a non-stick pan or PAM
6. preparing 4-8 oz servings of meat	prepare 2 to 3 oz servings of extra-lean meat and mix with whole grain rice, noodles, or vegetables.
7. frying, sautee in fats	bake, steam, broil, boil, or grill.
8. serving French fries with hamburgers	prepare baked potato with chives or cut potatoes into strips and bake on ungreased cookie sheet until brown and crispy.

People who wish to monitor fat intake more closely or people who count calories might want to count their weekly intake of fat grams. This method requires that a person know the approximate daily calorie intake. The maximum daily allotment of fat (30 percent of total calories) is determined by multiplying 0.30 times a person's daily calorie intake and dividing by 9 (fat contains 9 calories/gram). For example, a daily intake of 2,000 calories times 0.30 = 600, divided by 9 calories/1 gram of fat = 67 grams of fat/day. The number of grams of fat in various foods can be found in a variety of books available at most bookstores (Table 51).

Table 51
DETERMINING CALORIES FROM PROTEIN, CARBOHYDRATE, AND FAT

A serving of nonfat milk (90 calories) contains the following:

	Grams per serving		Calories per gram	Calories	Percentage of total Calories
Protein	9.3	X	4 calories/gram =	37.2	37.2 divided by 90 = 41 percent
Carbohydrate	12.5	X	4 calories/gram =	50	50 divided by 90 = 55 percent
Fat	0.4	X	9 calories/gram =	3.6	3.6 divided by 90 = 4 percent

Table 52
REDUCING FAT IN THE DIET: MILK PRODUCTS

Rather than...	*Choose to...*
1. using butter to saute	saute foods in defatted chicken stock, use non-stick pans or PAM.
2. putting butter on toast	use low-calorie jams or low-fat cottage cheese.
3. using sour cream	use nonfat yogurt with a dash of lemon or fat-free sour cream for dips.
4. using fruited yogurt	select plain, nonfat yogurt. Mix with fresh fruit.
5. using cream or whole milk	use nonfat milk with nonfat dry milk solids or evaporated nonfat milk. Partially frozen evaporated nonfat milk can be whipped into a foam for desserts or as a replacement for whipping cream.
6. using full amount of cheese	reduce portion of cheese in sauces to $1/3$ to $1/2$.
7. preparing fat and flour for "roux"	prepare cream sauces with cornstarch and nonfat milk, water, or juice.

Table 53
REMOVING FAT FROM THE DIET

Instead of...	Choose...
BREAKFAST	
Scrambled eggs and bacon	Oatmeal with low-fat milk, raisins, and nuts
Toast with butter	Whole wheat toast with low-sugar jam
Coffee with cream	Coffee with nonfat condensed milk
Orange drink	Orange juice
LUNCH	
Hamburger on bun with sauce	Broiled chicken sandwich, with lettuce, no mayonnaise
French fries	Tossed green salad with low-fat or fat-free dressing
Milkshake	Milk, nonfat or low-fat
Chocolate cake	Angel-food cake topped with fresh berries
DINNER	
Fried chicken	Baked or broiled chicken without the skin
Baked potato with sour cream and butter	Baked potato with butter substitute and chives
Sauteed vegetables	Steamed vegetables
Macaroni salad	Spinach salad with low-fat or fat-free dressing
Ice cream	Sherbet or plain low-fat yogurt with fruit

THE NEW FOODS: CONVENIENCE, FAST, AND SNACK

Since the 1940s thousands of new convenience foods have entered the marketplace. These new foods either attempt to replicate traditional homemade items, such as macaroni and cheese, or replace them, such as fruit drinks. Convenience foods are prepared at home from foods that already have been cooked or processed at the factory. These foods include:

- Cold breakfast cereals
- Powdered or condensed beverages
- Frozen entrees, breakfasts, vegetables, and other foods

- Pre-prepared meals and desserts that require the addition of water, milk, or another ingredient before serving
- Canned foods that require opening, possibly heating, and serving

In general, the more a food is processed, the higher its fat, salt, or sugar content and/or the lower its vitamin, mineral, and fiber content. For example, whole wheat bread made from 100 percent whole wheat flour is an excellent source of B vitamins, trace minerals, and fiber, while bread made from enriched white flour contains significantly less fiber, trace minerals (except iron), and many of the B vitamins. If the cornerstone of the diet is minimally processed foods, chances are good that the diet also is high in vitamins and minerals.

VITAMINS, MINERALS, AND HEALTH FOOD

All nutritious foods are health foods. People have a right to accessible, pure food that is not adulterated, contaminated with insecticides and other poisons or cancer-causing substances, or altered in any way as to compromise the nutritional or sanitary quality of the food. People also should be able to choose from extra-lean meats or milk products that are not exposed to steroid hormones, antibiotics, or other growth-promoting substances. Industrial waste products and toxic chemicals should not be allowed to contaminate the water supply and soil, thus entering the food chain. Food should not need to be labeled "health food" to be of this quality. In addition, many claims of "health food" are more promise than substance.

There is no evidence that "natural" or "organic" foods are more healthful or contain more vitamins and minerals than other foods. In fact, in many states there is no regulation or legal definition for these words; industry can use them on any item, regardless of its contents. It is assumed that organic foods are grown on soil fertilized with organic fertilizers and without chemical fertilizers or pesticides. However, pesticides from neighboring farms, added directly to the food, or remaining in the soil from past use are found in organic produce.

There is no evidence that foods grown on soil fertilized with compost, manure, or other natural fertilizers are more nutritious than foods grown on chemically fertilized soil. The nutrient content of foods depends on the variety of food, the climate, the nutrients available for growth, and the stage of maturation when the food is harvested. For example, the vitamin C content of oranges varies widely in different areas of the United States and at different times of the year.

There are no guarantees that foods labeled natural or organic are free from additives, preservatives, or other unnatural substances.

Many foods called natural are highly processed and often contain additives, colorings, synthetic flavorings, or preservatives.

Another disadvantage to health foods is that they usually cost more than the same food purchased in a supermarket. Even the foods placed in special health food sections of the supermarket cost more than similar foods found on other shelves.

Some health food companies are sincere in their attempts to provide quality foods, and some items in health food stores are an inexpensive alternative to more conventional items. Items sold in bulk bins, such as oatmeal, flour, nuts, beans, and dried fruits, are often less expensive than the same items prepackaged or sold in supermarket sales. However, avoid peanuts in bins or "grind-your-own" peanut-butter, since peanuts exposed to air can harbor a fungus that produces a potent cancer-causing substance called aflatoxin. Some distributors and growers provide legal statements that their foods are grown or handled according to organic principles. The consumer should request to see those statements prior to purchasing an item promoted as organic or natural.

Reading labels and finding a reputable health food store manager can assist the consumer in sorting fact from the fiction. For example, a store that promotes natural vitamin and mineral supplements over other supplements should be viewed with a suspicious eye, since in most cases natural is not better, only more expensive, than other brands.

Beware of the credibility of salespersons who promote items that are not usually found in the diet, such as bee pollen, algae, protein powders, enzymes (superoxide dismutase or digestive enzymes), and hormonal extracts, or who falsely promote a substance as a vitamin or essential nutrient, such as pangamic acid as vitamin B15 or bioflavonoids as vitamin P. (See Chapters 3 and 4 for a list and description of the essential vitamins and Chapter 8 for a detailed account of supplementation.) These people are often self-taught and are not credible or reliable sources of sound nutrition information.

The same principles for selecting foods and meal planning apply to health food purchases and conventional food purchases.

- Read labels and avoid products that contain excessive amounts of fats, sugars, salt, additives, or refined ingredients.
- Select foods that have been minimally processed.
- Choose foods from the Food Guide Pyramid: whole grain breads and cereals, fresh fruits and vegetables, cooked dried beans and peas, extra-lean meats, and low-fat or nonfat milk products.
- Avoid promotional claims that increase the price, but do not improve the nutritional quality of a food, such as organic, natural, or therapeutic.

- Comparison shop and choose the nutritionally best item for the least amount of money.

SPECIAL DIETS (Athletes, Vegetarian Diets, The Weight-Loss Diet)

The principles of menu and diet planning are consistent regardless of age, gender, the presence or absence of degenerative disorders such as heart disease or diabetes, or food preferences. However, certain conditions, lifestyle patterns, or food-intake patterns require minor adjustments or considerations for an individual to maintain optimal health. The three general categories presented here are athletes, people following vegetarian diets, and people on weight-loss diets.

Athletes

No group, except dieters, is more vulnerable to nutrition mythology than athletes. Runners are sure there is a certain food combination that will improve their endurance, wrestlers are convinced there is a pill or powder that will increase their strength, weight-lifters believe extra protein will increase muscle mass, and football players think zinc will make them tougher. The dangerous use of steroid hormones and other potentially harmful or even lethal substances in the attempt to improve athletic performance attests to the athlete's belief in the magical properties of foods, vitamins, and minerals.

In reality, athletes require the same nutrients as anyone else, although they sometimes require more calories or a little more of a few vitamins and minerals. It is seldom necessary to increase protein intake, even for athletes building muscle mass, since the American diet already contains two to four times more protein than most people need. Extra protein, as steak, raw eggs, or protein powders, does not build extra muscle—only training builds muscle.

FLUIDS AND SODIUM. A primary concern for athletes is adequate fluid intake. To guarantee adequate fluid intake, drink twice as much water as it takes to quench thirst. A minimum of 8 glasses of water should be consumed each day, in addition to other beverages such as low-fat or nonfat milk, fruit juices, tea, and soft drinks. Athletes should not take sodium or salt tablets, especially prior to first replacing fluid losses. Salt tablets increase the effects of dehydration on the body and are unnecessary since the minimal amounts of electrolytes, such as sodium and potassium, lost in perspiration are easily replaced in the normal diet. Salt tablets or electrolyte replacement beverages should be considered only if more than four quarts of water have been lost as perspiration (1 quart of water = 2 pounds of body weight, so a person must lose more than 8 pounds during an athletic event or training session to warrant consideration of salt replacement). A gram of sodium (usually the equivalent of one salt tablet) can be consumed for every quart of water lost above the initial four quarts. Athletes should always replace water first and electrolytes second and should begin an athletic event or training session fully hydrated.

ANTIOXIDANTS. Frequent exercise might deplete antioxidant vitamins and mineral stores, while some forms of muscle damage in athletes has been attributed to free-radical damage to muscle cell membranes. Optimal intake and body stores of antioxidants might decrease injury risk and increase endurance performance. For example, increased intake of vitamin E might help prevent muscle damage and soreness. Laboratory studies on animals support this finding and report that exercise increases the need for vitamin E to levels difficult to obtain from foods alone. Vitamin E and vitamin C might also improve endurance.

OTHER VITAMINS. Female bicyclists show an increased dietary need for vitamin B2 to maintain normal tissue and blood levels of the vitamin. Inadequate intake of vitamins B1 and vitamin B6 also can impair athletic performance.

IRON. Iron is a particular concern for athletes, especially females, engaged in endurance or weight-bearing sports. This important mineral is frequently low in athletes' diets; as many as 80 percent of exercising women are iron deficient. Iron deficiency can impact exercise performance, resulting in lowered muscle strength and endurance and longer recovery times. Blood iron levels appear to decrease in runners and is known as "sports anemia," although this is partially explained by the increased blood volume, which dilutes the concentration of red blood cells and gives a false reading for iron.

The common iron tests (i.e., hematocrit and hemoglobin tests), are not as accurate as the serum ferritin and total iron binding capacity (TIBC) tests, which are more sensitive indicators of tissue iron levels. A serum ferritin level less than 20ng/ml or a TIBC reading of 450mcg/dl are indicators of iron deficiency even in the absence of anemia. (See pages 116–118 for more information on iron and tests for iron deficiency.)

OTHER MINERALS. Mineral needs might be higher for some athletes. Strenuous exercise alters trace mineral metabolism and increases the loss of several minerals, such as chromium, copper, selenium, and zinc, in the urine and iron in sweat. Magnesium loss in the urine increases after endurance events and is associated with a brief increase in blood levels of the mineral, suggesting magnesium loss from damaged muscle tissues. Low blood levels of magnesium persist for several months following the athletic event. Calcium intake is low in many athletes; which might decrease bone mass and increase the risk for bone fractures. Preliminary studies from Bemidji State University and Louisiana State University show that supplementation with the mineral chromium in the form of chromium picolinate might improve the loss of body fat and help increase lean tissue.

AMINO ACIDS. Some evidence shows that a few amino acids might benefit the athlete. For example, branched-chain amino acids (BCAA)—isoleucine, leucine, and valine—are used for energy by the muscles when carbohydrate stores are low. In one study, muscle loss after exercise was prevented in athletes supplemented with extra BCAAs. These athletes actually gained muscle mass under heavy training conditions. However, the long-term effects of BCAAs are unclear and the athlete should use this supplement with caution. The amino acid L-carnitine transports fats to be used for energy and some research shows it improves performance by improving exercise metabolism. However, other studies found no benefit from this amino acid; so, supplementation with L-carnitine is still considered experimental.

Dietary Recommendations

The diets of athletes are not always optimal. For example, intake of vitamin B6, iron, magnesium, and zinc is reported to be below 70 percent of the RDA in many athletes and some athletes do not consume adequate amounts of calcium, iron, and vitamins A, D, E, B2, B12, C, and niacin. In addition, there are no adequate measurements of nutritional status in competition athletes or people who exercise frequently and intensely. The RDAs, designed for a "reference person," are a poor guideline for assessing adequate nutrient intake for the competition athlete who is a 280-pound football player, a 7-foot-tall basketball player, or a marathon runner with 5 percent body fat.

The same dietary guidelines outlined at the beginning of this chapter should be followed by all athletes, with more whole grains, fruits, and vegetables. For example, the carbohydrate needs are high for the endurance athlete, such as swimmers, runners, and bicyclists, because this form of energy is an important storage fuel source during long-distance events. Athletes often think they have a high-carbohydrate diet, but, in reality, most consume only 45 percent of their calories from carbohydrates. The Food Guide Pyramid recommends at least two-thirds of the diet to come from foods high in starch, such as whole grain breads and cereals, fresh fruits and vegetables, and cooked dried beans and peas. The daily diet for the endurance athlete will provide ample amounts of complex carbohydrate (starch) if this diet plan is followed.

An athlete must carefully plan the diet to meet all vitamin and mineral requirements (Table 54). Whole grain breads and cereals should be chosen, rather than refined varieties. Extra calories to meet the demands of exercise should be provided by additional servings of grains, vegetables, fruits, and other nutrient-dense foods, not highly processed foods. Minimally processed foods are usually the foods richest in vitamins and minerals. In some cases, a vitamin/mineral supplement might be useful (See pages 358–362 for guidelines on choosing a supplement); however, megadoses of vitamins and minerals do not improve athletic performance.

Table 54
20 POWER FOODS

The following foods give you an extra vitamin and mineral "punch" while being low in fat, sugar, and calories.

1. Brewer's Yeast: Not a typical inclusion in the daily menu for most people; however, a quarter cup serving of this nutritional yeast mixed into orange juice, contains more vitamin B1 than 27 pounds of extra-lean hamburger or 45 slices of vitamin B1-enriched bread, it also contains more folic acid than 12 cups of green peas. Brewer's yeast is equally high in the other B vitamins as well as being an excellent source of iron, calcium, selenium, and zinc. For that kind of nutritional punch, it might be worth getting used to the taste!

2. Broccoli: This relative to the cabbage is loaded with vitamin C, beta carotene, fiber, calcium, potassium, and folic acid. It also contains a group of compounds called "indoles" that help prevent cancer. All this for only 25 calories a cup!

3. Brown Rice: This whole grain puts "enriched" white rice to shame. One cup contains 45 grams of complex carbohydrates and more than 3 grams of fiber. It also is mineral-rich, including magnesium, selenium, the B vitamins, iron, and zinc. Brown rice contains another compound called oxyzanol that reduces the "bad" cholesterol called LDL and, thus, might help lower a person's risk for developing heart disease.

4. Cantaloupe: A cup of icy cold cantaloupe is not only a low-calorie, low-fat, sweet and refreshing snack, it also is bursting with the antioxidants vitamin C and beta carotene.

5. Carrots: Two carrots contain more than 24mg of beta carotene for only 60 calories. They also provide 5 grams of fiber and some folic acid, vitamin C, iron, magnesium, and selenium.

6. Evaporated nonfat milk: As a replacement for cream or whole milk in sauces or as the liquid used for cooking rice, this milk is 60 percent carbohydrate calories and is high in calcium, vitamin B2, magnesium, potassium, and zinc.

Table 54 (cont.)
20 POWER FOODS

7.Kidney Beans: One cup, sprinkled onto a salad, added to vegetable soup, or rolled into a tortilla with cheese adds complex carbohydrates, half the day's need for fiber and folic acid, and ample amounts of iron, calcium, magnesium, and zinc. In addition, beans contain a group of compounds called saponins that help lower blood cholesterol and reduce a person's risk for developing heart disease. All for only 225 calories!

8. Lentils: A bowl of lentil soup packs a carbohydrate punch, contains 10 grams of fiber, the day's requirement for folic acid, 40 percent of a woman's and 70 percent of a man's need for iron, and substantial amounts of magnesium, potassium, zinc, vitamin E, and B vitamins.

9. Mango: Chock-full of the antioxidants beta carotene and vitamin C, this fruit also provides fiber carbohydrates, and a refreshing taste (especially when sprinkled with lime juice).

10. Nonfat Yogurt: One cup of this creamy cousin to milk contains almost half the day's requirement for calcium and vitamin B2, and a healthy dose of magnesium, selenium, and zinc. Yogurt that contains Lactobacillus acidophilus are the best, since this bacteria helps maintain a healthy environment in the digestive tract and might help maintain low blood cholesterol levels.

11. Orange Juice: This vitamin C-packed juice also is an excellent source of folic acid and contains some calcium, magnesium, and B vitamins. A glass of orange juice with meals helps the body absorb iron from other foods, while a large glass of diluted OJ is an excellent way to replenish fluids and potassium after a workout.

12. Oysters: Eaten raw or lightly cooked in oyster stew, these mollusks are loaded with minerals. A half cup serving contains more than the entire week's requirement for zinc, more than 100 percent of your daily selenium and vitamin B12 needs, three times the daily need for copper, 45 percent to 88 percent of the daily iron requirement for a woman and man respectively, and ample amounts of calcium, B vitamins, and magnesium.

13. Red Bell Pepper: Two of these beautiful vegetables chopped and added to burritos or stuffed with a rice and bean mix contain nine times as much beta carotene and more than twice the vitamin C of green peppers.

14. Spinach: Two cups of this leafy green supplies only 25 calories yet provides 4 grams of fiber, more than half the daily need for folic acid, the calcium equivalent of a half cup of milk, and lots of iron, magnesium, potassium, and vitamin C.

15. Strawberries: A woman exerciser who consumes only 2,000 calories each day must consume approximately 1mg of iron for every 100 calories to ensure optimal iron intake. Strawberries are one juice fruit that exceeds this criteria, supplying 1.23mg of iron per 100 calorie serving (equal to about 2+ cups of fresh strawberries).

16. Sweet Potatoes: These starchy vegetables are a great source of carbohydrate and supply more fiber and lots more beta carotene than white or red potatoes. They also contain some vitamin C, vitamin E, and calcium.

Table 54 (cont.)

17. Wheat germ: This gold nugget of nutrition might be the closest thing to the perfect food. A half cup of wheat germ contains 8 grams of fiber, between 25 percent and 100 percent of the daily need for the B vitamins, and is high in protein, vitamin E, magnesium, iron, selenium, potassium, and zinc.

18. Whole Wheat Bagel: This chewy bread is more than 75 percent complex carbohydrates with a wide array of vitamins and minerals to help digest, store, and use that energy during exercise.

19. Whole Wheat Bread: Compared to "enriched" white bread, this whole grain contains 96 percent more vitamin E, 82 percent more vitamin B6, 78 percent more fiber and magnesium, 72 percent more chromium, 58 percent more copper, 52 percent more zinc, and 37 percent more folic acid.

20. Whole Wheat Pocket Bread: Like the other whole grains, this bread is packed with carbohydrates, fiber, vitamins, and minerals with little or no fat. It can be stuffed with anything from extra-lean sliced meats and lettuce or peanut butter and fruit to beans and tomatoes or low-fat cheese and salsa for a quick after-workout snack.

Wrestlers concerned about "making weight" for weekend wrestling matches or football players concerned about weight gain during the off-season should continue to follow the Food Guide Pyramid, but adjust calorie intake to gain or lose weight.

Calorie intake should never fall below 2,000 calories and no more than two pounds should be lost each week unless supervised by a physician. A faster weight loss means muscle tissue, rather than fat tissue, is being lost with the extra danger of dehydration and heat exhaustion. In addition, extreme weight loss, especially in women, is associated with cessation of the menses and bone loss.

Vegetarian Diets

Vegetarian diets are not new. Accounts of these diets date from 2,000 B.C. Some vegetarian diets might be more healthful than the conventional American diet. Numerous studies have found meat consumption linked to an increased risk for heart disease and other degenerative disorders, whereas a vegetarian diet reduces heart disease risk. The high fiber intake characteristic of the vegetarian diet also improves glucose tolerance in diabetics and lowers blood pressure. Finally, vegetarian diets tend to be low in sugar, which leaves more room for vitamin-and mineral-packed foods.

The vegetarian diet is actually a blanket term for a variety of diets. The vegan diet is the most restrictive and includes only foods of plant origin, such as nuts, seeds, vegetables, fruits, grains, and legumes. The lactovegetarian diet includes all the foods included in the vegan diet, plus milk products, such as cheese, milk, and yogurt. The lacto-ovo vegetarian diet includes all of the above foods plus eggs. Variations on the vegetarian diet include fruitarians who eat only fruit, nuts, olive oil, and honey, and the macrobiotic diet that includes seven progressively more restrictive diets with the final diet consisting only of brown rice. These latter diets are too restrictive to guarantee optimal intake of all vitamins, minerals, protein, and calories, and are not recommended. People who consume chicken or fish are not considered vegetarians.

A vegetarian diet, whether it be vegan, lactovegetarian, or lacto-ovo vegetarian, can supply all the necessary vitamins, minerals, protein, and other nutrients essential to health, if careful planning is followed. The more restrictive a diet is, the more likely nutrient deficiencies will result, especially in pregnant and lactating women and small children. For example, milk products supply as much as 50 percent of the daily need for calcium and vitamin B2. Other foods, such as dark green leafy vegetables and broccoli, are good sources of these nutrients, but large quantities must be consumed each day to meet the RDA levels. Children have small stomachs and finicky appetites, which makes it difficult for them to consume the RDA for calcium obtained from four to six cups of dark green leafy vegetables necessary in the vegan diet. Calcium-fortified soymilk can meet part of the calcium needs, but other nutrient deficiencies still are possible. In addition, vitamin E needs might be higher with these diets than with conventional diets, because of the increased intake of polyunsaturated fats from nuts, seeds, and vegetable oils.

THE VEGAN DIET. It is not recommended that children less than 18 years old follow a vegan diet, because of the high nutrient demands and either limited capacity to consume volumes of food or the sporadic eating habits of children. The nutrients most likely to be deficient in the vegan diets of adults include protein, calcium, vitamin B2, vitamin B12, iron, zinc, and calories.

The vegan diet must be planned carefully to include adequate amounts of protein. The 8 to 10 essential amino acids are found in protein-rich foods, such as lean meat, chicken, fish, eggs, milk, cheese, and yogurt. These foods are called high-quality protein foods because they provide all the essential amino acids in the proper ratio for optimal absorption and use. The vegan diet excludes these foods and individuals following this diet must combine lower quality protein foods, such as nuts, seeds, legumes, and grains, to obtain the proper amount and proportion of the essential amino acids. Each of these foods are excellent sources of amino acids, but usually are lacking in one or more of the essential amino acids.

A high-quality protein can be obtained by combining two or more of these foods. For example, legumes, such as kidney beans or split peas, are low in the amino acids methionine and cystine but are high in the amino acid lysine. Grains, such as corn or wheat, are high in lysine but low in methionine and cystine and are an excellent "complement" to the legumes. The combination of corn and beans, such as the corn tortilla and beans in a burrito, supply high-quality protein. Grains combined with nuts and seeds do not provide the complement of amino acids to constitute a high-quality protein source. Other complementary protein combinations include:

1. Legumes and Grains
   - peanut butter sandwich
   - baked beans and brown bread
   - lentil and rice soup
   - black beans and rice pilaf
2. Seeds/Nuts and Legumes
   - lentil and cashew loaf
   - tofu and sesame burgers
   - stuffed cabbage rolls, with split peas and sunflower seeds

Calcium needs are more difficult to meet on the vegan diet than on less restrictive diets that include milk products. A glass of milk provides 36 percent of the adult RDA for calcium; a cup of legumes provides only 12 percent; and nuts, seeds, and grains provide even less.

However, daily calcium needs can be met with planning. Dark green leafy vegetables, such as mustard greens, beet greens, collards, kale, and broccoli, are excellent sources of calcium and contain between 50 percent to 100 percent of the calcium in a glass of milk (300mg). Some greens, such as spinach, contain calcium, but the mineral is not well absorbed because of other calcium-binding substances, called oxalates, in spinach. Calcium-fortified soymilk is the best source of calcium for vegans. Soymilk can be included in the diet as a base for soups, as an ingredient in home-made breads, as the fluid for rice and other cereals, and as a beverage. Powdered calcium carbonate can be added to flour for baking or calcium supplements can be taken. A source of vitamin D also must be identified, since fortified milk is the only reliable dietary source of this essential vitamin.

A main source of vitamin B2 in American diets is milk products. The vegan must be particularly careful in diet planning to meet daily needs for this water-soluble vitamin. The foods of plant origin in the following list supply approximately the same amount of vitamin B2 as does one cup of milk (0.395mg), and a minimum of three servings each day should be consumed to meet the adult RDA.

- avocado, 1 medium
- fortified cereal, one ounce
- fresh mushrooms, 1¼ cups

- cooked turnip greens, 1¼ cups
- cooked broccoli, 1⅓ cups
- winter squash, 1½ cups
- cooked asparagus, 1¾ cups
- cooked spinach, 1¾ cups
- Brussels sprouts, 2 cups
- okra, 2¼ cups

The only reliable dietary sources of vitamin B12 are foods of animal origin. A few kinds of algae and some fermented soybean products, such as tempeh and miso, are the only plant sources of this vitamin, but contain varying amounts. Vitamin B12-fortified soymilk or supplements should be consumed regularly to prevent deficiencies.

Although many foods of plant origin are high in iron, the iron from these sources is not as well absorbed as the iron in meat (called "heme" iron). In addition, the high-fiber content of the vegan diet might interfere with optimal absorption of some trace minerals, such as iron and zinc. To increase absorption of iron, the vegan should consume a vitamin C-rich food with meals, cook in cast iron pots, and include several servings each day of iron-rich foods.

The best sources of zinc are extra-lean meats, oysters, herring, milk, and egg yolks. Whole grain breads and cereals are the best source of zinc in the vegan diet, but this form of zinc is poorly absorbed. Frequent daily servings of whole grain breads and cereals must be included in the vegan diet to increase zinc intake or a multivitamin/mineral supplement that includes zinc should be taken.

The Food Guide Pyramid must be adapted for the vegan diet. The daily food guide for people on this type of vegetarian diet is as follows:

Vegetables—4 to 6 servings
(At least 2 dark green leafy vegetables and 1 raw salad for calcium, vitamin B2, vitamin A, iron, and folic acid. A serving size is 1 cup.)
Fruits—4 to 6 servings
(At least 2 iron-rich selections and 1 vitamin C-rich selection. Servings include juice or whole fruit.)
Grains—8 to 12 servings
(Whole grain varieties only. A serving size is 2 slices of bread; 4 to 6 crackers; 1 cup cooked cereal, noodles, or rice; or 2 ounces of ready-to-eat cereal.)
Beans and Nuts, including soymilk—3 servings
(At least 1 cup calcium-fortified soymilk. Beans are preferable to nuts as a low-fat protein source. A serving size is 1 cup cooked beans, 2 cups soymilk, 6 ounces tofu, 2 ounces nuts, or 4 tablespoons peanut butter.)

THE LACTOVEGETARIAN AND THE LACTO-OVO VEGETARIAN DIETS. These vegetarian diets easily can meet the RDA for all vitamins, minerals, protein, and other nutrients. Inclusion of milk products guarantees adequate intake of protein, calcium, vitamin D, vitamin B12, and vitamin B2, and contributes to magnesium and zinc intake. The vegetarian should not rely too heavily on cheese as a source of calcium and protein, since it contains a high percentage of saturated fat and no vitamin D. Zinc and iron intake might be low since meat is not included in the diet.

In addition, combining the high-quality protein in eggs or low-fat or nonfat milk products with other plant sources of protein improves the quality of protein in beans, nuts, grains, and seeds. For example, the amino acids in eggs and milk products complement the plant proteins in the following foods:

- Cereals and milk..........whole grain breakfast cereal and milk
- Pasta and cheese ....macaroni and cheese
- Bread and cheese ....cheese sandwich on whole wheat bread
- Beans and cheese ....bean and cheese burrito
- Rice and milk ....brown rice pudding
- Bread and egg..............scrambled eggs and whole wheat toast
- Peanuts and milk.........peanut butter sandwich and yogurt

The Food Guide Pyramid plan remains the same for the lactovegetarian or lacto-ovo vegetarian. The only alteration is for the meat and legume group. Rather than the two to three recommended servings equally divided between extra-lean meats and legumes, now all servings each day must come from cooked dried beans and peas, nuts and seeds, or eggs. A serving of beans or peas is one cup, a serving of nuts or seeds is 2 ounces, and a serving of eggs is two eggs. The balanced diet for a lacto-ovo vegetarian might resemble the following:

- 2 to 3 servings low-fat or nonfat milk or milk products
- 3 to 4 servings protein-rich cooked dried beans and peas, peanut butter, seeds, or nuts
- 6 to 11 servings of whole grain breads and cereals
- 5 to 9 servings of fruits and vegetables, especially dark green leafy, orange, and citrus selections

The Weight-Loss Diet

Weight loss and weight maintenance are dependent on identifying and following a diet and exercise program that balances calories (energy) consumed with calories (energy) used. This regime will vary from individual to individual based on age, gender, history of dieting, genetic conditions, and hormonal or neurochemical variations. Not everyone can maintain the thin look promoted by today's fashion magazines and still remain healthy. But each person can find a personal and desirable weight that also maintains health.

There are no pills, powders, combination of foods or order of food intake, injections, individual foods, or machines that will produce long-term weight loss and maintenance. The only effective long-term eating pattern is a lifelong diet and exercise program. Some quick weight-loss techniques can be dangerous. Some herbal diet pills might cause overactive thyroid. Very-low-calorie diets (VLCD) that contain less than 800 calories must be monitored by a physician because of potential adverse changes in potassium. People who consume a diet that contains less than 2,000 calories also might be deficient in vitamin B1, vitamin B6, vitamin B12, calcium, chromium, iron, magnesium, and zinc. Finally, weight loss that exceeds two pounds a week results in loss of water and lean body tissue (muscle and internal organs) rather than fat tissue.

The best "diet" for weight loss is based on the Food Guide Pyramid plus a minimum of three aerobic exercise sessions each week (at least 30 minutes in length). The minimum number of servings (six whole grains, five fruits and vegetables, two nonfat milk, and two extra-lean meat or legume) provides as little as 1,400 calories, but does not guarantee optimal intake of all vitamins and minerals. The high fiber intake from these foods or from fiber products such as guar gum reduces hunger, possibly by reducing drastic fluctuations in blood sugar levels.

If weight is not lost on this diet, then exercise levels must be increased to either more or longer sessions each week. Further reductions in calorie intake only should be considered with the advice and supervision of a physician. Repeated weight loss and weight gain cycles—called "yo-yo dieting"—results in increasing body fat, making it more and more difficult to lose weight and maintain the weight loss. In other words, repeated unsuccessful attempts to lose weight make a person fatter.

Weight-loss diets must be followed at home and away from home. Suggestions for increasing the vitamin and mineral content and decreasing the fat content of meals ordered in restaurants include the following:

1. Eat something to take the edge off the appetite before leaving home.
2. Locate restaurants where the management will tailor their menu items to meet your needs and prepare each meal to order.

3. Order half-orders or split an order with a friend.
4. Order a la carte.
5. Focus on salad bars, but avoid marinated vegetables, pasta salads, and other ingredients mixed with mayonnaise or other fats.
6. Be assertive. Ask for foods steamed, baked, or broiled dry. Send orders back if they are not prepared to order.
7. Decide ahead of time what to order.
8. Order without looking at the menu.
9. Order mineral water, herb tea, or tomato juice to sip while waiting for the meal.
10. Ask for salad dressing on the side.
11. Avoid the following words: refried, sauteed, au gratin, gravied, fried, a la mode, prime, pot pie, au fromage, hollandaise, crispy, creamed, or cheese sauce.
12. Choose fresh fruit, steamed or raw vegetables, baked potatoes with chives, baked or boiled lean meats and fish, whole grain breads, consomme, barley or vegetable soups, seafood cocktails, pasta with marinara sauce, and fruit ices.
13. Call the local American Heart Association for a local guide to restaurants that serve low-calorie foods.
14. Pay more attention to the conversation than to the food or hors d'oeuvres.

Summary

Many variations on the conventional American diet still can provide adequate amounts of all the essential vitamins and minerals if planned carefully. All diets should contain a variety of foods and all foods should be consumed in moderation. Regardless of whether a diet for athletes, a vegetarian diet, a weight-loss diet, or a more conventional diet is desired, the foundation for food choices is a moderate calorie, nutrient-dense diet that is low in fat, low in cholesterol, low in sugar, low in salt, and high in fiber, vitamins, and minerals. A well-balanced supplement might be needed to guarantee optimal intake of all vitamins and minerals if the daily energy intake is less than 2,000 calories. (See pages 358–362 for guidelines in choosing a supplement.)

CHAPTER 8

Understanding Supplements

No other topic in nutrition has created such heated debates as vitamin-mineral supplements and the appropriateness of their inclusion in the diet. Everyone agrees the best place to obtain the daily needs for essential vitamins and minerals is from a well-balanced diet. However, not everyone is able or wants to consistently consume a diet based on the Food Guide Pyramid's recommendations, and vitamin-mineral status might suffer unless an alternative source of these nutrients is found.

UNDERSTANDING THE TERMINOLOGY

Vitamin-mineral supplements are a multi-billion dollar industry. The great variety of formulas, single-nutrients, or combination preparations in numerous dosages line an entire wall or aisle in many stores. This diversity and variation in products is more confusing than helpful to most shoppers. The hundreds of bottles, jars, individually-wrapped "packs," cans, and envelopes can be overwhelming to someone looking for a vitamin-mineral preparation to meet his or her needs. Words, such as "organic," "therapeutic," "natural," "buffered," or "time-released," further complicate the choice. Choosing a vitamin-mineral supplement to best meet individual needs is simple once the words are defined and a few guidelines for selecting a supplement are provided.

Dietary Supplements Versus Nonprescription Drugs

Most vitamin-mineral preparations are called dietary supplements. These products are designed to supplement a normal diet and to increase the total daily intake of one or more vitamins or minerals. The Food and Drug Administration (FDA) classifies a product as a nonprescription drug if it is promoted on the label or in accompanying literature to cure or treat health conditions, or if the ingredients produce dangerous side effects.

For example, FDA determined from the scientific literature that vitamin K could be dangerous for people on anticoagulant (blood thinning) medications. Consequently, supplementation with this fat-soluble vitamin is recommended only with the supervision of a physician. Therefore, vitamin K supplements are classified as a drug rather than a dietary supplement. Laetrile, a substance promoted to treat cancer and sold as vitamin B17, was banned by the FDA because of the therapeutic claims used to sell the substance and because laetrile contains potentially dangerous quantities of cyanide.

Megavitamin Supplements

Megavitamin therapy is the use of one or more vitamins in amounts exceeding the RDA by 10-fold or more. Megavitamin dosages became popular because of the misconception that if a small amount of a nutrient is good for health, more must be better.

Megavitamin therapy is usually unnecessary and can be expensive and potentially harmful. For example, many of the water-soluble vitamins perform specific functions, usually in conjunction with an enzyme made in the body. These vitamins have no recognized metabolic function by themselves. The amount of a vitamin-dependent enzyme that a cell can make in a day is limited. To consume more of the vitamin than can be used in the manufacture or use of the related enzyme will not stimulate a greater production of the enzyme; instead it will increase urinary excretion of the unused water-soluble vitamin.

Fat-soluble vitamins (A, D, E, and K) potentially can accumulate to toxic levels in the tissues because they are not readily excreted in the urine. Vitamins A and D have shown toxicity symptoms in healthy individuals and vitamin K might be toxic to people on anticoagulant medications when consumed in large amounts over long periods of time. Although megadoses of vitamin E have not been proven toxic, no benefits of large doses (i.e., >800IU) of this fat-soluble vitamin have been proven.

Large doses of certain minerals (several times the RDA) can be toxic if they accumulate in tissues or cause secondary deficiencies of other minerals, and only should be taken with the supervision of a physician and dietitian. For example, large doses of iron (more than 25mg) can cause constipation and other stomach or intestinal upsets and, in some people, can cause hemosiderosis, a disorder characterized by abnormal iron accumulation in the liver, pancreas, and other organs. Large doses of selenium (more than 600mcg) or copper (more than 10mg) also produce toxic symptoms, including nervous system disorders and liver or kidney malfunction. Long-term megadoses of zinc (50mg or more) can produce a copper deficiency because the two trace minerals compete in the small intestine for absorption.

In general, dietary intakes of no more than three times the RDA are probably safe. Doses of 10 to 1,000 times the RDA for long periods of time of even the water-soluble vitamins might have detrimental effects on health. For example, megadoses of:

- vitamin A (retinol) might cause liver damage
- vitamin D might contribute to atherosclerosis, liver damage, and kidney disease
- niacin (nicotinic acid) might cause liver damage
- vitamin B6 might cause irreversible nerve damage
- pantothenic acid might cause diarrhea
- folic acid can mask an underlying vitamin B12 deficiency and result in irreversible nerve damage
- vitamin C might encourage the formation of kidney stones and suppress the immune response
- iron can interfere with zinc absorption
- zinc can suppress the immune response

Size, genetic individuality, age, gender, and numerous other factors contribute to tolerance to megadoses of a nutrient. What is safe for one person could be toxic for another.

Buffered Vitamins

Some vitamins, especially vitamin C, are acidic and, although not strong acids like the hydrochloric acid in the stomach or sulfuric acid, they can irritate the digestive tract when consumed in megadoses. A compound that buffers or neutralizes the acidity of vitamin C can be added to a supplement to counteract the irritating effects. Ascorbate is a form of buffered vitamin C. Sodium ascorbate should be avoided by people who must restrict their salt (sodium) intake, such as people with high blood pressure.

Chelated Minerals

A chelated mineral is one attached to another substance, such as an amino acid, called a chelator. The chelator can be a natural or synthetic substance. Gluconate, as in zinc gluconate, is a common chelator. Chelated minerals are promoted as better absorbed and more available than other minerals. Supposedly, the attached substance, such as the amino acid, enhances the absorption of the mineral from the intestines into the bloodstream. This argument in favor of chelation is based on incomplete information and might be incorrect.

Chelation forms a weak bond between the mineral and the other compound or chelator. This bond is easily broken in the highly acidic environment of the stomach. Once detached from its chelator, the mineral floats freely and independently in the intestine and is absorbed no better (but no worse) than any other supplemental or dietary form of the mineral. The only benefit of chelated minerals, such as iron fumarate or zinc gluconate, is that they are less irritating to the stomach and intestine and less likely to cause stomach upsets or constipation than are other minerals, such as zinc sulfate or iron sulfate, when taken in large amounts. One exception to this general rule is chromium picolinate, which is a chelated form of chromium that is very well absorbed.

Chelation is less important to absorption and utilization of a mineral than are the circumstances associated with taking the supplement. Minerals, in general, are better absorbed if taken with a meal. The presence of other dietary ingredients, such as protein and carbohydrate, stimulate the release of digestive enzymes and juices that facilitate the breakdown and absorption of all nutrients, including minerals. An exception to this rule is iron, which is better absorbed on an empty stomach.

Chewable Vitamins

The most common vitamin available in chewable form is vitamin C. No harm will come from infrequent small doses of this form of the water-soluble vitamin. However, frequent exposure of the tooth enamel to an acidic substance, such as vitamin C, can wear away the enamel and increase the likelihood of dental cavities.

Parents should closely monitor children's consumption of chewable multivitamins. These supplements are sweetened, taste like candy to a child, and if consumed in quantities could approach toxic levels. Children are more susceptible than adults to vitamin toxicities and should not consume more than the RDAs from the combination of wholesome foods, fortified cereals and convenience foods, vitamin-mineral supplements, or other potential sources of nutrients.

Natural, Organic, or Synthetic Vitamins?

Despite the implied wholesomeness of the words "natural" and "organic," in most cases the quality or usefulness of a vitamin is not dependent on its source. The definitions and distinction between these words are either nonexistent or vague.

Vitamins and minerals do not exist alone. They are either manufactured by a plant or microorganism or are synthesized in a laboratory. In many cases both processes occur at one time. For example, vitamins or minerals often are synthesized by using bacteria or yeast to manufacture the substance or incorporate a nutrient from their environment into a more biologically available form. Selenomethionine and chromium from yeast grown on chromium-rich "soil", are the "natural" forms of selenium and chromium, yet are synthesized by yeast in the laboratory. Does that make them synthetic or natural?

Other "natural" vitamins are extracted from foods, such as wheatgerm, by exposure to numerous chemical solvents during both the removal from the original food source and the concentration of the vitamin into a tablet, capsule, or pill. For example, vitamin E is obtained from natural sources, such as the vegetable oils from soy beans, corn, or wheatgerm. Several chemical solvents are required to separate the vitamin from the oil and concentrate it in a capsule small enough to swallow. In addition, preservatives are included in many preparations to prevent decay of the capsule. What began as natural ends up a highly refined and processed product. Does that make them natural or synthetic?

In other cases, the word natural is used on a vitamin-mineral supplement, but the product is manufactured in the laboratory with only a small addition of the natural source. For example, small amounts of bioflavonoids and rose hips are added to large amounts of synthetic vitamin C and the product is called "natural." In reality, natural rose hips contain approximately 2 percent vitamin C and a vitamin C supplement that relied entirely on this source of the vitamin would be too big to swallow.

In contrast, some nutrients start out as synthetic vitamins added to a yeast or other natural base. Selenomethionine, a natural form of selenium, is only formed if selenium is added to the yeast culture and is absorbed and converted to the natural form within the yeast. However, inorganic selenium mixed with yeast is often mistakenly sold as a natural form of the mineral. Natural B vitamins also often are mis-labelled and sold this way.

Theoretically, supplements should be manufactured only from organic food sources. The lack of regulation, however, allows such a loose interpretation of the word that it becomes useless, especially in the case of supplements. Some credibility does exist for organically produced sources of supplemental selenium and chromium. The terms "organic" and "natural" are used to describe the process where these minerals are added to a yeast base where they are absorbed and incorporated into the structure of the yeast. These sources of selenium and chromium might be better absorbed and used by the human body. Otherwise, the term "organic" promises no more than increased cost.

In addition, no scientific evidence exists showing that the body uses organic vitamins and minerals better than it does synthetic forms. Except for selenium, chromium, and vitamin E, the nutrients are identical, and no reliable tests exist to discern a natural from a synthetic vitamin or mineral. The natural selenomethionine, chromium-rich yeast, and vitamin E (d-alpha-tocopherol) appear to be less toxic (in the case of selenium) and more potent (in the cases of chromium and vitamin E) than the synthetic or inorganic sodium selenite, chromic chloride, or dl-alpha-tocopherol.

Water-Solubilized Fat-Soluble Vitamins

The fat-soluble vitamins A, D, E, and K require small amounts of dietary fat, special fat-digesting enzymes from the pancreas, and bile from the liver and gallbladder to be digested and absorbed. The fat-soluble vitamins are easily absorbed by most people, but deficiencies can develop in people with intestinal diseases, such as celiac disease, tropical sprue, cystic fibrosis, or ulcerative colitis. In these disorders, a physician might recommend a water-solubi-lized form of vitamins A, D, E, or K. The vitamin is attached to a water-soluble compound that is easily absorbed in the intestine without the need for the fat-digesting enzymes and bile. Once in the bloodstream, the vitamin portion splits from the attached com-pound and is used like any other form of the vitamin. There is no evidence that this form of the fat-soluble vitamins is better used by healthy people.

Some fat-soluble vitamins, especially vitamin A, are available in an emulsified form. The emulsifier separates the fat-soluble vitamin into tiny beadlets that remain suspended in a watery base, much like the lecithin added to commercial salad dressings that keeps the oil and vinegar from separating. Emulsified vitamin A dissolves more readily in the watery medium of the intestine and is easier for people with the above mentioned intestinal disorders to digest and absorb. Emulsified vitamin A might be toxic at lower doses than other forms of the vitamin and no more than the RDA should be consumed unless monitored by a physician. Again, healthy people do not need to spend the extra money on emulsified fat-soluble vitamins.

Time-Released Supplements

The theory supporting time-released vitamins makes sense. In reality, however, time-released vitamins might be no better, and even might be less effective, than regular supplements.

The time-release theory is based on two important considerations about vitamin and mineral absorption:

1. Vitamin-mineral supplements taken in large doses cause blood levels of the nutrients to rise abruptly. A substantial amount of the nutrient is lost in the urine because the kidneys increase urinary excretion to remove the abnormally high blood concentrations.
2. Anything that slows the absorption of vitamins and minerals would eliminate the rapid rise in blood levels and more of the nutrient would be available for longer periods of time for use in body processes.

Time-released supplements were developed in an attempt to solve this problem. They were to dissolve slowly in the intestine, increase the amount of absorption of a vitamin or mineral, and hopefully reduce the dramatic fluctuations in blood levels. Vitamins and minerals are absorbed at very specific spots along the intestinal tract, however, and unless they dissolve and are available at that point of absorption, they continue to travel down the digestive tract and are excreted. It is chance that a time-release tablet requiring four to eight hours to dissolve will release each nutrient at the appropriate spot for absorption.

In reality, nutrients from time-release preparations are often poorly absorbed. In one study, when niacin as either a time-released or regular supplement was given to patients with high blood cholesterol levels, the regular niacin supplement was more effective in lowering blood cholesterol and other fats than was the time-released tablets. In some cases, therapeutic doses of time-released niacin were reported to be more toxic to the liver than similar doses of regular niacin.

SHOULD YOU SUPPLEMENT?

Most nutrition experts agree that food and the "balanced diet" are the best recommendations for obtaining optimal levels of all vitamins and minerals. Unfortunately, what sounds good in theory does not hold true in practice.

What Do National Nutrition Surveys Report?

People don't consume the "balanced diet." Only one in nine people eat the recommended number of servings of fruits and vegetables. Average calcium consumption in the United States and Canada is ²/₃ of the current recommended level of 800mg. People have increased their consumption of grains, but are more likely to grab a doughnut than a whole wheat bagel. Consequently, sugar and refined flour intake is up, but nutrient-packed whole grains are still low on the priority list.

Even when people follow the guidelines of a "balanced diet," they often make nutrient-poor choices. For example, according to researchers at UC Berkeley who reviewed the data from national nutrition surveys, people are more likely to select French fries than broccoli as a serving of vegetables; hot dogs rather than split peas for a high-protein source; white bread than whole wheat bread for a grain; and a soft drink than a glass of nonfat milk. In fact, sugar intake approaches 25 percent of total calories and fat (according to the latest National Health and Nutrition Examination Survey) approaches 34 percent; consequently 59 percent of our calories are coming from potentially nutrient-poor food sources. All of these food choices equate to sub-optimal vitamin and mineral status, which is supported by nutrition surveys that repeatedly report that Americans are not doing very well when it comes to nutrition (Table 55).

For example,

- Nine out of 10 diets are marginal in chromium.
- Many diets in the United States contain half the recommended amount of magnesium and folic acid.
- Only one person in five consumes adequate levels of vitamin B6.
- Up to 80 percent of exercising women are iron deficient.

Table 55
NATIONAL NUTRITION SURVEYS: WHAT DID THEY FIND?

Survey	Nutrients Low in the Diet
USDA Household Food Consumption Survey	A, C, Calcium
Ten State Nutrition Survey	A, C, B2, Calcium, Iron
NHANES I (1971-1972)	A, C, Calcium, Iron
NHANES II (1977-1978)	C, B1, B2, Iron
USDA Nationwide Food Consumption Survey	A, C, B6, Calcium, Iron, Magnesium
Total Diet Study (1982–1988)	Calcium, Copper, Iron, Magnesium, Zinc

Researchers from Tufts University and University of California at Berkeley report on the inadequate dietary intakes in the United States. For example, according to the National Health and Nutrition Examination Survey (NHANES II),

- only one in every three women reported eating a diet that contained at least one serving of each of the recommended food groups—fruit, vegetables, grains, milk, and extra-lean meat.
- almost one in every five women had two to three food groups missing;
- 46 percent of women consumed no fruit on any four consecutive days;
- 24 percent consumed no milk products;
- 71 percent did not regularly consume at least 2 servings of fruit and 4 servings of grain; and
- as few as 7 percent consumed one serving of dark green leafy vegetable on one of any four days.

As a result, the average iron intake is only 10.9mg/day and calcium intake is only 636mg/day. Half of all women in higher income brackets consume less than the recently lowered RDA for folic acid of 180mcg, while the majority of women in lower socio-economic groups fall far short of folic acid needs.

Women average less than 1,700 calories a day; an energy intake more appropriate for a toddler than an adult. Even with the best nutritional planning, there are no guarantees that the diet will meet the RDA for all nutrients when the calorie intake is below 1,600. For example, a woman must consume 3,000 calories to meet her daily need of 18mg; with calorie needs almost half this amount, it is no wonder women consume too little iron (Table 56).

Table 56
THE DAY'S TOTAL ENERGY NEEDS

The day's total energy use for the average, moderately active female or male could be divided approximately as follows:

FEMALE

Basal metabolism	1,200 calories
Physical activity	600
Digestion of food	200
(assuming food intake of	
approximately 2,000 calories)	
Total calories	**2,000**

MALE

Basal metabolism	1,620 calories
Physical activity	810
Digestion of food	270
(Assuming food intake of	
approximately 2,700 calories)	
Total calories	**2,700**

Beyond the RDAs

The issue has even expanded beyond just meeting the RDAs. While all nutrient deficiency diseases are prevented or cured by consuming even $2/3$ of the RDAs, the prevention or treatment of other disorders often benefit from nutrients supplied in amounts greater than RDA levels (Table 57). Recent evidence that nutrients, especially the antioxidant vitamins, can help prevent chronic disease and age-related disorders is very promising. Yet, some people continue to hold onto the belief that if you can't consume enough of a nutrient from the diet, then you don't need it.

A tidal wave of research in the past 10 years and in particular the past three years, has put the RDAs on the hot seat. Historically, these recommendations were based on the nutrient needs of healthy persons to prevent classic deficiency diseases. But, current research shows that many nutrients contribute to far more than their classic functions. The antioxidants do more than just prevent scurvy in the case of vitamin C, xerophthalmia in the case of beta carotene, or anemia and nerve damage in the case of vitamin E. In fact, the antioxidants may be a fundamental defense system against many chronic diseases and even premature aging.

Medication use, illness, and stress also increase nutrient needs to levels difficult to obtain from even the best diet. For example, oral contraceptives might increase a woman's need for vitamin B6, while stress raises requirements for magnesium, vitamin C, and zinc.

Table 57
THE ADULT RDAS VERSUS OPTIMAL INTAKES

The following RDA and optimal dietary intakes can be derived from diet with or without supplements (except for the optimal intake for vitamin E, which is impossible to obtain from diet alone).

Nutrient	RDA	Optimal Intake
VITAMINS		
Vitamin A/Beta Carotene	800RE–1,000RE	800RE from A 10mg–25mg beta carotene
Vitamin D	200IU–400IU	400IU
Vitamin E	12IU	100IU–400IU
Vitamin K	55–65mcg	65mcg
Vitamin B1	1.0–1.5mg	1.5–5mg
Vitamin B2	1.2–1.3mg	1.3–5mg
Niacin	13–19mg	20–25mg
Vitamin B6	1.5–2.0mg	2.0–10mg
Vitamin B12	2.0mcg	2.0–5.0mcg
Folic Acid	180–200mcg	400–800mcg
Biotin	30–100mcg	100mcg
Pantothenic Acid	4–7mg	7–10mg
Vitamin C	60mg	250–500mg
MINERALS		
Calcium	800–1,200mg	1,200–1,500mg
Chromium	50–200mcg	200mcg
Copper	1.5–3.0mg	3.0mg
Iron:		
men/postmenopausal women	10mg	10mg
premenopausal women	15mg	18–25mg
Magnesium	280–350mg	350–500mg
Manganese	2.0–5.0mg	5.0mg
Molybdenum	75–250mcg	250mcg
Selenium	55–70mcg	200mcg
Zinc	12–15mg	15–25mg

Nutritional Pharmacology

Beyond the issue of marginal deficiencies, or the RDA, or even therapeutic nutrition that attempts to correct nutrient deficiencies, is the realm of nutritional pharmacology. Nutritional pharmacology is the study of the use of nutrients, essential or nonessential, either in their natural chemical form or in a chemically modified form, to achieve a pharmacological effect rather than a nutritional effect. In other words, "Nutritional pharmacology is the study of substances found in foods that might have a pharmacological effect when fed in higher concentrations than normally found in the diet and/or chemically modified form." In this capacity, nutrients do not correct a deficiency but raise serum levels above normal limits.

The research here is quite new and with newness comes ambiguities, incomplete information, and hypothesis. However, much of the current research in nutrition has focused on the effects of pharmacological doses of certain nutrients, especially the antioxidants, in the treatment of certain disorders ranging from cancer to behavioral disorders.

In addition, many studies report that certain vitamins and minerals in amounts greater than current recommendations might help prevent many diseases. For instance, antioxidant nutrients (i.e., vitamin C, vitamin E, and beta carotene) might help prevent and aid in the treatment of heart disease, cancer, cataracts, and numerous other age-related diseases. High dose supplements of vitamin B6 might relieve symptoms of carpal tunnel syndrome, niacin lowers cholesterol, and optimal folic acid intake in the mother prevents neural tube defects.

The Bottom Line

Many people might benefit from a moderate-dose, well-balanced multiple vitamin and mineral supplement. Those that would benefit the most from this insurance include people who consume less than 2,000 calories a day, have irregular eating habits, skip meals, or make poor food choices. Supplements also might be a good choice for those at increased risk for developing nutrient deficiencies, such as pre-menopausal, pregnant, lactating, or dieting women; seniors; and anyone with a chronic illness. In addition, some people who might have increased nutrient needs that are difficult to meet with diet alone, such as people who abuse alcohol and other drugs or who use tobacco, people on long-term medications, under stress, or who have poor eating habits, might consider a supplement. Finally, a well-balanced supplement might fill in nutritional gaps or boost nutrient intake from "just adequate" to optimal levels for generally healthy people who cannot always eat the "perfect" diet.

CHOOSING A VITAMIN AND MINERAL SUPPLEMENT

Vitamin and mineral needs vary widely from one individual to another and even within the same person from week to week. Nutrient needs fluctuate depending on individual variation in the absorption and use of specific nutrients, the adequacy of the diet, age, sex, and confounding factors such as disease, medications, tobacco use, alcohol consumption, and stress (see sidebar below).

Do You Need to Supplement?

Answer the following questions to assess your supplement needs.

1. How often to you eat vitamin A or beta carotene-rich foods, such as spinach, kale, collard greens, broccoli, carrots or sweet potatoes?
   a. less than 5 times a week.
   b. once a day.
   c. two or more times a day.

2. How often do you eat vitamin C-rich foods, such as oranges, orange juice, grapefruit, strawberries, cantaloupe, or Brussels sprouts?
   a. less than 5 times a week.
   b. once a day.
   c. two or more times a day.

3. How often do you eat B vitamin-rich foods, such as nonfat milk, chicken, soybeans, wheatgerm, green peas, or fish?
   a. less than three times a day.
   b. three to five times a day.
   c. more than five times a day.

4. How often do you eat vitamin D-rich foods, such as vitamin D-fortified milk, sardines, salmon, or liver?
   a. once a day or less.
   b. one to two times a day.
   c. more than two times a day.

5. How often do you eat calcium-rich foods, such as milk products, tofu, collard greens, or salmon with the bones?
   a. less than once a day.
   b. one to two times a day.
   c. three or more times a day.

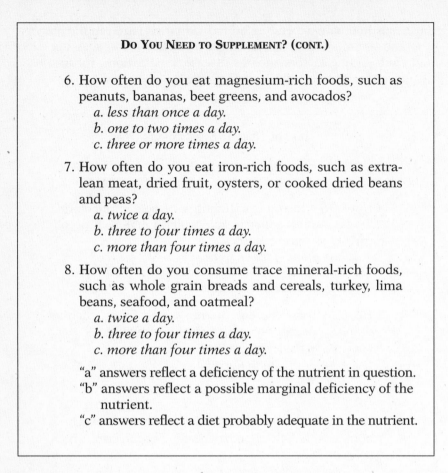

DO YOU NEED TO SUPPLEMENT? (CONT.)

6. How often do you eat magnesium-rich foods, such as peanuts, bananas, beet greens, and avocados?
   a. *less than once a day.*
   b. *one to two times a day.*
   c. *three or more times a day.*

7. How often do you eat iron-rich foods, such as extra-lean meat, dried fruit, oysters, or cooked dried beans and peas?
   a. *twice a day.*
   b. *three to four times a day.*
   c. *more than four times a day.*

8. How often do you consume trace mineral-rich foods, such as whole grain breads and cereals, turkey, lima beans, seafood, and oatmeal?
   a. *twice a day.*
   b. *three to four times a day.*
   c. *more than four times a day.*

"a" answers reflect a deficiency of the nutrient in question.
"b" answers reflect a possible marginal deficiency of the nutrient.
"c" answers reflect a diet probably adequate in the nutrient.

In general, a low-dose, broad-spectrum, multiple vitamin and mineral preparation would meet the needs of most people, would avoid the problems of supplement abuse and nutrient toxicities, and is a convenient, cost-efficient way to supply a balance of nutrients. The following guidelines are designed to guarantee safety and economy when choosing an all-purpose vitamin-mineral supplement.

1. Choose a multiple vitamin-mineral preparation and avoid numerous individual supplements that contain a few nutrients, unless individual nutrients are prescribed by a physician or dietitian. A multiple vitamin-mineral supplement should include the following:
   • the fat-soluble vitamins: A, D, E, and beta carotene
   • the water-soluble vitamins: B1, B2, B6, B12, niacin, pantothenic acid, biotin, folic acid, and vitamin C

- the minerals: chromium, copper, iron, manganese, molybdenum, selenium, and zinc

2. Multiple vitamin-mineral supplements usually do not provide adequate amounts of calcium and magnesium and a separate supplement that provides these minerals in a ratio of 2 parts calcium to 1 part magnesium (i.e., 1,000mg calcium and 500mg magnesium) might be needed if these two minerals are a concern in the diet.

3. Choose a supplement that provides approximately 100 percent (no more than 300 percent) of the RDA for all the vitamins and minerals listed. The delicate balance of nutrients necessary for optimal health is upset by both deficiencies and excesses. Although not always toxic, these excesses can negatively influence other nutrients.

   For example, a multiple preparation that supplies 50 times the RDA for pantothenic acid can increase niacin loss. Large intakes of either iron, copper, or zinc affects the absorption and use of the other two minerals. These nutrient-nutrient interactions can be avoided if a supplement is chosen that supplies approximately the same percentage of the RDA of each vitamin and mineral. Exceptions to the rule are the antioxidant nutrients, which might be beneficial in doses several times current RDA levels. For example, 250mg to 500mg of vitamin C, 100IU to 400IU of vitamin E (as d-alpha tocopherol), and 10mg to 25mg of beta carotene would provide safe levels of these antioxidant nutrients.

4. Avoid supplements that contain unrecognized substances, such as vitamin 15 or pangamic acid, bee pollen, cytochrome C, herbs, octacosanol, hormones, enzymes, or spirulina. Avoid supplements that provide nutrients in minute amounts (less than 15 percent of the RDA). If a substance is listed, such as bioflavonoids, but no amounts are given, assume little or none of the substance is contained in the product.

   Carefully read labels on supplement products and purchase only those products that contain the vitamins and minerals needed. Avoid extras, the vitamins or minerals not needed in a supplement, such as sodium, phosphorus, or chloride. Avoid potentially unsafe inclusions, such as glandular products, hormones, and desiccated organs, that increase the cost, but not the health benefits, of a product. In general, avoid promotional words such as "natural," "organic," "therapeutic," "sustained" or "time-released," or "super potency" or "stress formula." However, minute amounts of starch, sugar, or preservatives in a supplement are relatively harmless.

5. If you are willing to put up with the inconvenience, select a product that can be taken in several doses throughout the day, since nutrients supplied in small doses throughout the day are better absorbed than are one-shot supplements. Multi-dose multiples also provide flexibility; you can adjust the dose to meet your needs.
6. Except for iron, which is best absorbed on an empty stomach, take your supplement with food and without coffee or tea.

Table 58 is an example of a vitamin-mineral preparation that meets the above recommendations.

Table 58
SAMPLE MULTIPLE VITAMIN-MINERAL SUPPLEMENT

2 to 4 tablets daily provide the following nutrients:

Nutrient	Amount	percent of the USRDA
Vitamin A (retinol)	500RE	50
Beta Carotene	10mg	NA
Vitamin D	400IU	100
Vitamin E (d-alpha tocopherol)	200IU	666
Vitamin B1 (Thiamin)	1.5mg	100
Vitamin B2 (Riboflavin)	1.7mg	100
Niacin (Niacinamide)	20mg	100
Vitamin B6 (Pyridoxine)	2mg	100
Vitamin B12 (Cobalamin)	6mcg	100
Folic Acid (Folacin)	400mcg	100
Biotin	300mcg	100
Pantothenic Acid (Calcium Pantothenate)	10mg	100
Vitamin C (Ascorbate)	250mg	416
Calcium (Calcium carbonate)	162mg	15[1]
Chromium (GTF-Chromium)	200mcg	[3]
Copper	3mcg	[3]
Iron (Ferrous)	18mg	100[2]
Magnesium	60mg	15[1]
Manganese	5mg	[3]
Molybdenum	20–50mcg	[3]
Selenium (Selenomethionine)	200mcg	[3]
Zinc (Zinc gluconate)	15mg	100

[1]*This supplement would not supply adequate amounts of calcium and magnesium, and additional supplements of these two minerals might be necessary if calcium and magnesium intake is low in the diet.*

[2]*Men and most postmenopausal women do not need to take extra supplemental iron.*

[3]*No USRDA has been established for these nutrients. The amounts recommended are based on the Food and Nutrition Board's Safe and Adequate daily amounts.*

Supplementation: A Word of Caution

Supplements are considered foods, so the manufacturer is not required by the Food and Drug Administration (FDA) to prove safety and effectiveness. In addition, often supplements are sold by people with a limited understanding of nutritional science. Although FDA strictly regulates label claims, there is no way to regulate what sales-persons claim a product can do. So, a person must do some home-work before choosing a supplement in order to avoid purchasing a poorly made, expensive, ineffective, or unsafe one. The only health claims for supplements currently allowed by FDA are for folic acid in the prevention of birth defects and calcium in the prevention of osteoporosis.

Supplementing the diet with vitamins and minerals has its limita-tions. Supplements cannot substitute for a nutritious and wholesome diet, especially as many substances in foods, other than vitamins and minerals, have been and continue to be identified that promote health and protection against disease. For example, compounds called "indoles" found in vegetables in the cabbage family, such as broccoli, asparagus, and cauliflower, apparently protect against cer-tain forms of cancer. Substances in garlic might help lower blood cholesterol levels and aid in the prevention of heart disease and ath-erosclerosis. These non-nutrient substances are not found in supple-ments.

Supplements will not bestow immunity from disease or prevent premature aging in an otherwise unhealthy body. They are, however, an economical and practical way to ensure adequate nutrition when combined with a nutritious diet or during those times when a person cannot eat the perfect diet (see sidebar below).

YOUR PERSONALIZED SUPPLEMENTATION SHEET

Design a personalized supplementation program based on the analysis of your diet on pages 359–360 and the Sample Multiple Vitamin-Mineral Supplement on page 362. Review the guide-lines for choosing a vitamin and mineral supplement discussed on pages 358–362.

After completion of the Personalized Supplementation Sheet, visit the vitamin-mineral supplement section of the local drug store, supermarket, or health food store. Identify a multiple preparation or a combination of multiple and individ-ual supplements that provide approximately the amounts of each nutrient listed on the sheet. Use the suggested dosage on

---

YOUR PERSONALIZED SUPPLEMENTATION SHEET (CONT.)

the Sample Multiple Vitamin-Mineral Supplement table if an RDA is not listed on the supplement's label.

Nutrient	Amount (mg,mcg,IU)	USRDA	percent of the USRDA
FAT-SOLUBLE VITAMINS			
Vitamin A	_____	1,000RE	_____
Beta Carotene	_____	NA	
Vitamin D	_____	400IU	
Vitamin E	_____	30IU	_____
WATER-SOLUBLE VITAMINS			
Vitamin B1	_____	1.5mg	_____
Vitamin B2	_____	1.7mg	_____
Niacin	_____	20mg	_____
Vitamin B6	_____	2mg	_____
Vitamin B12	_____	6mcg	_____
Folic Acid	_____	400mcg	_____
Biotin	_____	300mcg	_____
Pantothenic Acid	_____	10mg	_____
Vitamin C	_____	60mg	_____
MINERALS			
Calcium	_____	1,000mg	_____
Chromium	_____	50-200mcg[1]	_____
Copper	_____	2mg	_____
Iron	_____	18mg	_____
Magnesium	_____	400mg	_____
Manganese	_____	5mg[1]	_____
Molybdenum	_____	15-50mcg[1]	_____
Selenium	_____	50-200mcg[1]	_____
Zinc	_____	15mg	_____

[1]*No USRDA has been established for these nutrients. The Safe and Adequate ranges determined by the Food and Nutrition Board, National Research Council are used instead.*

Appendix

BODY BASICS

Following is a brief overview of physiology and biochemistry as they relate to nutrition. This introduction is meant to provide a basic understanding of the terms, compounds, interrelationships, and processes involving vitamins and minerals discussed throughout the book.

Atoms and Molecules

The study of nutrition begins with the smallest component of life—the atom. A substance composed of only one atom is called an element. Examples of elements are oxygen, carbon, hydrogen, calcium, iron, and other minerals. The physical properties, such as smell, weight, taste, or color, of any material depend on the arrangement and composition of its atoms.

A molecule is the second smallest component of life and is formed when two or more atoms join. Examples of molecules are hormones, cholesterol, amino acids, fats, carbohydrates such as sugar and starch, all the vitamins, and any mineral joined to another compound such as calcium carbonate or sodium chloride (table salt).

Metabolism

Molecules that are also nutrients, such as vitamins, protein, and fats, are consumed in the diet and stored, broken down, and rebuilt in the body. In addition, other molecules, such as hormones, prostaglandins, neurotransmitters, and other body regulators are formed from dietary and stored nutrients. The total of all alterations in molecules that constitute growth, maintenance, and repair of body processes is called metabolism.

The word "metabolism" originates from the Greek word "metaballein," meaning to change or alter. In short, metabolism is all the processes that allow the body to take apart substances and put them back together in new ways as needed. Metabolic assembly lines composed of a few to thousands of chemical reactions are exact and interconnected and the accuracy of one system determines the outcome of others. The sequence of these reactions is called a metabolic pathway, and proceeds in a step-by-step manner, so a failure at one step affects all following steps.

For example, hemoglobin in red blood cells is a complex molecule comprised of many amino acids, iron, and other substances. The multi-stepped process of making hemoglobin includes one step where vitamin B6 serves as a helper. If vitamin B6 is in short supply, all reactions that follow this step are halted and the hemoglobin molecule is not made. Long-term deficiency of vitamin B6 would result in a reduction in red blood cells and the development of anemia. The efficiency of metabolism depends on the constant availability of all nutrients from both the diet and from body storage.

Energy

Many of the most important concepts in nutrition pertain to energy. Energy is defined as the capacity to do work. Heat, electricity, and movement are common forms of energy. There are two types of energy: active energy is used to perform work much like the active energy in a burning log or the movement of muscles, and stored energy is potential energy such as the stored energy in a wood pile or the fat tissue in the human body.

The ultimate source of energy is the sun. Chlorophyll in plants absorbs solar energy and converts it into chemical molecules, such as carbohydrates. This trapped energy is consumed by animals who further convert it to protein and fats and store these energy-containing nutrients in muscle and fat tissue. The stored energy can be converted to active energy to fuel all metabolic reactions; move muscles, digest foods, excrete waste products, or stimulate nerve cells. Humans ingest the stored energy in plants and animals and either use that energy to fuel metabolic reactions or store excess energy for later use.

Calories

The body is constantly using and producing energy. The unit in nutrition used to measure energy is the calorie (kcalorie or kcal). A calorie is equivalent to the amount of energy (heat) required to raise the temperature of one liter (1,000 grams) of water 1° C. All calories in the body originate from the diet and are supplied by four sources: protein (4 calories/gram), carbohydrates (4 calories/gram), fat (9 calories/gram), and alcohol (7 calories/gram). Vitamins, minerals, and other substances in foods do not supply calories and are not a source of energy.

Basal Metabolism

Most of the energy expended each day is used to maintain normal body processes, such as the beating of the heart, the inhaling of oxygen and the exhaling of carbon dioxide from the lungs, nerve transmission, the production of red blood cells and hormones, and the maintenance of body temperature. This involuntary energy expenditure is called basal metabolism and constitutes most of the daily energy requirement of the body. For the average woman, basal metabolism requires approximately 1,200 to 1,400 calories each day; a man's basal metabolic needs are higher. The basal metabolic rate (BMR) is influenced by many factors. The more muscle a person has and the taller he or she is, the greater will be the basal metabolic rate. Periods of rapid growth, such as pregnancy or puberty also increase BMR.

Physical activity accounts for the second greatest use of energy in the body and varies greatly between individuals. Moderate physical activity requires approximately 30 percent of the total day's use of calories, while the competition athlete may expend more than 60 percent of his or her daily energy in physical activity. This energy is used to move muscles and increase blood flow, heart rate, and breathing. The amount of energy expended during activity depends on the size of the individual and the duration and intensity of the activity. Extra calories are used or "burned" during exercise and for several hours following exercise when basal metabolism increases to repair damaged tissues, build muscle tissue, and return other body processes to pre-exercise conditions.

The third category of energy use by the body is the amount of calories used to digest food. Chewing, secretion of digestive juices, muscular movements of the gastrointestinal tract, and the activation of billions of cells that line the digestive tract account for approximately 10 percent of the day's total energy expenditure (Table 59).

Table 59
THE DAY'S TOTAL ENERGY NEEDS

The day's total energy use for the average, moderately active female or male could be divided approximately as follows:

FEMALE
Basal metabolism ....1,200 calories
Physical activity 600
Digestion of food...200
(assuming food intake of approximately 2,000 calories)

Total calories 2,000

MALE
Basal metabolism ....1,620 calories
Physical activity 810
Digestion of food...270
(Assuming food intake of approximately 2,700 calories)

Total calories 2,700

Enzymes

Metabolism of proteins, carbohydrates (sugar and starch), and fats is regulated by molecules called enzymes. Enzymes are molecules made from protein that catalyze or trigger the rate of chemical reactions. Enzymes are like the equipment on an automobile production line; they speed the assembly process without becoming part of the car. An enzyme assures the two substances connect properly and quickly, so a chemical reaction that might take hours or years to occur randomly will occur several thousand times in a split second with the aid of the enzyme.

Each enzyme is designed for only one type of reaction and each of the millions of reactions that constitute metabolism requires a different, specific enzyme. For example, large food particles from the diet are broken down to their individual molecules by digestive enzymes in the mouth, stomach, and small intestine. Specific enzymes called amylases convert carbohydrates into sugar, other enzymes called proteases convert protein into amino acids. Other enzymes in the body help manufacture hormones, break down substances for energy, and build numerous essential substances needed for life.

Many enzymes are activated or completed by a second molecule called a co-enzyme or co-factor. Many of the B vitamins and some minerals function as co-enzymes. For example, vitamin B1 and vitamin B2 each work with different enzymes in the breakdown of carbohydrates and proteins for energy. Vitamin B6 is a co-enzyme for one of the steps in the manufacture of hemoglobin, the molecule in red blood cells that carries oxygen to all the tissues. Selenium is a cofactor of an enzyme that protects the body against attack by damaging compounds called free radicals.

The Cell

The fundamental unit of the body is the cell. All processes of metabolism, including the breaking down and building up of every molecule and the extraction of energy from protein, carbohydrates, and fats, occur in the cell. Each cell is a minute factory, which processes nutrients for energy, growth, maintenance, and repair.

Cells reproduce and multiply by dividing. A cell grows to a specific size then divides to form two daughter cells. Six divisions later 128 cells have formed and an additional 6 divisions results in more than 8,000 cells. By this process a baby is formed, a child grows, and old or damaged tissues are repaired, while body processes monitor growth so that a person does not continue to grow uncontrollably. By the same process, abnormal and potentially cancerous cells grow and multiply into tumors.

The blueprint of cell division, and therefore the growth and maintenance of all body tissues, is the genetic code within the center or nucleus of each cell. Each cell contains all heredity material for the entire body, but activates only portions of the genetic code to maintain its specific processes. In this way, a kidney cell produces two kidney cells, whereas a liver cell divides to form two new liver cells. Normal functioning of the genetic code and cell replication requires the presence of several vitamins and minerals, including folic acid and vitamin B12.

Cells are organized into tissues (muscle, fat, connective, or nerve tissues), which are further organized into organs, such as the liver, kidney, pancreas, or heart, that may contain hundreds of different types of specialized cells and tissues. Organs that function together are organized into body systems, such as the digestive system containing the mouth, throat, stomach, small and large intestine, and secondary organs such as the gall bladder and liver; or the immune system containing the lymph nodes and vessels, the spleen, the thymus gland, and the bone marrow. Other systems include the reproductive, respiratory, nervous, skeletal, endocrine (hormones and their glands), and excretory (kidney, ureters, bladder, and urethra) systems.

These systems are intimately related and cooperate with each other to maintain health and functioning of the total body. For example, the cells, tissues, and organs of the digestive tract break down complex foods into minute molecules that are absorbed to feed the rest of the body's cells and tissues. All of these systems comprise the human body.

The Digestive System

The digestion and absorption of food occurs along the gastro (stomach) intestinal (small and large intestine) tract or GI tract. The GI tract is similar to a tube within the body that extends about 16.5 feet in length from mouth to anus. It includes the mouth, esophagus, stomach, small intestine, pancreas, gall bladder, liver, and large intestine (colon).

The digestion of food begins in the mouth. Chewing grinds the food into smaller particles and an enzyme called amylase in saliva begins the chemical breakdown of carbohydrates (starch and complex sugars) to simple sugars. The sweet taste sometimes experienced when starchy foods are chewed for a long time is caused by breaking down starch to its component part, sugar. The food is swallowed, travels down the esophagus, and enters the stomach where it mixes with stomach acid and another enzyme, called pepsin, that begins the digestion of protein.

Most digestion and absorption occurs in the small intestine. Food slowly enters the small intestine from the stomach and is mixed with digestive enzymes from the pancreas and intestinal lining, bile from the gall bladder and liver, and other digestive juices. The digestive juices neutralize the highly acidic stomach contents and activate intestinal enzymes. Bile is essential for the emulsification or breaking apart and holding in suspension of fat particles, such as cholesterol, fats, and the fat-soluble vitamins A, D, E, and K.

The small intestine is lined with billions of cells specialized to digest and absorb the end products of digestion—amino acids from protein, sugar from carbohydrates, fatty acids from fats, cholesterol, vitamins, and minerals. Every vitamin, mineral, and other essential nutrient must be recognized and transported across these cells in order to enter the bloodstream and be available to the cells of the body.

The material entering the large intestine is comprised of water, undigested fibers, end products of digestion that were not absorbed, minerals, bile, and other waste products. The large intestine serves primarily as a site for the absorption of water and sodium. No nutrients are absorbed here except for a few vitamins, such as biotin and vitamin K that are manufactured by bacteria living in the large intestine (Table 60).

Table 60
DIGESTION OF NUTRIENTS

Digestive Tract	Digestive Action
Mouth	Food mashed by teeth and mixed with saliva.Small amount of breakdown of carbohydrates to sugars.
Esophagus	No digestive action.
Stomach	Food mixed with hydrochloric acid and enzymes. Small amount of breakdown of protein to small protein fragments called polypeptides.
Small Intestine	Starch and sugar broken down to simple sugars (glucose, fructose, and galactose). Fat broken down to fatty acids, cholesterol, and small fat fragments. Protein and polypeptides broken down to amino acids. Vitamins and minerals released from food as protein, fat, and carbohydrates are broken down to basic parts. Final end products of digestion (sugar, fatty acids, cholesterol, amino acids, vitamins, and minerals) are absorbed.
Large Intestine	Fiber and unabsorbed nutrients excreted. Water reabsorbed into bloodstream. Bacteria synthesize biotin and vitamin K.

In general, if a nutrient is not recognized or absorbed in the small intestine it travels into the large intestine, is excreted, and is useless to the maintenance of a healthy body. For this reason, the GI tract is considered a separate tube within a tube (the body) and eating food does not always guarantee the nutrients will nourish the body.

The Circulatory System

Each of the billions of cells in the body needs a constant supply of oxygen, water, energy, and nutrients. Body fluids, such as the blood, lymph, and the fluid that bathes the individual cells (interstitial fluid) supply the cells with essential oxygen, water, and nutrients, and remove waste products such as carbon dioxide.

The blood is comprised of water, red blood cells, white blood cells, blood cell fragments called platelets, proteins, carriers of fat-soluble substances, minerals, vitamins, and numerous other compounds. Red blood cells are the carriers of oxygen in the blood. White blood cells are important components of the immune system, the body's natural defense system against disease. Platelets are cell fragments important for normal blood clotting and initiate the healing process after an injury such as a cut or a scraped knee.

The circulatory system, comprised of the heart and blood vessels (arteries, capillaries, and veins), is the carrier of blood and its nutrients. The heart pumps blood rich in oxygen and nutrients through the arteries into the tiny blood vessels called capillaries where oxygen and nutrients are released to the cells and the waste products of metabolism are absorbed into the blood. The "deoxygenated" blood is returned to the heart by way of the veins. This blood leaves the heart and is filtered through the tissues of the lungs where carbon dioxide is released and more oxygen is absorbed into the blood. The "oxygenated" blood returns to the heart and is again pumped out to the body to repeat the continuous cycle. The cycle of blood flow is as follows:

Heart ➜ body ➜ heart ➜ lungs ➜ heart ➜ body. . .

Some blood vessels pass by the digestive system and pick up nutrients entering from the small intestine. Water-soluble nutrients, such as the B vitamins and vitamin C, enter directly into the blood. The fat-soluble nutrients, such as vitamins A, D, E, and K, are packaged in water-soluble "bubbles" so they will remain suspended in the watery medium of the blood.

These nutrient-laden blood vessels stop at the liver, which filters the blood and releases only the proper amount of any one nutrient so a constant blood level of nutrients is maintained at all times. Excesses of nutrients are stored in the liver or are converted to other compounds for later release into the blood. This cycle of blood flow is as follows:

Heart ➜ digestive tract ➜ liver ➜ heart ➜ lungs ➜ heart ➜ digestive tract. . .

In addition to oxygen and nutrients, the blood also carries other molecules that function as messengers and regulators of body processes. Hormones, such as insulin, adrenaline, or estrogen, are chemicals produced and secreted from specialized glands in the body called endocrine glands, such as the pancreas, the adrenal glands, or the ovaries. Hormones are released into the blood and influence the activity of another tissue or organ. For example, insulin is released from the pancreas when blood sugar levels are too high. Insulin, with the help of chromium, stimulates the cells to absorb the excess blood sugar, supplies the cells with a usable form of energy, and returns blood sugar levels to normal.

Prostaglandins are compounds produced from fats, such as the fats in fish oils and vegetable oils. Prostaglandins are transported in the blood and regulate numerous body processes, including heart and muscle contraction and blood pressure.

The Excretory System

The body needs a system to dispose of waste products and nutrient excesses produced in the normal metabolism of foods and other body processes. The kidneys serve as the blood purifying and detoxifying system. Blood is constantly filtered through the sieve-like structures of the kidneys where waste products, such as urea, and excess water-soluble vitamins, potassium, and sodium, are removed and the purified blood is returned to the circulation. Waste products and excess fluids are held in the urinary bladder for periodic removal during urination.

The Nervous System

The nervous system is the body's telephone service. Messages from the brain are transported from one nerve cell to another, much like voices are carried through telephone wires. Messages also travel from the body back to the brain so that a constant communication system between the body and the brain is maintained. Touching a hot stove sends signals from the nerve cells at the tip of the finger to the brain and back to the finger, and, in a fraction of a second, the hand is pulled away from danger.

Neurotransmitters are chemicals that transport messages from one nerve cell to another or from a nerve cell to another tissue, such as a muscle. Neurotransmitters are powerful chemicals in the body responsible for numerous physical and behavioral processes, including sleep, pain, mood, and many of the stress responses including increased heartbeat and perspiration. An example of a neurotransmitter is serotonin. Several nutrients are needed to create the neurotransmitters, including vitamin B6.

Conclusion

Most of the body's work is conducted automatically with no help from the conscious mind. Sometimes, however, higher centers in the brain ignore body needs and it is important to do a routine check of the body's health by "listening" to how the body is feeling and acting. Paying attention to how the body responds to foods, the environment, other people, and internal processes, such as stress, is useful in determining the body's needs and in designing an individualized lifestyle that promotes optimal health.

Selected References

CHAPTER 1

Anderson R, Kozlovsky A: Chromium intake, absorption and excretion of subjects consuming self-selected diets. *Am J Clin N* 1985;41:1177–1183.

Dietary Intake Source Data: United States 1976-1980. Data from the National Health Survey, Series 11, No. 231, DHHS Publication No (PHS) 83–1681, March 1983.

Dietary levels of households in the United States, Spring 1965. Agriculture Research Service, US Department of Agriculture, 1968, pp 12–17.

First Health and Nutrition Examination Survey. Public Health Service, Health Resources Administration, US Department of Health, 1971–1972.

Morgan K, Stampley G, Zabik M, et al: Magnesium and calcium dietary intakes of the US population. *J Am Col N* 1985;4:195–206.

Nationwide Food Consumption Survey, Spring 1980. US Department of Agriculture, Science and Education Administration, Beltsville, MD.

Pennington J, Young B: Total diet study nutritional elements, 1982–1989. *J Am Diet A* 1991;91:179–183.

Pennington J, Young B, Wilson D, et al: Mineral content of foods and total diets: The selected minerals in foods survey, 1982–1984. *J Am Med A* 1986;86:876-891.

Polley D, Willis R, Folkers K: Dietary vitamin B6 in college women. *Nutr Rep In* 1985;31:281–285.

Ricketts C, Kies C, Garcia P, et al: Manganese and magnesium utilization of humans as affected by level and kind of dietary fat. *Fed Proc* 1985;44:1850.

Ten State Nutrition Survey. US Department of Health, Education, and Welfare, Health Series and Mental Health Administration Center for Disease Control. DHEW Publication No (HSM) 72-8130-8134, Atlanta, GA.

375

CHAPTER 2

Abou-Saleh M: The biology of folate in depression: Implications for nutritional hypotheses of the psychoses. *J Psych Res* 1986;20:91–101.

Altura B: Hypomagnesemia and vasoconstriction: Possible relationship to etiology of sudden death ischemic heart disease and hypertensive vascular diseases. *Artery* 1981;9:212–280.

Bistrain B, et al: Prevalence of malnutrition in general medical patients. *J Am Med A* 1976;235:1567–1570.

Block G, Abrams B: Vitamin and mineral status of women of childbearing potential. *Ann NY Acad* 1993;678:244–254.

Blumberg J: Nutrient requirements of the healthy elderly: Should there be specific RDAs? *Nutr Rev* 1994;52(8):S15–S18.

Borel M, Smith S, Brigham D, et al: The impact of varying degrees of iron nutriture on several functional consequences of iron deficiency in rats. *J Nutr* 1991;121:729–736.

Brozek J: Physiological effects of thiamine restriction and deprivation in young men. *Am J Clin N* 1973;26:150.

Grobbee D, Waal-Manning H: The role of calcium supplementation in the treatment of hypertension. *Drugs* 1990;39:7–18.

Hambidge K, Walravens P, Brown R, et al: Zinc nutrition of preschool children in the Denver Head Start Program. *Am J Clin N* 1976;29:734.

Pollitt E, Greenfield D, Leibel R: Behavioral effects of iron deficiency among preschool children in Cambridge, MA. *Fed Proc* 1976;37:487.

Potter J, Levin P, Anderson R, et al: Glucose *Metabolism* in glucose intolerant older people during chromium supplementation. *Metabolism* 1985;34:199–204.

Rabinowitz M, Gonick H, Levin S, et al: Clinical trial of chromium and yeast supplements on carbohydrate and lipid *Metabolism* in diabetic men. *Biol Tr El* 1983;5:449–466.

Roden D: Magnesium treatment of ventricular arrhythmias. *Am J Card* 1989;63:43G–46G.

Siminoff M: Chromium deficiency and cardiovascular risk: A review. *Cardio Res* 1984;18:591–596.

Sterner R, Price W: Restricted riboflavin: Within subject behavioral effects in humans. *Am J Clin N* 1973;26:150.

Stich H, Hornby A, Dunn B: Beta carotene levels in exfoliated mucosa cells of population groups at low and elevated risk for oral cancer. *Int J Canc* 1986;37:389–393.

Stryker W, Stampfer M, Stein E, et al: Diet, plasma levels of beta-carotene and alpha tocopherol, and risk of malignant melanoma. *Am J Epidem* 1990;131:597–611.

Willett W: Vitamin A and lung cancer. *Nutr Rev* 1990;48:201–211.

CHAPTER 3

Vitamin A

Barros J, Silveira F, Coelho R: Vitamin A in colon cancer. *Dig Dis Sci* 1986;31:172S.

Butler J, Havens P, Sowell A, et al: Measles severity and serum retinol (vitamin A) concentration among children in the United States. *Pediatrics* 1993;91:1176–1181.

Byers T, Graham S, Haughey B, et al: Diet and lung cancer risk: Findings from the Western New York Diet Study. *Am J Epidem* 1987;125:351–363.

Corbett J, Selhorst J, Waybright E, et al: Liver lover's headache: Pseudotumor cerebri and vitamin A intoxication. *J Am Med A* 1984;252:3365.

Edes T: Beta carotene and vitamin A: Casting separate shadows? *Nutr Rep* 1992;10(2):8,16.

Edes T, Gysbers D: Carcinogen-induced tissue vitamin A depletion. *Ann NY Acad* 1993;686:203–212.

Glasziou P, Mackerras D: Vitamin A supplementation in infectious diseases: A meta-analysis. *Br Med J* 1993;306:366–370.

Kizer K, Fan A, Bankowska J, et al: Vitamin A—A pregnancy hazard alert. *West J Med* 1990;152:78–81.

La Vecchia C, Franceschi S, Decarli A, et al: Dietary vitamin A and the risk of invasive cervical cancer. *Int J Canc* 1994;34:319–322.

Patty I, Benedek P, Deak G, et al: Cytoprotective effect of vitamin A and its clinical importance in the treatment of patients with chronic gastric ulcer. *Int J Tiss* 1983;5:301–305.

Solomons N, Russel R: The interaction of vitamin A and zinc: Implications for human nutrition. *Am J Clin N* 1980;33:2131–2140.

Stahelin H, Gey K, Eicholzer M, et al: Beta carotene and cancer prevention: The Basel Study. *Am J Clin N* 1991;53:265S–269S.

Stehr P, Gloninger F, Kuller L, et al: Dietary vitamin A deficiencies and stomach cancer. *Am J Epidem* 1985;121:65–70.

Verreault R, Chu J, Mandelson M, et al: A case-control study of diet and invasive cervical cancer. *Int J Canc* 1989;43:1050–1054.

Willett W, Hunter D: Vitamin A and cancers of breast, large bowel, and prostate: epidemiologic evidence. *Nutr Rev* 1994;52:S53–S59.

Beta Carotene

Albanes D, Heinonen O, Huttunen J, et al: The effect of vitamin E and beta carotene on the incidence of lung cancer and other cancers in male smokers. *N Eng J Med* 1994;330:1029–1035.

Albanes D, Virtamo J, Rautalahti M, et al: Serum beta carotene before and after beta carotene supplementation. *Eur J Clin N* 1992;46:15–24.

Greenberg E: Retinoids or carotenoids: Is there another choice? *Prev Med* 1993;22:723–727.

Hughes G: The effects of beta-carotene on the immune system in cancer. *Nutr Rep* 1992;10:1,4,8.

Micozzi M, Brown E, Edwards B, et al: Plasma carotenoid response to chronic intake of selected foods and beta carotene supplements in men. *Am J Clin N* 1992;55:1120–1125.

Omenn G, Goodman G, Thornquist M: The beta-carotene and retinol efficacy trial (CARET) for chemoprevention of lung cancer in high risk populations: Smokers and asbestos-exposed workers. *Cancer Res* 1994;54 (Suppl):2038–2043.

Palan P, Mikhail M, Basu J, et al: Beta carotene levels in exfoliated cervicovaginal epithelial cells in cervical intraepithelial neoplasia and cervical cancer. *Am J Obst G* 1992;167:1899–1903.

Palan P, Mikhail M, Romney S: Decreased B-carotene tissue levels in uterine leiomyomas and cancers of reproductive and nonreproductive organs. *Am J Obst G* 1989;161:1649–1652.

Rimm E: Smoking, alcohol, and antioxidants. *Nutr Rep* 1993;11:73,80.

Van Eenwyk J, Davis F, Bowen P: Dietary and serum carotenoids and cervical intraepithelial neoplasia. *Int J Canc* 1991;48:34–38.

Wolf G: Retinoids and carotenoids as inhibitors of carcinogenesis and inducers of cell–cell communication. *Nutr Rev* 1992;50:270–274.

Ziegler R: A review of epidemiologic evidence that carotenoids reduce the risk of cancer. *J Nutr* 1989;119:116–122.

Vitamin D

Abe J, Nakano T, Nishii Y, et al: A novel vitamin D3 analog, 22-oxa-1, 25-dihydroxyvitamin D3, inhibits the growth of human breast cancer in vitro and in vivo without causing hypercalcemia. *Endocrinol* 1991;129:832–837.

Agwu D, Holub B: The proaggregatory effect of 25- hydroxycholecalciferol (25-(OH)D3) on human platelets. *Nutr Res* 1984;4:823–827.

Anderson J, Toverud S: Diet and vitamin D: A review with an emphasis on human function. *J Nutr Bioc* 1994;5(2):58–65.

Brookes G: Vitamin D deficiency: A new cause of cochlear deafness. *J Laryng Ot* 1983;97:405–420.

Cunningham D, Gilchrist N, Cowan R, et al: Vitamin D as a modulator of tumor growth in low grade lymphoma. *Scot Med J* 1985;30:193.

DeLuca H: New concepts of vitamin D functions. *Ann NY Acad* 1992;669:59–69.

El-Azhary R, Peters M, Pittelkow M, et al: Efficacy of vitamin D3 derivatives in the treatment of psoriasis vulgaris: A preliminary report. *Mayo Clin P* 1993;68:835–841.

Feldman D, Skowronski R, Peehl D, et al: Vitamin D receptors and actions in cultured human prostate cancer cells. *J Cell Bioc* 1994;S18D:237.

Gerritsen M, Rulo H, Vlijmen Willems I, et al: Topical treatment of psoriatic plaques with 1,25 dihydroxyvitamin D3: A cell biological study. *Br J Derm* 1993;128:666–673.

Giannini S, Nobile M, Castrignano R, et al: Possible link between vitamin D and hyperoxaluria in patients with renal stone disease. *Clin Sci* 1993;84:51–54.

Irwin J: Hearing loss and calciferol deficiency. *J Laryng Ot* 1986;100:1245–1247.

Komar L, Nieves J, Cosman F, et al: Calcium homeostasis of an elderly population upon admission to a nursing home. *J Am Ger So* 1993;41:1057–1064.

Lointier P, Levin B, Wargovich M, et al: The effects of vitamin D on human colon carcinoma cells in vitro. *Gastroenty* 1986;90:1526.

MacLaughlin J, Holick M: Aging decreases the capacity of human skin to produce vitamin D3. *J Clin Inv* 1985;76:1536–1538.

Mahajan S, Abu-Hamdan D, Prasad A, et al: Zinc *Metabolism. Kidney Int* 1990;34:473.

Morrison N, Qi J, Tokita A, et al: Prediction of bone density from vitamin D receptor alleles. *Nature* 1994;367:284–287.

Need A, Morris H, Horowitz M, et al: Effects of skin thickness, age, body fat, and sunlight on serum 25-hydroxyvitamin D. *Am J Clin N* 1993;58:882–85.

Pence B, Buddingh F: Inhibition of dietary fat promotion of colon carcinogenesis by supplemental calcium and vitamin D. *P Am Assoc Ca* 1987;28:154.

Santos F, Smith M, Chan J: Hypercalciuria associated with long-term administration of calcitriol (1,25-dihydroxyvitamin D3). *Am J Dis Ch* 1986;140: 139–142.

Supplementation with vitamin D3 and calcium prevents hip fractures in elderly women. *Nutr Rev* 1993;51:183–185.

Tsoukas C: 1-25 dehydroxycholecalciferol vitamin D3: A novel immuno-regulatory hormone. *Science* 1984;224:1438.

Villareal D, Civitelli R, Chines A, et al: Subclinical vitamin D deficiency in postmenopausal women with low vertebral bone mass. *J Clin End* 1991;72:628–634.

Vitamin D and insulin. *Nutr Rev* 1982;40:221.

Vitamin D: New perspectives. *Dairy Council Digest* 1990;61(3):13–18.

Vitamin E

Ayres S: Vitamin E therapy and lupus erythematosus. *Nutr Rep* 1986;4:44–45.

Bierenbaum M, Noon F, Machlin L, et al: The effect of supplemental vitamin E on serum parameters in diabetic, post coronary and normal subjects. *Nutr Rep In* 1985;31:1171–1180.

Bjorneboe G, Johnsen J, Bjorneboe A, et al: Diminished serum concentration of vitamin E in alcoholics. *Ann Nutr Med* 1988;32:56–61.

Bunk M, Dnistrian A, Schwartz M: Dietary zinc deficiency lowers plasma concentration of vitamin E. *P Soc Exp M* 1989;4:379–384.

Calabrese E: Influence of dietary vitamin E on susceptibility to ozone exposure. *B Envir Con* 1985;34:417–422.

Chatelain E, Boscoboinik D, Bartoli G, et al: Inhibition of smooth muscle cell proliferation and protein kinase C activity by tocopherols and tocotrienols. *Bioc Biop* 1993;A1176:83–89.

Chuong C, Dawson E, Smith E: Vitamin E levels in Premenstrual Syndrome. *Am J Obst G* 1990;163:1591–1595.

Gridley G, McLaughlin J, Block G, et al: Vitamin supplement use and reduced risk of oral and pharyngeal cancer. *Am J Epidem* 1992;135:1083 –1092.

Haeger K: Long-time treatment of intermittent claudication with vitamin E. *Am J Clin N* 1974;27:1179.

Jandak J, Steiner M, Richardson P: Reduction of platelet adhesiveness by vitamin E supplements in humans. *Thromb Res* 1988;49:393–404.

Knekt P: Vitamin E and cancer: Epidemiology. *Ann NY Acad* 1992;669:269–279.

Kunisaki M, Umeda F, Inogucci B, et al: Vitamin E binds to specific binding sites and enhances prostacyclin production by cultured aortic endothelial cells. *Thromb Haem* 1992;68:744–751.

London R, Bradley L, Chiamori N: Effect of a nutritional supplement on premenstrual symptomatology in women with Premenstrual Syndrome: A double-blind longitudinal study. *J Am Col N* 1991;10:494–499.

Mayne S, Janerich D, Greewald P, et al: Dietary beta carotene and lung cancer risk in U.S. nonsmokers. *J Nat Canc* 1994;86:33–38.

Micronutrient Interactions: Vitamins, Minerals, and Hazardous Elements. Levander O, Cheng L, eds. New York, *Annals of the New York Academy of Sciences,* 1980, vol. 355. pp 249–266.

Munthe E, Aaseth J: Treatment of rheumatic arthritis with selenium and vitamin E. *Sc J Rheum* 1984;103:S53.

Omaye S: Heavy metal-nutrient interactions. Interaction between nutrients and toxicants. *Food Tech* 1982;October.

An overview of vitamin E efficacy in humans: Part 1. *Nutr Rep* 1993;11:17,24.

Paolisso G, DiMaro G, Galzerano D, et al: Pharmacological doses of vitamin E and insulin action in elderly subjects. *Am J Clin N* 1994;59:1291–1296.

Possible role of vitamin E in the conversion of cyanocobalamin to its coenzyme form. *Nutr Rev* 1979;37:332–333.

Reaven P, Witztum J: Comparison of supplementation of RRR-alpha-tocopherol and racemic alpha-tocopherol in humans. *Arter Throm* 1993;13:601–608.

Reddan P: Vitamin E and selenium in exercise-induced tissue damage. *Nutr Rep* 1993;11:9,16.

Rimm E, Stampfer M, Ascherio A, et al: Vitamin E consumption and risk of coronary heart disease in men. *N Eng J Med* 1993;328:1450–1456.

Shklar G, Schwartz J, Trickler D, et al: Regression of experimental cancer by oral administration of combined alpha tocopherol and beta-carotene. *Nutr Cancer* 1989;12:321–325.

Srivastava K: Vitamin E exerts anti-aggregatory effects without inhibiting the enzymes of the arachidonic acid cascade in platelets. *Pros Leuk E* 1986;21:177–185.

Stampfer M, Hennekens C, Manson J, et al: Vitamin E consumption and the risk of coronary disease in women. *N Eng J Med* 1993;328:1444–1449.

Trevithick J, Mitton K: Topical application and uptake of vitamin E acetate by the skin and conversion to free vitamin E. *Bioc Mol B* 1993;31:869–878.

Yau T, Weisel R, Mickle D, et al: Vitamin E for coronary bypass operations. *J Thor Surg* 1994;108:302–310.

Vitamin K

Chlebowski R, Dietrich M, Akman S, et al: Vitamin K3 inhibition of malignant murine cell growth and human tumor colony formation. *Canc Tr Rev* 1985;69:527–532.

Dowd P, Hershline R, Ham S, et al: Mechanism of action of vitamin K. *Nat Prod R* 1994;11:251–264.

Ferland G: Subclinical vitamin K deficiency: Recent development. *Nutr Rep* 1994;12:1–2.

Ferland G, Sadowski J, O'Brien M: Dietary induced subclinical vitamin K deficiency in normal human subjects. *J Clin Inv* 1993;91:1761–1768.

Lipsky J: Nutritional sources of vitamin K. *Mayo Clin P* 1994;69:462–466.

Noto V, Taper H, Yihua J, et al: Effects of sodium ascorbate (vitamin C) and 2-methyl-1-4-naphthaquinone (vitamin K) treatment on human tumor cell growth in vitro. *Cancer* 1989;63:901–906.

Suttie J: Vitamin K and human nutrition. *J Am Diet A* 1992;92:585–590.

Vitamin B1

Goswami S, Dhara P: Effects of vitamin B1 supplementation on reaction time in adult males. *Med Sci Res* 1994;22:279–280.

Lonsdale D, Shamberger R: Red cell transketolase as an indicator of nutritional deficiency. *Am J Clin N* 1980;33:205–211.

Meador K, Nichols M, Franke P, et al: Evidence for a central cholinergic effect of high-dose thiamine. *Ann Neurol* 1993;34:724–726.

Miller D, Hayes K: Vitamin excess and toxicity. In: Nutritional Toxicology. Hathcock J, ed. New York, Academic Press, 1982, vol 1, pp 81–133.

O'Keeffe S, Tormey W, Glasgow R, et al: Thiamine deficiency in hospitalized elderly patients. *Gerontology* 1994;40:18–24.

Powers J, Zimmer J, Meurer K, et al: Direct assay of vitamins B1, B2, and B6 in hospitalized patients: Relationship to level of intake. *J Parent En* 1993;17:315–316.

Ruenwonasa P, Pattanavibag S: Decrease in activities of thiamine pyrophosphate dependent enzymes in rat brain after prolonged tea consumption. *Nutr Rep In* 1983;27:713–721.

Vitamin B2

Bell I, Edman J, Morrow F, et al: Brief communication: Vitamin B1, B2, and B6 augmentation of tricyclic antidepressant treatment in geriatric depression with cognitive dysfunction. *J Am Col N* 1992;11:159–163.

Powers H: The relative effectiveness of iron and iron with riboflavin in correcting a microcytic anaemia in men and children in rural Gambia. *Human Nutr-Cl* 1983;37:413–425.

Kaul L, Heshmat M, Kovi J, et al: The role of diet in prostate cancer. *Nutr Cancer* 1987;9:123–128.

Prasad A, et al: Effect of oral contraceptive agents on nutrients. II: Vitamins. *Am J Clin N* 1975;28:385.

Belko A, Roe D: Exercise-riboflavin relationship. *Fed Proc* 1984;43:870.

Sauberlich H: Interactions of thiamin, riboflavin, and other B vitamins. In: Micronutrient Interactions: Vitamins, Minerals, and Hazardous Elements. Levander O, Cheng L, eds. New York, *Annals of the New York Academy of Sciences*, 1980, vol 355, pp 80–97.

Niacin

Bendich A: Vitamin supplement safety issues. *Nutr Rep* 1993;11:57,64.

Berge K, Canner P: Coronary Drug Project: Experience with niacin. *Eur J Cl Ph* 1991;40:549–551.

Bourgeois B, Dodson W, Ferrendelli J: Potentiation of the antiepileptic activity of phenobarbital by nicotinamide. *Epilepsia* 1983;24:238–244.

Cohen L, Morgan J: Effectiveness of individualized long-term therapy with niacin and probucol in reduction of serum cholesterol. *J Fam Pract* 1988;26:145–150.

The Coronary Drug Project Research Group: Clofibrate and niacin in coronary artery disease. *J Am Med A* 1975;231:360–381.

Odetti P, Cheli V, Carta G, et al: Effect of nicotinic acid associated with retinol and tocopherols on plasma lipids in hyperlipoproteinaemic patients. *Pharmathera* 1984;4:21–24.

Vitamin B6

Amadio P: Pyridoxine and carpal tunnel syndrome. *Nutr Rep* 1988;6:65,70,72.

Bartel P, Ubbink J, Delport R, et al: Vitamin B6 supplementation and theophylline-related effects in humans. *Am J Clin N* 1994;60:93–99.

Bassler K: Megavitamin therapy with pyridoxine. *Int J Vit N* 1988;58:105–118.

Chrisley B, Hendricks T, Driskell J: Vitamin B6 status of a group of cancer patients. *Nutr Res* 1986;6:1023–1029.

Deijen J, van der Beek E, Orlebeke J, et al: Vitamin B6 supplementation in elderly men: Effects on mood, memory, performance and mental effort. *Psychophar* 1992;109:489–496.

Driskell J, Wesley R, Hess I: Effectiveness of pyridoxine hydrochloride treatment on carpal tunnel syndrome patients. *Nutr Rep In* 1986;34:1031-1040.

Eastman C, Gullarte T: Vitamin B6, kynurenines, and central nervous system function: Developmental aspects. *J Nutr Bioc* 1992;3:618–631.

Gridley D, Shultz T, Stickney D, et al: In vivo and in vitro stimulation of cell-mediated immunity by vitamin B6. *Nutr Res* 1988;8:201–207.

Gridley D, Stickney D, Shultz T: Evaluation of cancer patients leukocyte responses in presence of physiologic and pharmacologic pyridoxine and pridoxal levels. *J Cl Lab An* 1989;3:95–100.

Guilarte T: Vitamin B6 and cognitive development: recent research findings from human and animal studies. *Nutr Rev* 1993;51:193–198.

Hagen I, Nesheim B, Tuntland T: No effect of vitamin B6 against premenstrual tension. *Acta Obst Sc* 1985;64:667–670.

Kang-Yoon S, Kirksey A: Relation of short-term pyridoxine-HCI supplementation to plasma vitamin B6 vitamers and amino acid concentrations in young women. *Am J Clin N* 1992;55:865–872.

Kok F, Schrijver J, Hofman A, et al: Low vitamin B6 status in patients with acute myocardial infarction. *Am J Card* 1989;63:513– 516.

Manore M, Vaughn L, Carroll S, et al: Plasma pyridoxal 5'- phosphate concentration and dietary vitamin B6 intake in free-living, low-income elderly people. *Am J Clin N* 1989;50:339–345.

McCullough A, Kirksey A, Wachs T, et al: Vitamin B6 status of Egyptian mothers: relation to infant behavior and maternal-infant interactions. *Am J Clin N* 1990;51:1067–1074.

Meydani S, Ribaya-Mercado J, Russell R, et al: Vitamin B6 deficiency impairs interleukin 2 production and lymphocyte proliferation in elderly adults. *Am J Clin N* 1991;53:1275–1280.

Reynolds R, Natta C: Depressed plasma pyridoxal phosphate concentrations in adult asthmatics. *Am J Clin N* 1985;41:684–688.

Schaeffer M: Excess dietary vitamin B6 alters startle behavior of rats. *J Nutr* 1993;123:1444–1452.

Stampfer M, Willett W: Homocysteine and marginal vitamin deficiency. *J Am Med A* 1993;270:2726–2727.

Turnlund J, Keyes W, Hudson C, et al: A stable-isotope study of zinc, copper, and iron absorption and retention by young women. *Am J Clin N* 1991;54:1059–1064.

Vermaak W, Ubbink J, Barnard H, et al: Vitamin B6 nutrition status and cigarette smoking. *Am J Clin N* 1990;51:1058–1061.

Watts R, Veall N, Purkiss P, et al: The effect of pyridoxine on oxalate dynamics in three cases of primary hyperoxaluria (with glycolic acid-uria). *Clin Sci* 1985;69:87–90.

Williams M, Harris R, Dean B, et al: Controlled trial of pyridoxine in the Premenstrual Syndrome. *J Int Med R* 1985;13:174– 179.

Yin S, Sato I, Yamaguchi K: Comparison of selenium level and glutathione peroxidase activity in tissues of vitamin B6-deficient rats fed sodium selenite or DL-selonomethionine. *J Nutr* Bioc 1992;3:633–643.

Vitamin B12

Allen R, Stabler S, Savage D, et al: Metabolic abnormalities in cobalamin (vitamin B12) and folate deficiency. *FASEB J* 1993;7:1344–1353.

Bell I, Edman J, Morrow F, et al: B complex vitamin patterns in geriatric and young adult inpatients with major depression. *J Am Ger So* 1991;39:252–257.

Bhatt H, Linnell J, Matthews D: Can faulty B12 (cobalamin) Metabolism produce diabetic neuropathy? *Lancet* 1983;II:572.

Freedman M, Tighe S, Amato D, et al: Vitamin B12 in Alzheimer's disease. *Can J Neur* 1986;13:183.

Lindenbaum J, Rosenberg I, Wilson P, et al: Prevalence of cobalamin deficiency in the Framingham elderly population. *Am J Clin N* 1994;60:2–11.

Lossos A, Argov Z: Orthostatic hypotension induced by vitamin B12 deficiency. *J Am Ger So* 1991;39:601–602.

O'Neill D, Barber R: Reversible dementia caused by vitamin B12 deficiency. *J Am Ger So* 1993;41:192–193.

Folic Acid

Bell I: Vitamin B12 and folate in acute geropsychiatric inpatients. *Nutr Rep* 1991;9:1,8.

Bower C, Stanley F, Nicol D: Maternal folate status and risk for neural tube defects. *Ann NY Acad* 1993;678:146–155.

Butterworth C: Folic acid and vitamin C in cervical dysplasia. *Am J Clin N* 1983;37:332.

Butterworth C: Folate-induced regression of cervical intraepithelial neoplasias in users of oral contraceptive agents. *Am J Clin N* 1980;32:926.

Check W: Folate for oral contraceptive users may reduce cervical cancer risk. *J Am Med A* 1980;244:633–634.

Folate deficiency, parenteral caffeine, and cytogenetic damage in mice. *Nutr Rev* 1991;49:285.

Godfrey P, Toone B, Carney M, et al: Enhancement of recovery from psychiatric illness by methylfolate. *Lancet* 1990;336:392–395.

Larroque B, Kaminski M, Lelong N, et al: Folate status during pregnancy: relationship with alcohol consumption, other maternal risk factors and pregnancy outcome. *Eur J Ob Gy* 1992;43:19–27.

Rush D: Periconceptional folate and neural tube defect. *Am J Clin N* 1994;59(Suppl):511S–516S.

Tamura T, Goldenberg R, Freeberg L, et al: Maternal serum folate and zinc concentrations and their relationships to pregnancy outcome. *Am J Clin N* 1992;56:365–370.

Van Allen M, Fraser F, Dallaire L, et al: Recommendations on the use of folic acid supplementation to prevent the recurrence of neural tube defects. *Can Med A J* 1993;149:1239–1243.

Werler M, Shapiro S, Mitchell A: Periconceptual folic acid exposure and risk of occurrent neural tube defects. *J Am Med A* 1993;269:1257–1261.

Biotin

Mock D, Johnson S, Holman R: Effects of biotin deficiency on serum fatty acid composition: Evidence for abnormalities in humans. *J Nutr* 1988;118:342–348.

Pantothenic Acid

Lacroix B, Didier E, Grenier J: Role of pantothenic acid and ascorbic acid in wound healing processes: In vitro study on fibroblasts. *Int J Vit N* 198;58:407–413.

Litoff D, Scherzer H, Harrison J: Effects of pantothenic acid on human exercise. *Med Sci Spt* 1985;17:287.

Vitamin C

Bielory L, Gandhi R: Asthma and vitamin C. *Ann Allergy* 1994;73:89–96.

Block G: Vitamin C status and cancer: Epidemiologic evidence of reduced risk. *Ann NY Acad* 1992;669:280–292.

Chandra D, Varma R, Ahmad S, et al: Vitamin C in the human aqueous humor and cataracts. *Int J Vit Nutr Res* 1986;56:165–168.

Chen J, Geissler C, Parpia B, et al: Antioxidant status and cancer mortality in China. *Int J Epidem* 1992;21:625–635.

Darr D, Combs S, Dunston S, et al: Topical vitamin C protects porcine skin from ultraviolet radiation-induced damage. *Br J Derm* 1992;127:247–253.

Darr D, Dunston S, Kamino H, et al: Effectiveness of a combination of vitamins C and E in inhibiting UV damage to porcine skin. *J Inv Derm* 1993;100:597.

Dawson E, Harris W, Powell L: Affect of vitamin C supplementation on sperm quality of heavy smokers. *FASEB J* 1991;5:A915.

Feldman E, Gold S, Greene J, et al: Ascorbic acid supplements and blood pressure. *Ann NY Acad* 1992;669:342–344.

Frei B: Ascorbic acid protects lipids in human plasma and low-density lipoprotein against oxidative damage. *Am J Clin N* 1991;54:1113S–1118S.

Frei B, England L, Ames B: Ascorbate is an outstanding antioxidant in human blood plasma. *P NAS US* 1989;86:6377–6381.

Gaziano J, Manson J, Buring J, et al: Dietary antioxidants and cardiovascular disease. *Ann NY Acad* 1992;669:249–259.

Gey K, Stahelin H, Eichholzer M: Poor plasma status of carotene and vitamin C is associated with higher mortality from ischemic heart disease and stroke: Basel Prospective Study. *Clin Invest* 1993;71:3–6.

Hallfrisch J, Singh V, Muller D, et al: High plasma vitamin C associated with high plasma HDL and HDL2 cholesterol. *Am J Clin N* 1994;60:100–105.

Hemila H: Does vitamin C alleviate the symptoms of the common cold? A review of current evidence. *Sc J In Dis* 1994;26:1–6.

Hunter D, Manson J, Colditz G, et al: A prospective study of the intake of vitamins C, E, and A and the risk of breast cancer. *N Eng J Med* 1993;329:234–240.

Jacques P: A cross-sectional study of vitamin C intake and blood pressure in the elderly. *Int J Vit N* 1992;62:252–255.

Jialal I, Grundy S: Effect of combined supplementation with alpha-tocopherol, ascorbate, and beta carotene on low-density lipoprotein oxidation. *Circulation* 1993;88:2780–2786.

Johnson M, Murphy C: Adverse effects of high dietary iron and ascorbic acid on copper status in copper-deficient and copper-adequate rats. *Am J Clin N* 1988;47:96–101.

Keith R, Lawson C: Effects of dietary ascorbic acid and exercise on plasma ascorbic acid, cortisol, serum enzymes, blood pressure, and heart rate response in trained cyclists (meeting abstract). *FASEB J* 1991;5:1655.

Manson J, Gaziano M, Jonas M, et al: Antioxidants and cardiovascular disease: A review. *J Am Col N* 1993;12:426–432.

Micronutrient Interactions: Vitamins, Minerals, and Hazardous Elements. Levander O, Cheng L, eds. New York, *Annals of the New York Academy of Sciences*, 1980, vol 355, pp 249–266.

Moran J, Cohen L, Greene J, et al: Plasma ascorbic acid concentrations related inversely to blood pressure in human subjects. *Am J Clin N* 1993;57:213–217.

Okunieff P: Interactions between ascorbic acid and the radiation of bone marrow, skin, and tumor. *Am J Clin N* 1991;54:1281S–1283S.

Oldroyd K, Dawes P: Clinically significant vitamin C deficiency in rheumatoid arthritis. *Br J Rheum* 1985;24:362–363.

Paolisso G, D'Amore A, Balbi V, et al: Plasma vitamin C affects glucose homeostasis in healthy subjects and in non-insulin-dependent diabetics. *Am J Physl* 1994;266:E261–E268.

Papaioannou R, Sohler A, Pfeiffer C: Effect of ascorbic acid and other adjuvants on manganese absorption. *Fed Proc* 1986;45:484.

Pennington E, Kies C, Fox H: Thiamin and ascorbic acid status of humans as affected by use of calcium carbonate, calcium phosphate and manganese gluconate supplements. *Fed Proc* 1986;45:820.

Peters E, Goetzsche J, Grobbelaar B, et al: Vitamin C supplementation reduces the incidence of postrace symptoms of upper-respiratory-tract infection in ultramarathon runners. *Am J Clin N* 1993;57:170–174.

Pru C, Eaton J, Kjellstrand C: Vitamin C intoxication and hyperoxalemia in chronic hemodialysis patients. *Nephron* 1985;39:112–116.

Robinson M, Huemmer P: Effect of a megadose of ascorbic acid, a meal and orange juice on the absorption of selenium as sodium selenite. *NZ Med J* 1985;98:627–629.

Schectman G: Estimating ascorbic-acid requirements for cigarette smokers. *Ann NY Acad* 1993;686:333–346.

Sinclair A, Girling A, Gray L, et al: Disturbed handling of ascorbic acid in diabetic patients with and without microangiopathy during high dose ascorbate supplementation. *Diabetol* 1991;34:171–175.

Stahelin H, Gey F, Eichholzer M, et al: Plasma antioxidant vitamins and subsequent cancer mortality in the 12-year follow-up of the prospective Basel study. *Am J Epidem* 1991;131:766–775.

Trout D: Vitamin C and cardiovascular risk factors. *Am J Clin N* 1991;53:322S–325S.

Vinson J, Possanza C, Drack A: The effect of ascorbic acid on galactose-induced cataracts. *Nutr Rep In* 1986;33:665-668.

Vitamin-Like Factors

Alpha tocopherol, Beta Carotene Cancer Prevention Study Group: The effect of vitamin E and beta carotene on the incidence of lung cancer and other cancers in male smokers. *N Eng J Med* 1994;330:1029–1035.

Bobek P, Ginter E, Jarcovicova M, et al: Cholesterol-lowering effect of the mushroom pleurotus ostreatus in hereditary hypercholesterolemic rats. *Ann Nutr M* 1991;35:191–195.

Cara L, Armand M, Borel P, et al: Long-term wheat germ intake beneficially affects plasma lipids and lipoproteins in hypercholesterolemic human subjects. *J Nutr* 1992;122:317–326.

Clements R, DeJesus P, Winegrad A: Raised plasma myoinositol level in uraemic and experimental neuropathy. *Lancet* 1973;I:1137.

Dietary flavonoids and risk of coronary heart disease. *Nutr Rev* 1994; 52:59–68.

Frankel E, Kanner J, German J, et al: Inhibition of oxidation of human low-density lipoprotein by phenolic substances in red wine. *Lancet* 1993;341:454–456.

Hanaki Y, Sugiyama S, Ozawa T, et al: Ratio of low-density lipoprotein cholesterol to ubiquinone as a coronary risk factor. *N Eng J Med* 1991;325: 814–815.

Helser M, Hotchkiss J, Roe D: Influence of fruits and vegetable juices on the endogenous formation of N-nitrosoproline and N-nitrotheazolidine-4-carboxylic acid in humans on controlled diets. *Carcinogene* 1992;13(12): 2277–2280.

Hertog M, Feskens E, Hollman P, et al: dietary antioxidant flavonoids and risk of coronary heart disease: The Zutphen Elderly Study. *Lancet* 1993;342:1007–1011.

Roe A, Janezic S: The role of dietary phytosterols in colon carcinogenesis. *Nutr Cancer* 1992;18:43–52.

Stavric B, Matula T, Klassen R, et al: Effect of flavonoids on mutagenicity and bioavailability of xenobiotics in foods. *Acs Symp S* 1992;507:239–249.

Tazaki Y, Sakai F, Otomo E, et al: Treatment of acute cerebral infarction with a choline precursor in a multicenter double-blind placebo-controlled study. *Stroke* 1988;19:211–216.

Vinson J, Bose P: Comparative bioavailability to humans of ascorbic acid alone or in a citrus extract. *Am J Clin N* 1988;48:601.

Wattenberg L: Inhibition of carcinogenesis by minor dietary constituents. *Cancer Res* 1992;52(Suppl):2085S–2091S.

Woodbury M, Woodbury M: Neuropsychiatric development: Two case reports about the use of dietary fish oils and/or choline supplementation in children. *J Am Col N* 1993;12:239–245.

Yuting C, Rongliang Z, Zhongjian J, et al: Flavonoids as superoxide scavengers and antioxidants. *Free Rad B* 1990;9:19–21.

Zeisel S, Blusztajak J: Choline and human nutrition. *Ann R Nutr* 1994;14:269–296.

Zeisel S, Da Costa K, Franklin P, et al: Choline, an essential nutrient for humans. *FASEB J* 1991;5:2096–2098.

CHAPTER 4

Boron

Beattie J, Peace H: The influence of a low-boron diet and boron supplementation on bone, major mineral and sex steroid metabolism in postmenopausal women. *Br J Nutr* 1993;69:871–884.

Elliot M, Edwards H: Studies to determine whether an interaction exists among boron, calcium, and cholecalciferol on the skeletal development of broiler chickens. *Poult Sci* 1992;71:677–690.

Fairbrother A, Fix M, O'Hara T, et al: Impairment of growth and immune function of avocet chicks from sites with elevated selenium arsenic, and boron. *J Wildl Dis* 1994;30:222–233.

Ferrando A, Green N: The effect of boron supplementation on lean body mass, plasma testosterone levels, and strength in male bodybuilders. *Int J Sport N* 1993;3:140–149.

Herbel J, Hunt C: Interactions between dietary boron and thiamine affect lipid metabolism. *FASEB J* 1991;5:A1310.

Hunt C, Herbel J, Idso J: Dietary boron modifies the effects of vitamin D3 nutrition on indices of energy substrate utilization and mineral metabolism in the chick. *J Bone Min* 1994;9:171–182.

Naghii M, Samman S: The role of boron in nutrition and metabolism. *Prog Food N* 1993;17:331–349.

Nielsen F: Ultratrace elements of possible importance for human health: An update. *Prog Clin Bio* 1993;380:355–376.

Nielsen F, Shuler T: Studies of the interaction between boron and calcium, and its modification by magnesium and potassium, in rats: Effects on growth, blood variables, and bone mineral composition. *Biol Tr El* 1992;35:225–237.

Volpe S, Taper L, Meacham S: The relationship between boron and magnesium status and bone mineral density in the human: A review. *Magnes Res* 1993;6:291–296.

Calcium

Argiratos V, Samman S: The effect of calcium carbonate and calcium citrate on the absorption of zinc in healthy female subjects. *Eur J Cl N* 1994;48(3):198–204.

Bostick R, Potter J, Sellers T, et al: Relation of calcium, vitamin D, and dairy food intake to incidence of colon cancer among older women. *Am J Epidem* 1993;137:1302–1317.

Bourgoin B, Evans D, Cornett J, et al: Lead content in 70 brands of dietary calcium supplements. *Am J Pub He* 1993;83:1155–1160.

Carroll K, Jacobson E, Eckel L, et al: Calcium and carcinogenesis of the mammary gland. *Am J Clin N* 1991;54:206S–208S.

Denke M, Fox M, Schulte M: Short-term dietary calcium fortification increases fecal saturated fat content and reduces serum lipids in men. *J Nutr* 1993;123:1047–1053.

Levy J, Gavin J, Sowers J: Diabetes Mellitus: A disease of abnormal cellular calcium Metabolism? *Am J Med* 1994;96:260–270.

Lipkin M, Newmark H: Calcium and colon cancer. *Nutr Rev* 1993;51:213.

Licata A, Jones-Gall D: Effect of supplemental calcium on serum and urinary calcium in osteoporosis patients. *J Am Col N* 1992;11:164–167.

Matkovie V, Ilich J: Calcium requirements for growth: Are current recommendations adequate? *Nutr Rev* 1993;51:171–180.

McCarron D, Morris C, Bukoski R: The calcium paradox of essential hypertension. *Am J Med* 1987;82:27–33.

McCarron K, Reusser M: The integrated effects of electrolytes on blood pressure. *Nutr Rep* 1991;9:57,62,64.

Nolan C, DeGoes J, Alfrey A: Aluminum and lead absorption from dietary sources in women ingesting calcium citrate. *South Med J* 1994;87(9): 894–898.

Slob I, Lambregts J, Schuit A, et al: Calcium intake and 28-year gastro-intestinal cancer mortality in Dutch civil servants. *Int J Canc* 1993;54:20–25.

Spencer H, Kramer L: NIH Concensus Conference: Osteoporosis. *J Nutr* 1986;116:316–319.

Stemmerman G, Nomura A, Chyou P: The influence of dairy and non-dairy calcium on subsite large-bowel cancer risk. *Dis Colon Rec* 1990;33:190–194.

Weaver C: Age related calcium requirements due to changes in absorption and utlilization. *J Nutr* 1994;124:1418–1425.

Whiting S: Safety of some calcium supplements questioned. *Nutr Rev* 1994;52:95–97.

Whittaker P, Cook J: The effect of calcium supplementation on iron absorption in healthy subjects. *Am J Clin N* 1988;47:773.

Chromium

Abraham A, Brooks B, Eylath U: The effects of chromium supplementation on serum glucose and lipids in patients with and without non-insulin-dependent diabetes. *Metabolism* 1992;41:768–771.

Anderson R: Chromium and its role in lean body mass and weight reduction. *Nutr Rep* 1993;11:41,46,48.

Anderson R, Kozlovsky A, Moser P: Effects of diets high in simple sugars on urinary chromium excretion of humans. *Fed Proc* 1985;44:751.

Cohen M, Kargacin B, Klein C, et al: Mechanisms of chromium carcinogenicity and toxicity. *Cr R Toxic* 1993;23:255–281.

Katz S, Salem H: The toxicology of chromium with respect to its chemical speciation: A review. *J Appl Toxicol* 1993;13:217–224.

Kuligowski J, Halperin K: Stainless steel cookware as a significant source of nickel, chromium, and iron. *Arch Env C* 1992;23:211–215.

Mertz W: Chromium in human nutrition: A review. *J Nutr* 1993;123:626–633.

Mertz W: Chromium history and nutritional importance. *Biol Tr El* 1992;32:3–7.

Morris B, Blumsohn A, MacNeil S, et al: The trace element chromium—a role in glucose homeostasis. *Am J Clin N* 1992;55:989–991.

Copper

Harris E: Copper as a cofactor and regulator of copper, zinc, superoxide dismutase. *J Nutr* 1992;122:636–640.

He J, Tell G, Tang Y, et al: Relation of serum zinc and copper to lipids and lipoproteins: The Yi people study. *J Am Col N* 1992;11:74–78.

Hoffman H, Phyliky R, Flemming C: Zinc-induced copper deficiency. *Am J Clin N* 1988;94:508–512.

Koo S, Lee C, Stone W, et al: Effect of copper deficiency on the plasma clearance of native and acetylated human low density lipoproteins. *J Nutr Bioc* 1992;3:45–50.

Lampi K, Mathias M, Allen K: The role of dietary copper in prostaglandin synthesis. *Fed Proc* 1986;45:237.

Medeiros D, Davidson J, Jenkins J: A unified perspective on copper deficiency and cardiomyopathy. *P Soc Exp M* 1993;203:262–273.

Oleske J: Plasma zinc and copper in primary and secondary immunodeficiency disorders. *Biol Tr El* 1983;5:189–194.

Olin K, Walter R, Keen C: Copper deficiency affects selenoglutathione peroxidase and selenodeiodinase activities and antioxidant defense in weanling rats. *Am J Clin N* 1994;59:654–658.

Rayssiguier Y, Gueux E, Bussiere L, et al: Copper deficiency increases the susceptibilty of lipoproteins and tissues to peroxidation in rats. *J Nutr* 1993;123:1343–1348.

Salonen J, Salonen R, Korpela H, et al: Serum copper and the risk of acute myocardial infarction: A prospective population study in men in eastern Finland. *Am J Epidem* 1991;134:268–276.

Strause L, Andon M, Howard G, et al: Dietary calcium intake, serum copper concentration, and bone density in postmenopausal women. *FASEB J* 1991;5:A576.

Sun S, O'Sell B: Low copper status of rats affects polyunsaturated fatty acid composition of brain phospholipids unrelated to neuropathology. *J Nutr* 1992;122:65–73.

The Electrolytes: Sodium, Potassium, and Chloride

Bell R, Eldrid M, Watson F: The influence of NaCl and KCl on urinary calcium excretion in healthy young women. *Nutr Res* 1992;12:17–26.

Elliott P: Observational studies of salt and blood pressure. *Hypertensio* 1991;17:I1–I3.

He J, Tell G, Tang Y, et al: Effect of dietary electrolytes upon calcium excretion: The Yi People Study. *J Hyperten* 1992;10:671–676

Langford H: Sodium-potassium interaction in hypertension and hypertensive cardiovascular disease. *Hypertension* 1991;17(suppl):I155–I157.

Norbiato G, Bevilacqua M, Meroni R, et al: Effects of potassium supplementation on insulin binding and insulin action in human obesity: Protein-modified fast and refeeding. *Eur J Cl In* 1984;14:414–419.

Reppert M, Diehl J, Kolloch R, et al: Short-term dietary sodium restriction increase serum lipids and insulin in salt-sensitive and salt-resistant normotensive adults. *Klin Woch* 1991;69(Suppl XXV):51–57.

Fluoride

Dambacher M, Ittner J, Ruegsegger P: Long-term fluoride therapy of postmenopausal osteoporosis. *Bone* 1986;7:199–205.

Iron

Ascherio A, Willett W, Rimm E, et al: Dietary iron intake and risk of coronary disease among men. *Circulation* 1994;89:969–974.

Beard J, Connor J, Jones B: Iron in the brain. *Nutr Rev* 1993;51:157–170.

Beard J: Are we at risk for heart disease because of normal iron status? *Nutr Rev* 1992;51:112–115.

Finch C: Regulators of iron balance in humans. *Blood* 1994;84(6):1697–1702.

Fordy J, Benton D: Does low iron status influence psychological functioning? *J Hum Nu D* 1994;7:127–133.

Gavin M, McCarthy D, Garry P: Evidence that iron stores regulate iron absorption—a setpoint theory. *Am J Clin N* 1994;59:1376–1380.

Hallberg L, Rossander-Hulten L: Iron requirements in menstruating women. *Am J Clin N* 1991;54:1047–1058.

Hunt J, Gallagher S, Johnson L: Effect of ascorbic acid on apparent iron absorption by women with low iron stores. *Am J Clin N* 1994;59:1381–1385.

Hunt J, Zito C, Erjavec J, et al: Severe or marginal iron deficiency affects spontaneous physical activity in rats. *Am J Clin N* 1994;59:413–418.

Idjradinata P, Pollitt E: Reversal of developmental delays in iron-deficient anaemic infants treated with iron. *Lancet* 1993;341:1–4.

Lozoff B, Jimenez E, Wolf A: Long-term developmental outcome of infants with iron deficiency. *N Eng J Med* 1991;325;687–694.

Newhouse I, Clement D, Lai C: Effects of iron supplementation and discontinuation on serum copper, zinc, calcium, and magnesium levels in women. *Med Sci Spt* 1993;25:562–571.

Pollitt E: Iron deficiency and cognitive function. *Ann R Nutr* 1993;13:521–537.

Rimm E, Ascherio A, Stampfer M, et al: Dietary iron and risk of coronary disease among men (Meeting Abstract). *Circulation* 1993;87:692.

Salonen J, Nyyssonen K, Korpela H, et al: High stored iron levels are associated with excess risk of myocardial infarction in Eastern Finnish men. *Circulation* 1992;86:803–811.

Stevens R, Graubard B, Micozzi M, et al: Moderate elevation of body iron level and increased risk of cancer occurrence and death. *Int J Canc* 1994;56:364–369.

Thibault H, Galan P, Selz F, et al: The immune response in iron-deficient young children: Effect of iron supplementation on cell mediated iummunity. *Eur J Ped* 1993;152:120–124.

Willis W, Gohil K, Brooks G, et al: Iron deficiency: Improved exercise performance within 15 hours of iron treatment in rats. *J Nutr* 1990;120:909–916.

Magnesium

Abraham G, Lubran M: Serum and red cell magnesium levels in patients with premenstrual tension. *Am J Clin N* 1981;34:2364–2366.

England M, Gordon G, Salem M, et al: Magnesium administration and dysrhythmias after cardiac surgery. *J Am Med A* 1992;268:2395–2402.

Ericsson Y, Angmar-Mansson B, Flores M: Urinary mineral ion loss after sugar ingestion. *Bone Miner* 1990;9:233–237.

Fischer P, Belonje B, Giroux: Magnesium status and excretion in age-matched subjects with normal and elevated blood pressures. *Clin Bioch* 1993;26:207–211.

Landon R, Young E: Role of magnesium in regulation of lung function. *J Am Diet A* 1993;93:674–677.

Morgan K, Stampley G, Zabik M, et al: Magnesium and calcium dietary intakes of the US population. *J Am Col N* 1985;4:195–206.

Neglen P, Qvarfordt P, Eklof B: Peroral magnesium hydroxide therapy and intermittent claudication. *VASA* 1985;14:285–288.

Orlov M, Brodsky M, Douban S: A review of magnesium, acute myocardial infarction and arrhythmia. *J Am Col N* 1994;13:127–132.

Seelig M: Cardiovascular consequences of magnesium deficiency and loss: Pathogenesis, prevalence and manifestations—magnesium and chloride loss in refractory potassium repletion. *Am J Card* 1989;63:4G–20G.

Shechter M, Kaplinsky E, Rabinowitz B: The rationale of magnesium supplementation in acute myocardial infarction. *Arch In Med* 1992;152:2189–2194.

Sherwood R, Rocks B, Stewart A, et al: Magnesium and the Premenstrual Syndrome. *Ann Clin Bi* 1986;23:667–670.

Whang R, Whang D, Ryan M: Refractory potassium repletion. *Arch In Med* 1992;152:40–45.

Witteman J, Grobbee D, Derkx F, et al: Reduction of blood pressure with oral magnesium supplementation in women with mild to moderate hypertension. *Am J Clin N* 1994;60:129–135.

Manganese

Baly D, Schneiderman J, Garcia-Welsh A: Effect of manganese deficiency on insulin binding, glucose transport and metabolism in rat adipocytes. *J Nutr* 1990;120:1075–1079.

Davis C, Greger J: Longitudinal changes on manganese-dependent superoxide dismutase and other indices of manganese and iron status in women. *Am J Clin N* 1992;55:747–752.

Saltman P, Strause L: The role of manganese in bone metabolism. *Nutr Rep* 1987;5:33,40.

Selenium

Benton D, Cook R: The impact of selenium supplementation on mood. *Biol Psychi* 1991;29:1092–1098.

Burke K, Combs G, Gross E, et al: The effects of topical and oral L-selenomé-thionine on pigmentation and skin cancer induced by ultraviolet irradiation. *Nutr Cancer* 1992;17:123–137.

Cahill R, O'Sullivan K, Beattie S, et al: Long term beneficial effects of selenium and vitamin C on colonic crypt cell proliferation. *Gastroenty* 1993;104:1032.

Combs G: Essentiality and toxicity of selenium with respect to recommended dietary allowances and reference doses. *Sc J Work E* 1993;19:119–121.

Kok F, Hoffman A, Witteman J, et al: Decreased selenium levels in acute myocardial infarction. *J Am Med A* 1989;261:1161–1164.

Maloney G, Salbe A, Levander O: Selenium (Se) as sodium selanate (NaSeO4) is more toxic than selenium as L-selenomethionine (SeMet) in methionine deficiency rats. *Clin Res* 1988;36:A763.

Peretz A, Neve J, Famaey J: Selenium in rheumatic disease. *Sem Arth Rheum* 1991;20:305–316.

Salonen J, Salonen R, Seppanen K, et al: Relationship of serum Se and antioxidants to plasma lipoproteins, platelet aggregability and prevalent ischemic heart disease in Eastern Finnish men. *Atheroscler* 1988;70:155–160.

Thomson O, Robinson M, Butler J, et al: Long-term supplementation with selenate and selenomethionine: Selenium and glutathione peroxidase in blood components of New Zealand women. *Br J Nutr* 1993;69:577–588.

Thuluvath P, Triger D: Selenium and chronic liver disease. *J Hepatol* 1992;14:176.

van 't Veer P, van der Wielen R, Kok F, et al: Selenium in diet, blood, and toenails in relation to breast cancer: A case-control study. *Am J Epidem* 1990;131:987–994.

Zinc

Eby G: Reduction in duration of common colds by zinc gluconate lozenges in a double blind study. *Antimicrobial Agents and Chemotherapy* 1984;25:20–24.

Johnson J, Walker P: Zinc and iron utilization in young women consuming a beef-based diet. *J Am Diet A* 1992;92:1474–1478.

Keen C, Taubeneck M, Daston G, et al: Primary and secondary zinc deficiency as factors underlying abnormal CNS development. *Ann NY Acad* 1993;678:37–47.

McClain C, Stuart M, Vivian B, et al: Zinc status before and after zinc supplementation of eating disorder patients. *J Am Col N* 1992;11:694–700.

Nakamura T, Nishiyama S, Furagolshi-Suginohara Y, et al: Mild-to-moderate zinc-deficiency in short children: Effects of zinc supplementation on linear growth velocity. *J Pediat* 1993;123:65–69.

Prasad A: Essentiality and toxicity of zinc. *Sc J Work E* 1993;19 (suppl 1):134–136.

Sandstead H: Zinc requirements, the recommended dietary allowance and the reference dose. *Sc J Work E* 1993;19(suppl 1):128–131.

Sandstead H: Zinc deficiency: A public health problem? *Am J Dis Ch* 1991;145:853–859.

Siewicki T, Sydlowski J, Van Dolah F, et al: Influence of dietary zinc and cadmium on iron bioavailability in mice and rats: Oyster versus salt sources. *J Nutr* 1986;116:281–289.

Singh K, Zaldi S, Ralsuddin S, et al: Effect of zinc on immune function and host resistance against infection and tumor challenge. *Immunoph Im* 1992;14:813–840.

Walsh C, Sandstead H, Prasad A, et al: Zinc: Health effects and research priorities for the 1990s. *Envir H Per* 1994;102:5–46.

Additional Trace Minerals

Allen V, Robinson K, Hembry F: Effects of ingested aluminum sulfate on serum magnesium and the possible relationship to hypomagnesemic tetany. *Nutr Rep In* 1984;29:107.

Lione A, Allen P, Smith J: Aluminum coffee percolators as a source of dietary aluminum. *Food Chem T* 1984;22:265–268.

Eggleston D: Effect of dental amalgam and nickel alloys on T-lymphocytes: Preliminary report. *J Pros Dent* 1984;51:617.

Abraham J: The effect of dental amalgam restorations on blood mercury levels. *J Dent Res* 1984;63:71–73.

Carlisle E: Biochemical and morphological changes associated with long bone abnormalities in silicon deficiency. *J Nutr* 1980;110:1046–1055.

Carlisle E: A silicon requirement for normal skull formation. *J Nutr* 1980;110:352–359.

French R, Jones P: Role of vanadium in nutrition: metabolism, essentiality and dietary considerations. *Life Sci* 1993;52:339–346.

Hegsted M, Keenan M, Siver F, et al: Effect of boron on vitamin D deficient rats. *Biol Tr El* 1991;28:243.

Hunt C, Herbel J, Idso J: Dietary boron modifies the effects of vitamin D3 nutrition on indices of energy substrate utilization and mineral metabolism in the chick. *J Bone Min* 1994;9:171–181.

Nielsen F: Ultratrace elements of possible importance for human health: An update. *Prog Clin Bio* 1993;380:355–376.

Uthus E, Nielsen F: Determination of the possible requirement and reference dose levels for arsenic in humans. *Sc J Work E* 1993;19(suppl 1):137–138.

CHAPTER 5

Introduction

Allard J, Royall D, Kurian R: Effects of beta carotene supplementation on lipid peroxidation in humans. *Am J Clin N* 1994;59:884–890.

Ames B, Shigenaga M, Hagen T: Oxidants, antioxidants, and the degenerative disease of aging. *P NAS US* 1993;90:7915–7922.

Diplock A: Antioxidant nutrients and disease prevention: An overview. *Am J Clin N* 1991;53:189S–193S.

Herbaczynska-Cedro K, Wartanowicz M, Panczenko-Kresowska B, et al: Inhibitory effect of vitamin C and vitamin E on the oxygen free-radical production in human polymorphonuclear leucocytes. *Eur J Cl In* 1994;24:316–319.

Pandey D, Shekelle R, Tangney C, et al: Dietary vitamin C and beta carotene and risk of death in middle-aged men: The Western Electric Study. *Am J Epidem* 1994;139:S56.

Sies H, Stahl W, Sundquist A: Antioxidant functions of vitamins: vitamins E and C, beta carotene, and other carotenoids. *Ann NY Acad* 1992;669:7–20.

Weikinger K, Eckl P: Vitamin C and vitamin E acetate efficiently reduce oxidative chromosome damage. *Mutat Res* 1993;291:284–285.

Vitamins, Minerals, and the Immune System

Bendich A: Beta carotene and the immune response. *P Nutr Soc* 1991;50:263–274.

Chandra R, Kumari S: Nutrition and immunity: An overview. *J Nutr* 1994;124:1433S–1435S.

Chandra R: Symposium on "Nutrition and immunity in serious illness." *P Nutr Soc* 1993;52:77–84.

Chandra R: Effect of vitamin and trace-element supplementation on immune responses and infection in elderly subjects. *Lancet* 1992;340:1124–1127.

Glasziou P, Mackerras D: Vitamin A supplementation in infectious diseases: A meta-analysis. *Br Med J* 1993;306:366–370.

Jacob R, Kelley D, Pianalto F, et al: Immunocompetence and oxidant defense during ascorbate depletion of healthy men. *Am J Clin N* 1991;54:1302S–1309S.

Kusaka Y, Kondou H, Morimoto K: Healthy lifestyles are associated with higher natural killer cell activity. *Prev Med* 1992;21:602–615.

Pasatiempo A, Abaza M, Taylor C, et al: Effects of timing and dose of vitamin A on tissue retinol concentrations and antibody production in the previously vitamin A-depleted rats. *Am J Clin N* 1992;55:443–451.

Rall L, Meydani S: Vitamin B6 and immune competence. *Nutr Rev* 1993;51:217–225.

Ross A: Vitamin A status: Relationship to immunity and the antibody response. *P Soc Exp M* 1992;200:303–320.

Semba R: Vitamin A, immunity, and infection. *Clin Inf D* 1994;19(3): 489–499.

Sherman A: Zinc, copper, and iron nutriture and immunity. *J Nutr* 1992;122:604–609.

Tanaka S, Inoue S, Isoda F, et al: Impaired immunity in obesity: Suppressed but reversible lymphocyte responsiveness. *Int J Obes* 1993;17:631–636.

Umegaki K, Ikegami S, Inoue K, et al: Beta carotene prevents x-ray induction of micronuclei in human lymphocytes. *Am J Clin N* 1994;59:409–412.

van Poppel G, Spanhaak S, Ockhuizen T: Effect of beta carotene on immunological indexes in healthy male smokers. *Am J Clin N* 1993;57:402–407.

Yang S, Smith C, Prahl J, et al: Vitamin D deficiency suppresses cell-mediated immunity in vivo. *Arch Bioch* 1993;303:98–106.

Zinc and immunity. *Nutr* 1994;10:79–80.

Acne

Rebello T, Atherton D, Holden C: The effect of oral zinc administration on sebum free fatty acids in acne vulgaris. *Act Der Ven* 1986;55:305–310.

Acquired Immunodeficiency Syndrome (AIDS)

Baker D: Cellular antioxidant status and human immunodeficiency virus replication. *Nutr Rev* 1992;50:15–17.

Baum M, Cassetti L, Bonvehi P, et al: Inadequate dietary intake and altered nutrition status in early HIV-1 infection. *Appl Nutr Inv* 1994;10:16–20.

Butterworth R, Gaudreau C, Vincelette J, et al: Thiamine deficiency in AIDS. *Lancet* 1991;338:1086.

Baum M, Shor-Posner G, Bonvehi P, et al: Influence of HIV infection on vitamin status and requirements. *Ann NY Acad* 1992;669:165–174.

Calabrese L, LaPerriere A: Human immunodeficiency virus infection, exercise, and athletics. *Sport Med* 1993;15:6–12.

Cirelli A, Ciardi M, De Simone C, et al: Serum selenium concentration and disease progress in patients with HIV infection. *Clin Bioch* 1991;24:211–214.

Coodley G, Coodley M, Nelson H: Micronutrient concentrations in the HIV wasting syndrome. *AIDS* 1993;7:1595–1600.

Dowling S, Lambe J, Mulcahy F: Vitamin B12 and folate status in human immunodeficiency virus infection. *Eur J Clin N* 1993;47:803–807.

Sworkin B: Selenium deficiency in HIV-infection and the acquired immunodeficiency syndrome (AIDS). *Chem-Bio In* 1994;91(2–3):181–186.

Favier A, Sappey C, LeClerc P, et al: Antioxidant status and lipid peroxidation in patients infected with HIV. *Chem-Bio In* 1994;91(2–3):165–180.

Garewal H, Ampel N, Watson R, et al: A preliminary trial of beta-carotene in subjects infected with the human immunodeficiency virus. *J Nutr* 1992;122:728–732.

Herzlich B, Schiano T: Reversal of apparent AIDS dementia complex following treatment with vitamin B12. *J Intern M* 1993;233:495–497.

Jain V, Chandra R: Does nutritional deficiency predispose to acquired immune deficiency syndrome? *Nutr Res* 1984;4:537–543.

Kemp F, Skurnick J, Baker H, et al: Antioxidant nutrition in HIV infection. *FASEB J* 1994;8:A949.

Kieburtz K, Giang D, Schiffer R, et al: Abnormal vitamin B12 metabolism in human immunodeficiency virus infection. *Arch Neurol* 1991;48:312–314.

Odeh M: The role of zinc in acquired immunodeficiency syndrome. *J Int Med* 1992;231:463–469.

Semba R, Graham N, Calalla W, et al: Increased mortality associated with vitamin A deficiency during human immunodeficiency virus type 1 infection. *Arch In Med* 1993;153:2149–2154.

Summerbell C: Nutrition and HIV infection. *Practition* 1994;238:558–562.

Tang A, Graham N, Kirby A, et al: Dietary micronutrient intake and risk of progression to acquired immunodeficiency syndrome (AIDS) in human immunodeficiency virus type 1 (HIV-1)-infected homosexual men. *Am J Epidem* 1993;138:937–951.

Ullrich R, Schneider T, Heise W, et al: Serum carotene deficiency in HIV-infected patients. *AIDS* 1994;8:661–665.

Wang Y, Watson R: Ethanol, immune responses, and murine AIDS: The role of vitamin E as an immunostimulant and antioxidant. *Alcohol* 1994;11:75–84.

Watson R: Nutrition, immunomodulation and AIDS: An overview. *J Nutr* 1992;122:715.

Allergies

Chandra R, Gill B, Kumari S: Food allergy and atopic disease: Pathogenesis, diagnosis, prediction of high risk, and prevention. *Ann Allergy* 1993;71:495–504.

Chandra R: Food allergy: 1992 and beyond. *Nutr Res* 1992;12:93–99.

Joneja J: Management of food allergy: Personal perspectives of an allergy dietitian. *J Can Diet* 1993;54:15–16.

Parker S, Krondi M, Coleman P: Foods perceived by adults as causing adverse reactions. *J Am Diet A* 1993;93:40–44.

Sampson H, Metcalfe D: Food allergies. *J Am Med A* 1992;268:2840–2844.

Taylor S: Food allergy and sensitivities. *J Am Diet A* 1986;86:601–608.

Alzheimer's Disease

Berthon G, Dayde S: Why aluminum phosphate is less toxic than aluminum hydroxide. *J Am Col N* 1992;11:340–348.

Burns A, Holland T: Vitamin E deficiency. *Lancet* 1986;I:805–806.

Imagawa M, Naruse S, Tsuji S, et al: Coenzyme Q10, iron, and vitamin B6 in genetically-confirmed Alzheimer's disease. *Lancet* 1992;340:671.

Levitt A, Karlinsky H: Folate, vitamin B12, and cognitive impairment in patients with Alzheimer's disease. *Act Psyc Sc* 1992;86:301–305.

Lewis J: Vitamin A and Alzheimer's disease. *Neuroep* 1992;11:163–168.

Meador K, Loring D, Nichols M, et al: Preliminary findings of high-dose thiamine in dementia of Alzheimer's type. *J Ger Psy N* 1993;6:222–229.

Moon J, Davison A, Bandy B: Vitamin D and aluminum absorption. *Can Med A J* 1992;147:1308–1309.

Priest N: Satellite symposium on "Alzheimer's disease and dietary aluminium." *P Nutr Soc* 1993;52:231–240.

Rosenberg G, Davis K: The use of cholinergic precursors in neuropsychiatric diseases. *Am J Clin N* 1982;36:709–720.

Zaman Z, Roche S, Fielden P, et al: Plasma concentrations of vitamins A and E and carotenoids in Alzheimer's disease. *Age Aging* 1992;21:91–98.

Anemia

Bezwoda W, Torrance J, Bothwell T, et al: Iron absorption from red and white wines. *Sc J Haemat* 1985;34:121–127.

Kim I, Yetley E, Calvo M: Variations in iron-status measures during the menstrual cycle. *Am J Clin N* 1993;58:705–709.

LaManca J, Haymes E: Effects of iron repletion on VO2max, endurance, and blood lactate in women. *Med Sci Spt* 1993;25:1386–1392.

Magazanik A, Weinstein Y, Abarbanel J, et al: Effect of an iron supplement on body iron status and aerobic capacity of young training women. *Eur J A Phy* 1991;62:317–323.

Ono K: Effects of large dose vitamin E supplementation on anemia in hemodialysis patients. *Nephron* 1985;40:440–445.

(Also see Chapter 4—Iron)

Arthritis

Darlington L, Ramsey N, Mansfield J: Placebo controlled, blind study of dietary manipulation therapy in rheumatoid arthritis. *Lancet* 1986;I:236–238.

DiSilvestro R, Marten J, Skehan M: Effects of copper supplementation on ceruloplasmin and copper-zinc superoxide dismutase in free-living rheumatoid arthritis patients. *J Am Col N* 1992;11:177–180.

Haugen M, Hoyeraal H, Larsen S, et al: Nutrient intake and nutritional status in children with juvenile chronic arthritis. *Sc J Rheum* 1992;21:165–170.

Kjeldsen-Kragh J, Haugen M, Borchgrevink C, et al: Controlled trial of fasting and one-year vegetarian diet in rheumatoid arthritis. *Lancet* 1991;338:899–902.

Kjeldsen-Kragh J, Lund J, Riise T, et al: Dietary omega-3 fatty acid supplementation and naproxen treatment in patients with rheumatoid arthritis. *J Rheumatol* 1992;19:1521–1536.

Kroger H, Penulla I, Alhava E: Low serum vitamin D metabolites in women with rheumatoid arthritis. *Sc J Rheum* 1993;22:172–177.

Makela A, Hyora H, Vuorinen K, et al: Trace elements (Fe, Zn, Cu, and Se) in serum of rheumatic children living in western Finland. *Sc J Rheum* 1984;S53:94.

Tarp U, Overvad K, Hansen J, et al: Low selenium level in severe rheumatoid arthritis. *Sc J Rheum* 1985;14:97–101.

UK, General Practitioner Research Group: Calcium pantothenate in arthritis conditions. *Practition* 1980;224:208–211.

Asthma

Gomaa H, Hussein H, Madkour E, et al: Plasma cortisol and vitamin C in asthmatic patients. *Ann Allergy* 1985;55:236.

Lindahl O, Lindwall L, Spangberg A, et al: Vegan regimen with reduced medication in the treatment of bronchial asthma. *J Asthma* 1985;22:45–55.

Stone J, Hinks L, Beasley R, et al: Reduced selenium status of patients with asthma. *Clin Sci* 1989;77:495–500.

Burns

Kohen I: Hypogeusia, anorexia and altered zinc metabolism following thermal burn. *J Am Med A* 1973;223:914.

Sandstead H: Zinc and wound healing. *Am J Clin N* 1970;23:514.

Cancer

Allen J, Bell E, Oken M, et al: Zinc deficiency, hyperzincuria and immune dysfunction in lung cancer patients. *Am J Clin N* 1983;37:720.

Allinger V, Johnasson G, Gustafsson J, et al: Shift from a mixed to a lactovegetarian diet: Influence on acidic lipid in fecal water: A potential risk factor for colon cancer. *Am J Clin N* 1989;50:992–996.

Baghurst P, Rohan T: High-fiber diets and reduced risk of breast cancer. *Int J Canc* 1994;56:173–176.

Block G: The data support a role for antioxidants in reducing cancer risk. *Nutr Rev* 1992;50:207–213.

Block G: Vitamin C status and cancer: Epidemiologic evidence of reduced risk. *Ann NY Acad* 1992;669:280–292.

Blot W, Li J, Taylor P, et al: Nutritional intervention trials in Linxian, China: Supplementation with specific vitamin/mineral combinations, cancer incidence, and disease-specific mortality in the general population. *J Nat Canc* 1993;85:1483–1491.

Bostick R, Potter J, McKenzie D, et al: Reduced risk of colon cancer with high intake of vitamin E: The Iowa Women's Health Study. *Cancer Res* 1993;53:4230–4237.

Bristol J, Emmett P, Heaton K, et al: Sugar, fat, and the risk of colorectal cancer. *Br Med J* 1985;291:1467–1470.

Dichter C: Risk estimates of liver cancer due to aflatoxin exposure from peanuts and peanut products. *Food Chem T* 1984;22:431–437.

Diplock A, Rice-Evans C, Burdon R: Is there a significant role for lipid peroxidation in the causation of malignancy and for antioxidants in cancer prevention. *Cancer Res* 1994;54:1954–1956.

Dorant E, van den Brandt P, Goldbohm R, et al: Garlic and its significance for the prevention of cancer in humans: A critical view. *Br J Canc* 1993;67:424–429.

Dyke G, Craven J, Hall R, et al: Effect of vitamin C supplementation on gastric mucosal DNA damage. *Carcinogene* 1994;15:291–295.

El-Mofty M, Sakr S, Essawy A, et al: Preventive action of garlic on aflatoxin B1-induced carcinogenesis in the toad Bufo regularis. *Nutr Cancer* 1994;21:95–100.

Fariss M: Oxygen toxicity: Unique cytoprotective properties of vitamin E succinate in hepatocytes. *Fr Rad B* 1990;9:333–343.

Garewal G: Potential role of beta-carotene and antioxidant vitamins in the prevention of oral cancer. *Ann NY Acad* 1992;669:260–268.

Garland C, Shekelle R, Barrett-Connor E, et al: Dietary vitamin D and calcium and risk of colorectal cancer: A 19-year prospective study in men. *Lancet* 1985;I:307–309.

Giovannucci E, Rimm E, Stampfer M, et al: Intake of fat, meat, and fiber in relation to risk of colon cancer in men. *Cancer Res* 1994;54:2390–2397.

Greenberg E, Baron J, Tosteson T, et al: A clinical trial of antioxidant vitamins to prevent colorectal adenoma. *N Eng J Med* 1994;331:141–147.

Herbert J, Landon J, Miller D: Consumption of meat and fruit in relation to oral and esophageal cancer: A cross-national study. *Nutr Cancer* 1993;19:169–179.

Ingram D: Diet and subsequent survival in women with breast cancer. *Br J Cancer* 1994;69:592–595.

La Vecchia C, Negri E, Franceschi S, et al: Tea consumption and cancer risk. *Nutr Cancer* 1992;17:27–31.

Lupulescu A: The role of vitamins A, beta carotene, E, and C in cancer cell biology. *Int J Vit N* 1994;64:3–14.

Mobarhan S: Micronutrient supplementation trials and the reduction of cancer and cerebrovascular incidence and mortality. *Nutr Rev* 1994;52:102–105.

Rose D, Connolly J: Effects of dietary omega-3 fatty acids on human breast cancer growth and metastases in nude mice. *J Nat Canc* 1993;85:1743–1747.

Rose D: Dietary fiber, phytoestrogens, and breast cancer. *Nutrition* 1992;8:47–51.

Taylor P, Li B, Dawsey S, et al: Prevention of esophageal cancer: The nutrition intervention trials in Linxian, China. *Cancer Res* 1994;54:2029–2031.

Thomas M, Tebbutt S, Williamson R: Vitamin D and its metabolites inhibit cell proliferation in human rectal mucosa and a colon cancer cell line. *Gut* 1992;33:1660–1663.

Van Antwerpen L, Theron A, Myer M, et al: Cigarette smoke-mediated oxidant stress phagocytes, vitamin C, vitamin E, and tissue injury. *Ann NY Acad* 1993;686:53–65.

Wynder E, Cohen L, Rose D, et al: Dietary fat and breast cancer: Where do we stand on the evidence. *J Clin Epid* 1994;47:217–222.

Cardiovascular Disease (CVD)

Abbey M, Nestel P, Baghurst P: Antioxidant vitamins and low-density-lipoprotein oxidation. *Am J Clin N* 1993;58:525–532.

Byers T: Vitamin E supplements and coronary heart disease. *Nutr Rev* 1993;51:333–345.

Chasan-Taber L, Selhub J, Rosenberg I, et al: Prospective study of folate and vitamin B6 and risk of myocardial infarction. *Am J Epidem* 1993;138:603.

Coghian J, Flitter W, Clutton S, et al: Lipid peroxidation and changes in vitamin E levels during coronary artery bypass grafting. *J Thor Surg* 1993;106:268–274.

Gey K, Moser U, Jordan P, et al: Increased risk of cardiovascular disease at suboptimal plasma concentrations of essential antioxidants: An epidemiological update with special attention to carotene and vitamin C. *Am J Clin N* 1993;57(suppl):787S–797S.

Hennig B, McClain C, Diana J: Function of vitamin E and zinc in maintaining endothelial integrity: Implications in atherosclerosis. *Ann NY Acad* 1993;686:99–111.

Hulley S: The US National Cholesterol Education Program: Adult treatment guidelines. *Drugs* 1988;36(supple 3):100–104.

Knekt P, Reunanen A, Jarvinen R, et al: Antioxidant vitamin intake and coronary mortality in a longitudinal population study. *Am J Epidem* 1994;139:1180–1189.

Korpela H: Hypothesis: Increased calcium and decreased magnesium in heart muscle and liver in pigs dying suddenly of microangiopathy (Mulberry Heart Disease): An animal model for the study of oxidative damage. *J Am Col N* 1991;10:127–131.

Leng G, Horrobin D, Fowkes F, et al: Plasma essential fatty acids, cigarette smoking, and dietary antioxidants in peripheral arterial disease. *Arter Throm* 1994;14:471–478.

Lipid Research Clinics Program: The Lipid Research Clinics Coronary Primary Prevention Trial results: The relationship of reduction in incidence of coronary heart disease to cholesterol lowering. *J Am Med A* 1984;25:365.

Mukhopadhyay M, Mukhopadhyay C, Chatterrjee I: Protective effect of ascorbic acid against lipid peroxidation and oxidative damage in cardiac microsomes. *Mol C Bioch* 1993;126:69–75.

Prasad K, Kaira J: Oxygen free radicals and hypercholesterolemic atherosclerosis: Effect of vitamin E. *Am Heart J* 1993;125:958–973.

Report of AHA Nutrition Committee: Rationale of the diet-heart statement of the American Heart Association. *Arterioscle* 1982;2:177–191.

Riemersma R: Epidemiology and the role of antioxidants in preventing coronary heart disease: A brief overview. *P Nutr Soc* 1994;53:59–65.

Salonen J, Nyyssonen K, Korpela H, et al: High stored iron levels are associated with excess risk of myocardial infarction in Eastern Finnish men. *Circulation* 1992;86:803–811.

Schaefer E, Lamon-Fava S, Jenner J, et al: Lipoprotein(a) levels and risk of coronary heart disease in men. *J Am Med A* 1994;271:999–1003.

Silagy C, Neil A: Garlic as a lipid lowering agent: A meta- analysis. *J Roy Col P* 1994;28:39–45.

Simon J: Vitamin C and cardiovascular disease: A review. *J Am Col N* 1992;11:107–125.

Strain J: Putative role of dietary trace elements in coronary heart disease and cancer. *Br J Biomed* 1994;51(3):241–251.

Street D, Comstock G, Salkeld R, et al: Serum antioxidants and myocardial infarction. *Circulation* 1994;90(3):1154–1161.

Suadicani P, Hein H, Gyntelberg F: Serum selenium concentration and risk of ischaemic heart disease in a prospective cohort study of 3,000 males. *Atheroscler* 1992;96:33–42.

Yeh Y, Yeh S: Garlic reduces plasma lipids by inhibiting hepatic cholesterol and triacylglycerol synthesis. *Lipids* 1994;29:189–193.

(Also see Chapter 3—Vitamins A, E, and Beta Carotene; Chapter 4—Chromium, Copper, Iron, Magnesium, Selenium, and Zinc; Chapter 5—Antioxidants)

Carpal Tunnel Syndrome (CTS)

Bernstein A, Dinesen J: Brief communication: Effect of pharmacologic doses of vitamin B6 on carpal tunnel syndrome, electroencephalographic results, and pain. *J Am Col N* 1993;12:73–76.

Copeland D, Stoukides C: Pyridoxine in carpal tunnel syndrome. *Ann Pharmac* 1994;28(9):1042–1044.

(Also see Chapter 3—Vitamin B6)

The Common Cold

Banic S: Immunostimulation by vitamin C. *Int J Vit N* 1982;23:49–53.

Carr A, Einstein R, Lai L, et al: Vitamin C and the common cold: Using identical twins as controls. *Med J Aust* 1981;2:411–412.

Hemila H: Vitamin C and the common cold. *Br J Nutr* 1992;67:3–16.

Hemila H: Vitamin C, neutrophils and the symptoms of the common cold. *Pediat Inf* 1992;11:779.

Peters E, Goetzsche J, Grobbelaar B, et al: Vitamin C supplementation reduces the incidence of postrace symptoms of upper-respiratory tract infection in ultramarathon runners. *Am J Clin N* 1993;57:170–174.

Cystic Fibrosis

Dworkin B, Newman L, Berezin S, et al: Low blood selenium levels in patients with cystic fibrosis compared to controls and healthy adults. *J Parent En* 1987;11:38–41.

Jacob R: Zinc status and vitamin A transport in cystic fibrosis. *Am J Clin N* 1978;31:638–644.

Palin D: The effect of oral zinc supplements on plasma levels of vitamin A and retinol-binding protein in cystic fibrosis. *Am J Clin N* 1979;32:1253–1259.

Shepherd R, Thomas B, Bennett D, et al: Changes in body composition and muscle protein degradation during nutritional supplementation in nutritionally growth-retarded children with cystic fibrosis. *J Ped Gastr* 1983;2:439–444.

Stead R: Selenium deficiency, cystic fibrosis, and pancreatic cancer. *Lancet* 1985;II:862–863.

Dermatitis

Rackett S, Rothe M, Grant-Kels J: Diet dermatology. *J Am Acad D* 1993;29:447–461.

Schaffer H: Essential fatty acids and eicosanoids in cutaneous inflammation. *Int J Derm* 1989;28:281–290.

Diabetes Mellitus

Anderson R, Polansky M, Bryden N, et al: Supplemental-chromium effects glucose, insulin, glucagon, and urinary chromium losses in subjects consuming controlled low-chromium diets. *Am J Clin N* 1991;54:909–916.

Beaulieu C, Kestekian R, Havrankova J, et al: Calcium is essential in normalizing intolerance to glucose that accompanies vitamin D depletion in vivo. *Diabetes* 1993;42:35–43.

Caballero B: Vitamin E improves the action of insulin. *Nutr Rev* 1993;51:339–340.

Faure P, Roussel A, Coudray C, et al: Zinc and insulin sensitivity. *Biol Tr El* 1992;32:305.

Helmrich S, Ragland D, Paffenbarger R: Prevention of non-insulin-dependent diabetes mellitus with physical activity. *Med Sci Spt* 1994;26:824–830

Lysy J, Zimmerman J: Ascorbic acid status in diabetes mellitus. *Nutr Res* 1992;12:713–720.

Mooradian A, Failla M, Hoogwerf B, et al: Selected vitamins and minerals in diabetes. *Diabet Care* 1994;17:464–479.

Paolisso G, D'Amore A, Galzerano D, et al: Daily vitamin E supplements improve metabolic control but not insulin secretion in elderly type II diabetic patients. *Diabet Care* 1993;16:1433–1437.

Paolisso G, Sgambato S, Gambardella A, et al: Daily magnesium supplements improve glucose handling in elderly subjects. *Am J Clin N* 1992;55:1161–1167.

Rogers K, Mohan C: Vitamin B6 metabolism and diabetes. *Bioch Med M* 1994;52(1):10–17.

Rohn R, Pleban P, Jenkins L: Magnesium, zinc, and copper in plasma and blood cellular components in children with IDDM. *Clin Chim A* 1993;215:21–28.

Sinclair A, Girling A, Gray L, et al: Disturbed handling of ascorbic acid in diabetic patients with and without microangiopathy during high dose ascorbate supplementation. *Diabetol* 1991;34:171–175.

White J, Campbell R: Magnesium and diabetes-A review. *Am J Clin N* 1993;27:775–780.

Eczema

Neild V, Marsden R, Bailes J, et al: Egg and milk exclusion diets in atopic eczema. *Br J Derm* 1986;114:117–123.

Emotional Disorders

Byrne A, Byrne D: The effect of exercise on depression, anxiety and other mood states: A review. *J Psychosom R* 1993;37:565–574.

Castano A, Cano J, Machado A: Low selenium diet affects monoamine turnover differentially in substantia nigra and striatum. *J Neuroch* 1993;61:1302–1307.

Deijen J, van der Beek E, Orlebeke J, et al: Vitamin B-6 supplementation in elderly men: Effects on mood, memory, performance and mental effort. *Psychophar* 1992;109:489–496.

Greenblatt J, Huffman L, Reiss A: Folic acid in neurodevelopment and child psychiatry. *Prog Neur-P* 1994;18(4):647–660.

Grunewald R: Ascorbic acid in the brain. *Brain Res R* 1993;18:123–133.

Guilarte T: Vitamin B6 and cognitive development: Recent research findings from human and animal studies. *Nutr Rev* 1993;51:193–198.

Heseker H, Kubler W, Pudel V, et al: Psychological disorders as early symptoms of a mild-to-moderate vitamin deficiency. *Ann NY Acad* 1992;669:352–357.

Joyal C, Lalonde R, Vikis-Freibergs V, et al: Are age-related behavioral disorders improved by folate administration? *Exp Aging R* 1993;19:367–376.

Kohlschutter A: Vitamin E and neurological problems in childhood: A curable neurodegenerative process. *Develop Med* 1993;35:642–646.

Pirttila T, Salo J, Laippala P, et al: Effect of advanced brain atrophy and vitamin deficiency on cognitive functions in non-demented subjects. *Act Neur Sc* 1993;87:161–166.

Pollitt E: Iron deficiency and cognitive function. *Ann R Nutr* 1993;13:521–537.

Preuss H: A review of persistent, low-grade lead challenge: Neurological and cardiovascular consequences. *J Am Col N* 1993;12:246–254.

Wood S, Hendricks D, Schvaneveldt N, et al: A longitudinal study of the influence of iron status on mental and motor development of infants and toddlers. *Nutr Res* 1993;13:1367–1378.

Epilepsy

Raju G, Behari M, Prasad K, et al: Randomized, double-blind, placebo-controlled, clinical trial of d-alpha-tocopherol (vitamin E) as add-on therapy in uncontrolled epilepsy. *Epilepsia* 1994;35:368–372.

Eye Disorders

Berson E, Rosner B, Sandberg M, et al: A randomized trial of vitamin A and vitamin E supplementation for retinitis pigmentosa. *Arch Ophth* 1993;111:761–772.

Bhat K: Nutritional status of thiamine, riboflavin, and pyridoxine in cataract patients. *Nutr Rep In* 1987;36:685–692.

Brady W, Mares-Perlman J, Lyle B, et al: Correlates of individual serum carotenoids in the nutritional factors in eye disease study. *Am J Epidem* 1994;139:S18.

Bunce G: Evaluation of the impact of nutrition intervention on cataract prevalence in China. *Nutr Rev* 1994;52:99–101.

Eckhert C, Hsu M, Pang N: Photoreceptor damage following exposure to excess riboflavin. *Experientia* 1993;49:1084–1087.

Garland D: Ascorbic acid and the eye. *Am J Clin N* 1991;54(Suppl):1198S–1202S.

Innes S, Nelson C, Rioux M, et al: Development of visual acuity in relation to plasma and erythrocyte omega-6 and omega-3 fatty acids in healthy term gestation infants. *Am J Clin N* 1994;60:347–352.

Mares-Perlman J, Klein R, Klein B, et al: Relationship between age-related maculopathy and intake of vitamin and mineral supplements (Meeting Abstract). *Inv Ophth V* 1993;34:1133.

Newsome D, Miceli M, Liles M, et al: Antioxidants in the retinal pigment epithelium. *Prog Ret Ey* 1994;13:101–123.

Seddon J, Christen W, Manson J, et al: The use of vitamin supplements and the risk of cataract among US male physicians. *Am J Pub He* 1994;84: 788–792.

Seddon J, Hennekens C: Vitamins, minerals, and macular degeneration. *Arch Ophth* 1994;112:176–179.

Taylor A: Role of nutrients in delaying cataracts. *Ann NY Acad* 1992;669:111–124.

Telkari J: Prevention of cataract with alpha tocopherol (vitamin E) and beta carotene. *Inv Ophth V* 1992;33:1307.

West S, Vitale S, Hallfrisch J, et al: Are antioxidants or supplements protective for age-related macular degeneration? *Arch Ophth* 1994;112:222–227.

Zinc and macular degeneration. *Nutr Rev* 1990;48:285–287.

Fatigue

Barclay C, Loiselle D: Dependence of muscle fatigue on stimulation protocol: Effect of hypocaloric diet. *J Appl Physl* 1992;72:2278–2284.

Costill D, Hargreaves M: Carbohydrate nutrition and fatigue. *Sports Med* 1992;13:86–92.

Cox I, Campbell J, Dowson D: Red blood cell magnesium and chronic fatigue syndrome. *Lancet* 1991;337:757–760.

Horswill C, Hickner R, Scott J, et al: Weight loss, dietary carbohydrate modifications, and high intensity physical performance. *Med Sci Spt* 1990;22:470–476.

Schwartz J, Jandorf L, Krupp L: The measurement of fatigue: A new instrument. *J Psychosom* 1993;37:753–762.

Wilson A, Hickie I, Lloyd A, et al: Longitudinal study of outcome of chronic fatigue syndrome. *Br Med J* 1994;308:756–759.

Fibrocystic Breast Disease (FBD)

London S, Connolly J, Schmitt S, et al: A prospective study of benign breast disease and the risk of breast cancer. *J Am Med A* 1992;267:941–944.

London S, Stein E, Henderson C, et al: Carotenoids, retinol, and vitamin E, and risk of proliferative benign breast disease and breast cancer. *Canc Causes Cont* 1992;3:503–512.

Meyer E, Sommers D, Reitz C, et al: Vitamin E and benign breast disease. *Surgery* 1990;107:549–551.

Rohan T, Cook M, McMichael A: Methylxanthines and benign proliferative epithelial disorders of the breast in women. *Int J Epid* 1989;18:626–633.

Gum and Tooth Disorders

Albanese A, Lorenze E, Edelson A, et al: Calcium nutrition and skeletal and alveolar bone health. *Nutr Rep In* 1985;31:741–755.

Albanese A, Edelson A, Lorenze E, et al: Problems of bone health in the elderly: A ten year study. *NYS J Med* 1975;75:326.

Hair Problems

Gummer C: Diet and hair loss. *Sem Derm* 1985;4:35–39.

Headaches

Bernstein A: Vitamin B6 in clinical neurology. *Ann NY Acad* 1990;585:250–260.

Cornwell N, Clarke L, VanNunen S: Intolerance to dietary chemicals in recurrent idiopathic headache. *Clin Pharm* 1987;41:201.

de Belleroche J, Cook G, Das I, et al: Erythrocyte choline concentrations and cluster headaches. *Br Med J* 1984;288:268–270.

Gallai V, Sarchielli P, Morucci P, et al: Magnesium content of mononuclear blood cells in migraine patients. *Headache* 1994;34(4):160–165.

Harrison D: Copper as a factor in the dietary precipitation of migraine. *Headache* 1986;26:248–250.

Lipton R, Newman L, Cohen J, et al: Aspartame as a dietary trigger of headache. *Headache* 1989;29:90–92.

Martin P, Phil D, Soon K: The relationship between perceived stress, social support and chronic headaches. *Headache* 1993;33:307–314.

Martin P, Phil D, Theunissen C, et al: The role of life event stress, coping, and social support in chronic headaches. *Headache* 1993;33:301–306.

McCarron T, Hitzemann R, Smith R, et al: Amelioration of severe migraine by fish oil (omega 3) fatty acids. *Am J Clin N* 1986;43:710.

Hearing Disorders

Davis M, Kane R, Valentine J: Impaired hearing in X-linked hypophosphataemic (vitamin D-resistant) osteomalacia. *Ann Int Med* 1984;100:230–232.

Wang Y, Yang S: Improvement in hearing among otherwise normal school children in iodine-deficient areas of China. *Lancet* 1985;II:518–520.

Herpes Simplex

Thein D, Hurt W: Lysine as a prophylactic agent in the treatment of recurrent herpes simplex labialis. *Oral Surg* 1984;58:659–666.

Armstrong E, Elenbaas J: Lysine for herpes simplex virus. *Drug Intel Clin Pha* 1983;39:186.

Hypertension

Basta L: Regression of atherosclerotic stenosing lesions of the renal arteries and spontaneous cure of systemic hypertension through control of hyperlipidemia. *Am J Med* 1976;61:420–421.

Berchtold P: Obesity and hypertension: Conclusions and recommendations. *Int J Obes* 1981;5(suppl 1):183.

Fisher P, Belonje B, Giroux A: Magnesium status and excretion in age-matched subjects with normal and elevated blood pressures. *Clin Bioch* 1993;26:207–211.

Gillman M, Oliveria S, Moore L, et al: Inverse association of dietary calcium with systolic blood pressure in young children. *J Am Med A* 1992;267:2340–2343.

Itoh R, Oka J, Echizen H, et al: The interrelation of urinary calcium and sodium intake in healthy elderly Japanese. *Int J Vit N* 1991;61:159–165.

Kurtz T, Albander H, Morris R: Dietary chloride as a possible determinant of NaCl-sensitive essential-hypertension in man. *Kidney Int* 1986;29:250.

Osilesi O, Trout D, Ogunwole J, et al: Blood pressure and plasma lipids during ascorbic acid supplementation in borderline hypertensive and normotensive adults. *Nutr Res* 1991;11:405–412.

Simopoulos A: Omega-3 fatty acids in health and disease and in growth and development. *Am J Clin N* 1991;54:438–463.

Singh B, Hollenberg N, Poole-Wilson P, et al: Diuretic-induced potassium and magnesium deficiency: Relation to drug-induced QT prolongation, cardiac arrhythmias and sudden death. *J Hypertens* 1992;10:301–316.

Witteman J, Grobbee D, Derkx F, et al: Reduction of blood pressure with oral magnesium supplementation in women with mild to moderate hypertension. *Am J Clin N* 1994;60:129–135.

Insomnia

Akata T, Sekiguchi S, Takahashi M, et al: Successful combined treatment with vitamin B12 and bright artificial light of one case with delayed sleep phase syndrome. *Jpn J Psy N* 1993;47:439–440.

Driver H, Rogers G, Mitchell D, et al: Prolonged endurance exercise and sleep disruption. *Med Sci Spt* 1994;26:903–907.

Lucero K, Hicks R: Relationship between habitual sleep duration and diet. *Perc Mot Sk* 1990;71:1377–1378.

Neumann M, Jacobs K: Relationship between dietary components and aspects of sleep. *Perc Mot Sk* 1992;75:873–874.

Ohta T, Ando K, Iwata T, et al: Treatment of persistent sleep-wake schedule disorders in adolescents with methylcobalamin (vitamin B12). *Sleep* 1991;14:414–418.

Okawa M, Mishima K, Nanami T, et al: Vitamin B12 treatment for sleep-wake rhythm disorders. *Sleep* 1990;13:15–23.

Smidt L, Cremin F, Grivetti L, et al: Influence of thiamin supplementation on the health and general well–being of an elderly Irish population with marginal thiamin deficiency. *J Gerontol* 1991;46:M16–22.

Kidney Disorders

Ono K: Reduced osmotic hemolysis and improvement of anemia by large dose vitamin E supplementation in regular hemodialysis patients. *Kidney Int* 1984;26:583.

Vathsala R, Sindhu S, Sachidev K, et al: Pyridoxine in the long-term follow-up of crystalluric patients. *Urol Res* 1988;16:249.

Liver Disorders

McKenney J, Proctor J, Harris S, et al: A comparison of the efficacy and toxic effects of sustained- vs. immediate-release niacin in hypercholesterolemic patients. *J Am Med A* 1994;271:672–677.

Parola M, Leonarduzzi G, Biasi F, et al: Vitamin E dietary supplementation protects against carbon tetrachloride-induced chronic liver damage and cirrhosis. *Hepatology* 1992;16:1014–1021.

Rocchi E, Borghi A, Paolillo F, et al: Carotenoids and liposoluble vitamins in liver cirrhosis. *J La Cl Med* 1991;118:176–185.

Senoo H, Wake K: Suppression of experimental hepatic fibrosis by administration of vitamin A. *Lab Inv* 1985;52:182–194.

Thuluvath P, Triger D: Selenium and chronic liver disease. *J Hepatol* 1992;14:176.

von Herbay A, de Groot H, Hegi U, et al: Low vitamin E content in plasma of patients with alcoholic liver disease, hemochromatosis, and Wilson's disease. *J Hepatol* 1994;20:41–46.

Lung Disorders

Bai T, Martin J: Effects of indomethacin and ascorbic acid on histamine induced bronchoconstriction. *NZ Med J* 1986;99:163.

Copper deficiency and developmental emphysema. *Nutr Rev* 1983;41:318–420.

Gerhardsson L, Brune D, Nordberg I, et al: Protective effect of selenium on lung cancer in smelter workers. *Br J Ind Me* 1985;42:617–626.

Heinonen O, Huttunen J, Albanes D, et al: The effect of vitamin E and beta carotene on the incidence of lung cancer and other cancers in male smokers. *N Eng J Med* 1994;330:1029–1035.

Kamei T, Kohno T, Ohwada H, et al: Experimental study of the therapeutic effects of folate, vitamin A, and vitamin B12 on squamous metaplasia of the bronchial epithelium. *Cancer* 1993;71:2477–2483.

Landon R, Young E: Role of magnesium in regulation of lung function. *J Am Diet A* 1993;93:674–677.

Mayne S, Janerich D, Greenwald P, et al: Dietary beta carotene and lung cancer risk in U.S. nonsmokers. *J Nat Canc* 1994;86:33–38.

Omenn G, Goodman G, Thornquist M, et al: The beta-carotene and retinol efficacy trial (CARET) for chemoprevention of lung cancer in high risk populations: smokers and asbestos-exposed workers. *Cancer Res* 1994;54:2038–2043.

Pastorino U, Infante M, Maioli M, et al: Adjuvant treatment of stage I lung cancer with high-dose vitamin A. *J Clin Oncol* 1993;11:1216–1222.

Schwartz J, Weiss S: Relationship between dietary vitamin C intake and pulmonary function in the First National Health and Nutrition Examination (NHANES I). *Am J Clin N* 1994;59:110–114.

Shariff R, Hoshino E, Allard J, et al: Vitamin E supplementation in smokers. *Clin Res* 1988;36:A770.

Shenai J, Rush M, Stahlman M, et al: Vitamin A supplementation and bronchopulmonary dysplasia-revisited. *J Pediat* 1992;121:399–401.

van den Brandt P, Goldbohm A, van 't Veer P, et al: A prospective cohort study on selenium status and the risk of lung cancer. *Cancer Res* 1993;53:4860–4865.

Lupus Erythematosus

Ayres S, Mihan R: Lupus erythematosus and vitamin E: An effective and nontoxic therapy. *Cutis* 1972;23:49–53.

Tappel A: Vitamin E as the biological lipid antioxidant. Symposium on vitamin E and metabolism, Zurich, Switzerland. *Vitam Horm* 1962;20:493.

Vien C, Gonzalez-Cabello R, Bodo I, et al: Effect of vitamin A treatment on the immune reactivity of patients with systemic lupus erythematosus. *J Clin Lab* 1988;26:33–35.

Osteomalacia

Omdahl J, Garry P, Hunsaker L, et al: Nutritional status in a healthy elderly population: Vitamin D. *Am J Clin N* 1982;36:1225–1233.

Rudolf M, Arulanantham K, Greenstein R: Unsuspected nutritional rickets. *Pediatrics* 1980;66:72.

Osteoporosis

Bikle D: Role of vitamin D, its metabolites, and analogs in the management of osteoporosis. *Rheum Dis C* 1994;20(3):759–775.

Brautbar N, Gruber H: Magnesium and bone disease. *Nephron* 1986;44:1–7.

Dawson-Hughes B, Dallal G, Krall E, et al: Effect of vitamin D supplementation on wintertime and overall bone loss in healthy postmenopausal women. *Ann Int Med* 1991;115:505–512.

Dodds R, Catterall A, Bitensky L, et al: Osteolytic retardation of early stages of fracture healing by vitamin B6 deficiency. *Clin Sci* 1985;68:21P.

Dubbelman R, Jonxis J, Muskiet F, et al: Age-dependent vitamin D status and vertebral condition of white women living in Curacao (The Netherlands Antilles) as compared with their counterparts in The Netherlands. *Am J Clin N* 1993;58:106–109.

Gunnes M: Bone mineral density in the cortical and trabecular distal forearm in healthy children and adolescents. *Act Paediat* 1994;83:463–467.

Hillman L, Cassidy J, Johnson L, et al: Vitamin D metabolism and bone mineralization in children with juvenile rheumatoid arthritis. *J Pediat* 1994;124:910–916.

Kanis J: Treatment of symptomatic osteoporosis with fluoride. *Am J Med* 1993;95:53S.

Melhus H, Kindmark A, Amer S, et al: Vitamin D receptor genotypes in osteoporosis. *Lancet* 1994;344:949–950.

Morrison N, Qi J, Tokita A, et al: Prediction of bone density from vitamin D receptor alleles. *Nature* 1994;367:284–287.

Osteoporosis-consensus Conference: *J Am Med A* 1984;252:799–802.

Pak C, Sakhaee K, Piziak V, et al: Slow-release sodium fluoride in the management of postmenopausal osteoporosis. *Ann Int Med* 1994;120:625–632.

Ramsdale S, Bassey E, Pye D: Dietary calcium intake relates to bone mineral density in premenopausal women. *Br J Nutr* 1994;71:77–84.

Saltman P, Strause L: The role of trace minerals in osteoporosis. *J Am Col N* 1993;12:384–389.

Soroko S, Barrett-Connor E, Edelstein S, et al: Family history of osteoporosis and bone mineral density at the axial skeleton: The Rancho Bernardo study. *J Bone Min* 1994;9:761–769.

Sowers M: Epidemiology of calcium and vitamin D in bone loss. *J Nutr* 1993;123:413–417.

Stallings V, Oddleifson N, Negrini B, et al: Bone mineral content and dietary calcium intake in children prescribed a low-lactose diet. *J Ped Gastr* 1994;18:440–445.

Tilyard M, Spears G, Thomson J, et al: Treatment of postmenopausal osteoporosis with calcitriol or calcium. *N Eng J Med* 1992;326:357–362.

Welten D, Kemper H, Post G, et al: Weight-bearing activity during youth is a more important factor for peak bone mass than calcium intake. *J Bone Min* 1994;9:1089–1096.

Premenstrual Syndrome (PMS)

Block E: The use of vitamin A in premenstrual tension. *Act Obst Sc* 1960;39:586.

Chuong C, Dawson E, Smith E: Vitamin E levels in Premenstrual Syndrome. *Am J Obst G* 1990;163:1591–1595.

London R, Bradley L, Chiamori N: Effect of a nutritional supplement on premenstrual symptomatology in women with Premenstrual Syndrome: A double-blind longitudinal study. *J Am Col N* 1991;10:494–499.

Penland J, Hunt J: Nutritional status and menstrual-related symptomatology (Meeting Abstract). *FASEB J* 1993;7:A379.

Penland J, Johnson P: Dietary calcium and manganese effects on menstrual cycle symptoms. *Am J Obst G* 1993;168:1417–1423.

Rogers P, Edwards S, Green M, et al: Nutritional influences on mood and cognitive performance: The menstrual cycle, caffeine, and dieting. *P Nutr Soc* 1992;51:343–351.

Rossignol A, Bonnlander H: Prevalence and severity of the Premenstrual Syndrome: Effects of food and beverages that are sweet or high in sugar content. *J Repro Med* 1991;36:131–136.

Seelig M: Interrelationship of magnesium and estrogen in cardiovascular and bone disorders, eclampsia, migraine, and Premenstrual Syndrome. *J Am Col N* 1993;12:442–458.

Psoriasis

Allen B, Maurice P, Goodfield M, et al: The effects on psoriasis of dietary supplementation with eicosapentaenoic acid. *Br J Derm* 1985;113:777.

Burton C: Disappearance of psoriatic lesions in 73-year-old man treated by rice diet for 8 weeks. *NC Med J* 1986;47:255.

Lowe K, Normal A: Vitamin D and psoriasis. *Nutr Rev* 1992;50:138–142.

Prystowsky J, Orologa A, Taylor S: Update on nutrition and psoriasis. *Int J Derm* 1993;32:582–586.

Sickle Cell Anemia

Heyman M, Katz R, Hurst D, et al: Growth retardation in sickle cell disease treated by nutritional support. *Lancet* 1985;1:903–906.

Jain S, Williams D: Reduced levels of plasma ascorbic acid (vitamin C) in sickle cell disease patients: Its possible role in oxidant damage to sickle cells in vivo. *Clin Chem A* 1985;149:257–261.

Skin Disorders

Gensler H, Magdaleno M: Topical vitamin E inhibition of immunosuppression and tumorigenesis induced by ultraviolet irradiation. *Nutr Cancer* 1991;15:97–106.

Gerrish K, Gensler H: Prevention of photocarcinogenesis by dietary vitamin E. *Nutr Cancer* 1993;19:125–133.

Halperin E, Gaspar L, George S, et al: A double-blind, randomized, prospective trial to evaluate topical vitamin C solution for the prevention of radiation dermatitis. *Int J Rad O* 1993;26:413–416.

Kune, G, Bannerman S, Field B, et al: Diet, alcohol, smoking, serum beta carotene, and vitamin A in nonmelanocyte skin cancer patients and controls. *Nutr Cancer* 1992;18:237–244.

Pence B, Delver E, Dunn D: Effects of dietary selenium on UVB-induced skin carcinogenesis and epidermal antioxidant status. *J Inves Der* 1994;102:759–761.

Record I, Dreosti I, Konstanitinopoulos M, et al: The influence of topical and systemic vitamin E on ultraviolet light-induced skin damage in hairless mice. *Nutr Cancer* 1991;16:219–225.

Trevithick J, Shum D, Redae S, et al: Reduction of sunburn damage to skin by topical application of vitamin E acetate following exposure to ultraviolet B radiation: Effect of delaying application or of reducing concentration of vitamin E acetate applied. *Scanning Microsc* 1993;7:1269–1281.

Vieth R, Milojecvic S: Application of vitamin D to the skin is a viable alternative to its oral nutrition (Meeting Abstract). *J Bone Min* 1993;8:S224.

Stress

Anderson R, Polansky M, Bryden N: Strenuous running: Acute effects of chromium, copper, zinc and selected clinical variables in urine and serum of male runners. *Biol Tr El* 1984;6:327–336.

Boosalis M, Konstantinides L, Salem F, et al: Vitamin balance in trauma/surgery: Are current multivitamin preparations adequate? *Fed Proc* 1987;46:1010.

Fine K, Santa Ana C, Porter J, et al: Intestinal absorption of magnesium from food and supplements. *J Clin Inv* 1991;88:396–402.

Kallner A: Influence of vitamin C status on the urinary excretion of catecholamines in stress. *Hum Nutr-Cl* 1983;37:405–411.

McMurtry C, Young S, Downs R, et al: Mild vitamin D deficiency and secondary hyperparathyroidism in nursing home patients receiving adequate dietary vitamin D. *J Am Ger So* 1992;40:343–347.

Nakano K, Mizutani R: Decreased responsiveness of pituitary-adrenal axis to stress in vitamin A-depleted rats. *J Nutr Sci* 1983;29:353–363.

Pryor W: Can vitamin E protect humans against the pathological effects of ozone in smog? *Am J Clin N* 1991;53:702–722.

Suzuki S, Nakano K: Decrease in urinary excretion of ascorbic acid and histamine in rats after repeated immobilization stress. *J Nutr* 1984;114:441–446.

Thyroid Disorders

Dolev E, Deuster P, Solomen B, et al: Alterations in magnesium and zinc metabolism in thyroid disease. *Metabolism* 1988;37:61–67.

Yeast Infection

Agelli M, Delcorso L: Vitamin C and vitamin B supplements helped prevent recurrence of urinary and vaginal tract infections (Meeting Abstract). *Clin Res* 1994;42:A346.

Almekinders L, Greene W: Vertebral Candida infections: A case report and review of the literature. *Clin Orthop* 1991;267:174–178.

McKenzie H, Main J, Pennington C, et al: Antibody to selected strains of saccharomyces cerevisiae (baker's and brewer's yeast) and Candida albincans in Crohn's disease. *Gut* 1990;31:536–538.

Hilton E, Isenberg H, Alperstein P, et al: Ingestion of yogurt containing Lactobacillus acidophilus as prophylaxis for Candida vaginitis. *Ann Int Med* 1992;116:353–357.

Klig L, Friedli L, Schmid E: Phospholipid biosynthesis in Candida albincans: Regulation by the precursors inositol and choline. *J Bact* 1990;172:4407–4414.

Sohnle P, Collins-Lech C, Wiessner J: The zinc-reversible antimicrobial activity of neutrophil lysates and abscess fluid supernatants. *J Infect Dis* 1991;164:137–142.

CHAPTER 6

Overview

Mehta S: Malnutrition and drugs: Clinical implications. *Dev Pharm T* 1991;15:159–165.

Stewart R, Moore M, May F, et al: Changing patterns of therapeutic agents in the elderly: A ten-year overview. *Age Aging* 1991;20:182–188.

Teresi M, Morgan D: Attitudes of healthcare professionals toward patient counseling on drug-nutrient interactions. *Ann Pharm* 1994;28: 576–580.

Alcohol

Collipp P, Kris V, Castro-Magana M, et al: The effects of dietary zinc deficiency on voluntary alcohol drinking in rats. *Alc Clin Ex* 1984;8: 556–559.

Dworkin B, Rosenthal W, Jankowski R, et al: Low blood selenium levels in alcoholics with and without advanced liver disease: Correlations with clinical and nutritional status. *Dig Dis Sci* 1985;30:838–844.

Grummer M, Erdman J: Effect of chronic alcohol consumption and moderate fat diet on vitamin A status in rats fed either vitamin A or beta carotene. *J Nutr* 1983;113:350–364.

Halsted C: Folate requirements and metabolism in alcoholic liver disease. *Nutr Res* 1994;14(9):1439–1456.

Milne D, Canfield W, Gallagher S, et al: metabolism of ethanol in postmenopausal women fed a diet marginal in zinc. *Clin Res* 1986;34: A801.

Ward R, Peters T: The antioxidant status of patients with either alcohol-induced liver damage or myopathy. *Alc Alcohol* 1992;27:359–365.

Watzl B, Watson R: Role of nutrients in alcohol-induced immunomodulation. *Alc Alcohol* 1993;28:89–95.

Antacids

Blood W, Flinchum D: Osteomalacia with pseudofractures caused by the ingestion of aluminum hydroxide. *J Am Med A* 1960;174:1327.

Goulding A, McIntosh J, Campbell D: Effect of sodium bicarbonate and 1,25 dihydroxycholecalciferol on calcium and phosphorus balances in the rat. *J Nutr* 1984;114:653–659.

McGuigan J: A consideration of the adverse effect of cimetidine. *Gastroenty* 1980;80:181.

Seaborn C, Stoecker B: Effects of antacid or ascorbic acid on tissue accumulation and urinary excretion of chromium. *Nutr Res* 1990;10:1401–1407.

Spencer H, Norris C, Coffey F, et al: Effect of small amounts of antacids on calcium, phosphorus and fluoride metabolism in man. *Gastroenty* 1975;68:990.

Antibiotics

Amabile-Cuevas C, Pina-Zentella R, Wah-Laborde M: Decreased resistance to antibiotics and plasmid loss in plasmid-carrying strains of staphylococcus aureus treated with ascorbic acid. *Nutr Res* 1991;264: 119–125.

Anticonvulsants

Fincham R, Berg M, Ebert B, et al: The effect of various doses of phenytoin on folic acid serum concentrations in normal volunteers. *Epilepsia* 1986;27:592–593.

Gough H, Bissesar A, Goggin T, et al: Factors associated with the biochemical changes in vitamin D and calcium metabolism in institutionalized patients with epilepsy. *Irish J Med* 1986;155:181–189.

Roe D: Drug-food and drug-nutrient interactions. *J Env P Tox* 1985;5: 115–135.

Stewart J: Phenelzine-induced pyridoxine deficiency. *J Clin Psychopharm* 1984;4:225–226.

Werther C, Cloud H, Ohtake M, et al: Effect of long term administration of anticonvulsants on copper, zinc, and ceruloplasmin levels. *Drug Nutr* 1986;4:269–274.

Aspirin, Pain-Killers, and Anti-Inflammatory Medications

Boudreaux J, Hayes D, Mizrahi S, et al: Use of water-soluble liquid vitamin E to enhance cyclosporine absorption in children after liver transplant. *Transplan* 1993;25:1875.

Franklin J, Roseberg I: Impaired folic acid absorption in inflammatory bowel disease: Effects of salicylazosulfapyridine (Azulfidine). *Gastroenty* 1973;64:517–525.

Murray J, Healy M: Drug-mineral interactions: A new responsibility for the hospital dietitian. *J Am Diet A* 1991;91:66–73.

Rettura G, Stratford F, Padawer J, et al: Vitamin A protects against aspirin toxicity. *J Am Col N* 1984;3:291–292.

Cancer Medications

Dudrick S, O'Donnell J, Claque M: Nutritional rehabilitation of the cancer patient. 13th International Cancer Congress, Part K- Research and Treatment, 1983, pp 161–170.

Klein S, Simes J, Blackburn G: Total parenteral nutrition and cancer clinical trials. *Cancer* 1986;58:1378–1386.

Schreurs W, Egger R, Wedel M, et al: The influence of radiotherapy and chemotherapy on the vitamin status of cancer patients. *Int J Vit N* 1985;55:425–432.

Van Eys J: Effect of nutrition on response to therapy. *Cancer Res* 1982;42:7475.

Medications for Cardiovascular Disease

Brown B, Albers J, Brunzell J: Normalization of elevated apoliprotein-B with niacin plus colestipol in subjects with familial-combined hyperlipidemia. *Atheroscler* 1983;3:A477.

Hoogwerf B, Hibbard D, Hunninghake D: Effects of long-term cholestyramine administration on vitamin D and parathormone levels in middle-aged men with hypercholesterolemia. *J La Cl Med* 1992;119:407–411.

Medications for Hyperactivity

Safer D, Allan R, Barr E: Depression of growth in hyperactive children on stimulant drugs. *N Eng J Med* 1972;287:217–220.

Hypertensive Medications

Demartini F, Briscoe A, Ragan C: Effect of ethacrynic acid on calcium and magnesium excretion. *P Soc Exp M* 1967;124:320–324.

Lim P, Jacob E: Magnesium deficiency in patients on long-term diuretic therapy for heart failure. *Br Med J* 1972;3:620–622.

McLean C, Williams R, Aviv A, et al: Effect of captopril on the metabolism of some trace elements in the rat. *Tr El Med* 1985;2:175–178.

Seligmann H, Halkin H, Rauchfleisch, et al: Thiamine deficiency in patients with congestive heart failure receiving long-term furosemide therapy: A pilot study. *Am J Med* 1991;91:151.

Wester P: Zinc during diuretic treatment. *Lancet* 1975;I:578.

Wirell M, Wester P, Stegmayr B: Nutritional dose of magnesium in hypertensive patients on beta blockers lowers systolic blood pressure: A double-blind, cross-over study. *J Intern M* 1994;236:189–195.

Oral Contraceptives

Adams P: Effect of pyridoxine hydrochloride (vitamin B6) upon depression associated with oral contraception. *Lancet* 1973;I:897–904.

Baumblatt M, Winston F: Pyridoxine and the pill. *Lancet* 1970;I:832–833.

Harper J, Levine A, Rosenthal D, et al: Erythrocyte folate levels, oral contraceptive use and abnormal cervical cytology. *Acta Cytol* 1994;38:324–330.

Steegers-Theunissen R, Van Rossum J, Steegers E, et al: Sub-50 oral contraceptives affect folate kinetics. *Gynecol Obs* 1993;36:230–233.

Zamah N, Humpel M, Kuhnz W, et al: Absence of an effect of high vitamin C dosage on the systemic availability of ethinyl estradiol in women using a combination oral contraceptive. *Contracept* 1993;48:377–391.

Steroid Medications

Breslau N: Calcium, estrogen, and progestin in the treatment of osteoporosis. *Rheum Dis C* 1994;20(3):691–716.

Tobacco

Bolton-Smith C: Antioxidant vitamin intakes in Scottish smokers and non-smokers. *Ann NY Acad* 1993;686:347–360.

Bolton-Smith C, Casey C, Gey K, et al: Antioxidant vitamin intakes assessed using a food-frequency questionnaire: Correlation with biochemical status in smokers and nonsmokers. *Br J Nutr* 1991;65:337–346.

Bui M, Sauty A, Collet F, et al: Dietary vitamin C intake and concentrations in the body fluids and cells of male smokers and nonsmokers. *J Nutr* 1992;122:312–316.

Hoshino E, Shariff R, Van Gossum A, et al: Vitamin E suppresses increased lipid peroxidation in cigarette smokers. *J Parent Ent Nutr* 1990;14:300–305.

Levin E, Behm F, Carnahan E, et al: Clinical trials using ascorbic acid aerosol to aid smoking cessation. *Drug Al Dep* 1993;33:211–223.

Margetts B, Jackson A: Interactions between people's diet and their smoking habits. The dietary and nutritional survey of British adults. *Br Med J* 1993;307:1381–1384.

Ortega R, Lopez-Sobaler A, Gonzalez-Gross M, et al: Influence of smoking on folate intake and blood folate concentrations in a group of elderly Spanish men. *J Am Col N* 1994;13:68–72.

Rimm E, Colditz G: Smoking, alcohol, and plasma levels of carotenes and vitamin E. *Ann NY Acad* 1993;686:323–334.

Schectman G, Byrd J, Hoffmann R: Ascorbic acid requirements for smokers: Analysis of a population survey. *Am J Clin N* 1991;53:1466–1470.

Stegmayr B, Johansson I, Huhtasaori F, et al: Use of smokeless tobacco and cigarettes—effects on plasma levels of antioxidant vitamins. *Int J Vit N* 1993;63:195–200.

Vermaak W, Ubbink J, Barnard H, et al: Vitamin B-6 nutrition status and cigarette smoking. *Am J Clin N* 1990;51:1058–1061.

Weight Control "Diet" Medications

Alger S, Larson K, Boyce V, et al: Effect of phenylpropanolamine on energy expenditure and weight loss in overweight women. *Am J Clin N* 1993;57:120–126.

Atkinson R, Hubbard V: Report on the NIH workshop on pharmacologic treatment of obesity. *Am J Clin N* 1994;60:153–156.

Bray G: Use and abuse of appetite-suppressant drugs in the treatment of obesity. *Ann Int Med* 1993;119:707–713.

Buemann B, Marckmann P, Christensen N, et al: The effect of ephedrine plus caffeine on plasma lipids and lipoproteins during a 4.2 MJ/day diet. *Int J Obes* 1994;18:329–332.

de Zwaan M, Mitchell J: Opiate antagonists and eating behavior in humans: A review. *J Clin Phar* 1992;32:1060–1072.

Drent M, van der Veen E: Lipase inhibition: A novel concept in the treatment of obesity. *Int J Obes* 1993;17:241–244.

Frewin D: Phenylpropanolamine: How safe is it? *Med J Aust* 1983;July 23:54–55.

Schteingart D: Effectiveness of phenylpropanolamine in the management of moderate obesity. *Int J Obes* 1992;16:487–493.

Stallone D, Levitsky D: Chronic fenfluramine treatment: Effects on body weight, food intake and energy expenditure. *Int J Obes* 1994;18:679–685.

Weintraub M: Long-term weight control: The National Heart, Lung, and Blood Institute funded multimodal intervention study. *Clin Pharm* 1992;51:581–646.

CHAPTER 7

Achterberg C, McDonnell E, Bagby R: How to put the Food Guide Pyramid into practice. *J Am Diet A* 1994;94:1030–1035.

Barnett D, Conlee R: The effects of a commercial dietary supplement on human performance. *Am J Clin N* 1984;40:586–590.

Bloomstrand E, Hassmen P, Ekblom B, et al: Administration of branch-chain amino acids during sustained exercise: Effects on performance and on plasma concentration of some amino acids. *Int J Spt N* 1992;2:191–195.

Bone loss and amenorrheic athletes. *Nutr Rev* 1986;44:361–363.

Brilla L, Haley T: Effect of magnesium supplementation on strength training in humans. *J Am Col N* 1992;11:326–329.

Buczynski A, Kedziora J, Tkaczewski W, et al: Effect of submaximal physical exercise on antioxidant protection of human blood platelets. *Int J Spt M* 1991;12:52–54.

Chen T, Shao Q, Heath H, et al: An update on the vitamin D content of fortified milk from the United States and Canada. *N Eng J Med* 1993;329:1507.

Deuster P, Singh A: Responses of plasma magnesium and other cations to fluid replacement during exercise. *J Am Col N* 1993;12:286–293.

Haeckel R, Kaiser E, Oellerich M, et al: Carnitine: metabolism, function, and clinical application. *J Clin Chem* 1990;28:291–295.

Hasten D, Rome E, Franks B, et al: Effects of chromium picolinate on beginning weight training students. *Int J Spt N* 1992;2:343–350.

Lefavi R, Anderson R, Keith R, et al: Efficacy of chromium supplementation in athletes: Emphasis on anabolism. *Int J Spt N* 1992;2:111–122.

Pattini A, Schena F: Effects of training and iron supplementation on iron status of cross-country skiers. *J Sport Med* 1990;30:347–353.

Robertson J, Maughan R, Duthie G, et al: Increased blood antioxidant systems of runners in response to training load. *Clin Sci* 1991;80: 611–618.

van der Beek B, van Dokkum W, Schrijver J, et al: Impact of marginal vitamin intake on physical performance in healthy young men. *P Nutr Soc* 1985;44:A27.

van Erp-Baart A, Saris W, Binkhorst R, et al: Nationwide survey on nutritional habits in elite athletes. II: Mineral and vitamin intake. *Int J Spt M* 1989;10:S11–S16.

van Rij A, Hall M, Dohm G, et al: Changes in zinc metabolism following exercise in human subjects. *Biol Tr El* 1986;10:99–105.

Vorster H, Lotter A, Odendaal I: Effects of an oats fiber tablet and wheat bran in healthy volunteers. *S Afr Med J* 1986;69:435–438.

CHAPTER 8

Baker H, Bhagavan H, Machlin L: Biological activities of d and dl forms of vitamin E: Comparison of plasma tocopherol levels following oral administration in humans. *Fed Proc* 1985;44:935.

Bendich A: Safety issues regarding the use of vitamin supplements. *Ann NY Acad* 1992;669:300–312.

Bogden J, Bendich A, Kemp F, et al: Daily micronutrient supplements enhance delayed-hypersensitivity skin tests repsonses in older peole. *Am J Clin N* 1994;60(3):437–447.

Castillo-Duran C, Garcias H, Venegas P, et al: Zinc supplementation increases growth velocity of male children and adolescents with short stature. *Act Paediat* 1994;83(8):833–837.

Chavance M, Herbeth B, Lemoine A, et al: Does multivitamin supplementation prevent infections in healthy elderly subjects? A controlled trial. *Int J Vit N* 1993;63:11–16.

Clarke J, Kies C: Niacin nutritional status of adolescent humans fed high-dosage of pantothenic acid supplements. *Nutr Rep In* 1985;31:1271–1279.

Dietary supplements: Rationale for regulation. *Nutr Rev* 1993;51(10):310–312.

Fine K, Santa Ana C, Porter J, et al: Intestinal absorption of magnesium from food and supplements. *J Clin Inv* 1991;88:396–402.

Knopp R, Ginsaber J, Albers J, et al: Contrasting effects of unmodified and time-release forms of niacin on lipoproteins in hyperlipidemic subjects: Clues to mechanism of action of niacin. *Metabolism* 1985;34:642–650.

LaChance P: To supplement or not to supplement: Is it a question? *J Am Col N* 1994;13:113–115.

Olson J: Vitamins: The tortuous path from needs to fantasies. *J Nutr* 1994;124(9):1771–1776.

Pennington J: Total Diet Study: Nutritional Elements. *Nutr Rep* 1992;10:33,40.

Reaven P, Witztum J: Comparison of supplementation of RRR-alpha-tocopherol and racemic alpha-tocopherol in humans. *Arter Throm* 1993;13:601–608.

Reynolds R: Vitamin supplements: Current controversies. *J Am Col N* 1994;13:118–126.

Rosenberg I: Nutrient requirements for optimal health: What does that mean? *J Nutr* 1994;124:1777S–1779S.

Shaw S, Jayatilleke E, Herbert V: Evidence against antioxidant-prooxidant vitamin C supplements protecting against cancer. *Clin Res* 1994;42:A172.

Glossary

Acetylcholine: A neurotransmitter associated with the regulation of numerous body processes including memory.

Acid: A chemical substance that contains hydrogen atoms and usually tastes sour. Hydrochloric acid in the stomach, vinegar, and acetic acid are examples of acids. An acid has a pH of less than 7.0.

Acid-Base Balance: The equilibrium between acids and bases (alkaline) in the body.

Acidosis: A disorder caused by low alkalinity of the blood and the body where the normal pH falls below 7.0.

Acromegaly: A disease of the pituitary gland that results in excessive growth of the bones.

Acquired Immunodeficiency Syndrome (AIDS): A deadly, progressive disease caused by a virus and resulting in suppressed immune function.

Acute: Sharp and severe onset of disease.

Additive: A chemical substance added to food, either intentionally or unintentionally.

Adrenal Gland: A ductless gland located near the kidneys, which produces/secretes hormones, including adrenalin and the corticosteroid hormone cortisone.

Adrenalin: A hormone secreted by the adrenal glands that aids in the release of stored sugar in the liver, contraction of muscles, and increased blood supply to the muscles—all in response to stress.

Aerobic: In the presence of oxygen. Aerobic exercise is any slow, steady exercise, such as walking, jogging, swimming, or bicycling, that requires constant long-term use of large muscle groups.

Aflatoxin: A carcinogenic mold found in stale peanuts and other foods.

Alkaline: A chemical substance called a base that will neutralize an acid to form a salt. Baking soda is an example of an alkaline substance. Alkaline compounds have a pH of more than 7.0.

Alkalosis: A disturbance of the body's natural acid-base balance that results in sweating, vomiting, and diarrhea.

Alveolar: The jaw bone where the sockets of the teeth are situated.

Alveoli: Tiny air-filled sacs in the lungs.

Alzheimer's Disease: A progressive, degenerative brain disease that results in severe memory loss.

Amino Acid: A building block or precursor of protein. More than 20 amino acids are used by the body to manufacture different proteins in hair, skin, blood, and other tissues.

Amphetamine: A synthetic drug used to stimulate the nervous system, reduce appetite, and increase blood pressure.

Amylase: An enzyme in saliva that aids in the digestion of carbohydrates.

Anabolic Steroids: Hormones, such as testosterone, that encourage muscle development.

Anabolism: The portion of metabolism where simple molecules are combined to form complex structures. For example, the joining of numerous amino acids to form a protein is an anabolic process.

Analgesic: A medication that relieves pain.

Anaphylactic Shock: An immediate and severe allergic reaction, which results in collapse of an individual and sometimes death.

Anencephaly: Condition in which an infant is born with all or most of the brain missing.

Anemia: A reduction in the size, number, or color of red blood cells that results in reduced oxygen-carrying capacity of the blood.

Anemia Tests: Hemoglobin and hematocrit tests provide information on the final stages of iron deficiency-anemia.

Angina Pectoris: Chest pain after mild to vigorous exercise or excitement, caused by reduced blood supply to the heart from obstruction of the arteries.

Anorexia: The lack or loss of appetite for food, associated with weight loss and muscle wastage.

Anthropometric: Measurements of the body, such as height, weight, and skin fold.

Antibiotic: A substance that inhibits the growth of or destroys microorganisms. Medications used to treat infectious diseases in plants, animals, and humans.

Antibody: A substance in body fluids that is a component of the immune system and protects the body against disease and infection.

Anticoagulant: A substance that slows or prevents blood clotting.

Anticonvulsant: An agent that prevents or relieves convulsions.

Antineuritic: A substance that prevents or treats nervous system disorders.

Antioxidant: A compound that protects other compounds or tissues from free radicals, often oxygen fragments.

Apathy: Showing little feeling or emotion. Indifferent.

Apnea: A pause or cessation in breathing.

Appetite: The desire to eat that normally accompanies hunger.

Arrhythmia: Irregular heart beat.

Arteriosclerosis: A general term for hardening and thickening of the arteries.

Artery: A blood vessel that supplies blood, oxygen, and nutrients to the tissues.

Ascorbic Acid: Vitamin C.

Atherosclerosis: A form of arteriosclerosis, characterized by the accumulation of fat in the artery wall. It is the underlying cause of cardiovascular disease.

Atom: The smallest particle of nature that can exist and still retain the chemical characteristics of an element.

Autism: A condition where the individual is socially withdrawn.

Autoimmunity: A condition where the immune system attacks organs or tissues of the body as if they were foreign invaders.

Avidin: A protein in raw egg white that binds biotin in the small intestine and reduces its absorption.

B Lymphocyte (B Cell): A specialized white blood cell of the immune system that produces antibodies.

Bacteria: Microscopic one-celled organism found in food, the body, and all living matter.

Balanced Diet: A diet that supplies optimal amounts in appropriate ratios to each other of all the known essential nutrients.

Basal Metabolism: Energy used for internal or cellular work, including the heart beat and the repair and maintenance of tissues. Also called basal metabolic rate.

Base: An alkaline substance.

Beriberi: A disease caused by a deficiency of vitamin B1 (thiamin) and characterized by nerve disorders, weakness, mental disturbances, dermatitis, and heart failure.

Beta Carotene: One of several hundred carotenoids and also the building block for vitamin A found in dark green and orange vegetables and fruits.

Beta Cells: Specific cells in the pancreas that produce insulin.

Bile: An emulsifying fluid produced from cholesterol in the liver and stored in the gall bladder to be secreted into the intestine as a digestive aid when fatty food is present.

Biological Activity or Bioavailability: The potency of a vitamin or mineral within the body.

Blood Brain Barrier: A semi-permeable series of barriers that acts as a gatekeeper to monitor and separate the body and its supply of substances and nutrients from the brain.

Branched-Chain Amino Acids (BCAA): The amino acids isoleucine, leucine, and valine that are sometimes used by muscles for energy.

Bronchial Tubes: The two main branches of the trachea leading to the lungs.

Bronchitis: Inflammation of the mucous membranes in the lungs.

Bulimia: An eating disorder characterized by excessive food intake followed by vomiting, laxative use, or fasting.

Calcify: The deposition of calcium into a tissue.

Calorie: A measurement of heat. In nutrition, calorie actually refers to kilocalorie (kcalorie) and signifies the amount of energy contained in food.

Candidiasis: An infection by a fungus called candida. The infection can occur in the lungs, heart, vagina, gastrointestinal tract, skin, nails, or other tissues.

Capillary: A tiny blood vessel that joins arteries and veins. Capillaries are the site in the blood vessel system where oxygen and nutrients are released from the blood into the tissues.

Carbohydrate: The starches and sugars in the diet.

Carbon Dioxide: One of the waste products of cellular metabolism that is carried from the cells by the blood through the veins back to the heart to be exhaled through the lungs.

Carcinogen: A substance that causes cancer.

Cardiomyopathy: Damage to the heart.

Cardiovascular Disease: A disease of the heart and blood vessels often caused by the accumulation of cholesterol in the lining of the blood vessels.

Carpal Tunnel Syndrome (CTS): A disorder caused by a compressed nerve in the hand and resulting in disturbed sensation, pain, and swelling.

Catabolism: The breakdown of complex substances to simple molecules and atoms and the release of energy. For example, glucose is catabolized to water, carbon dioxide, and energy.

Carotene: The building block for vitamin A, called a provitamin, found in dark green and orange vegetables. See beta carotene.

Cataracts: A milky film that forms over the eye and is one of the most common forms of visual loss.

Celiac Disease: An intestinal disorder brought on by a sensitivity to a protein called gliadin, and characterized by diarrhea, weight loss, anemia, and bone pain. Celiac disease requires lifelong diet therapy.

Cell-Mediated Immunity: The aspect of the immune response that occurs in the tissues and includes T lymphocytes and interferon.

Cell Membrane: The outer covering of each cell composed of fats, proteins, and other cell structures.

Cellulose: A plant-derived carbohydrate composed of glucose, which is indigestible to humans.

Cervical Intra-Epithelial Neoplasia (CIN): Precancerous changes to the cells of the cervix.

Cervix: The neck or opening to the uterus.

Chelate: To combine a metal with another compound.

Chemotherapy: The treatment of a disorder with medication; usually refers to cancer therapy.

Chlorophyll: The green color in plants where photosynthesis takes place. Chlorophyll is essential to the formation of carbohydrates in plants.

Cholesterol: A type of fat found in foods from animal origin and produced in the liver. High levels of cholesterol in the blood are associated with an increased risk for cardiovascular disease. Cholesterol, unlike other fats, does not supply calories.

Chronic: Long-term. Cardiovascular disease and diabetes are chronic diseases.

Chronic Fatigue Syndrome (CFS): A persistent condition of decreased activity levels, mood swings, and muscle aches and pains.

Cilia: Hair-like projections that protrude from cell membranes of the lungs and intestine and which move in a rhythmic fashion to propel substances either out of the lungs or along the intestinal tract.

Circadian Rhythm: Cycles that occur approximately every 24 hours in the body.

Cirrhosis: Inflammation or fatty infiltration of the liver, usually as a result of alcohol or drug abuse.

Clinical: Pertaining to the observable signs of a disease.

Cobalamin: Vitamin B12.

Cochlea: A fundamental organ of hearing located within the ear and shaped like a snail shell.

Co-enzyme: A compound required in order for an enzyme to function. Many of the B vitamins are co-enzymes.

Collagen: A protein in connective tissues and the organ substance in teeth and bones.

Colostrum: A thin fluid secreted from the mother's breast for the first few days after birth prior to full lactation.

Complex Carbohydrate: Starches and carbohydrate-like fibers.

Complimentary Protein: Two or more proteins whose amino acid composition complement each other so that the essential amino acids missing from one are supplied by the other. Examples include whole wheat bread and cooked dried beans.

Congestive Heart Failure: A condition where the efficiency of the circulatory system declines as a result of heart failure.

Conjunctivitis: Inflammation of the mucous membrane covering the outer surface of the eye.

Connective Tissue: A web-like tissue located in every organ that binds and supports the various tissues within the organ.

Cornea: The exposed and transparent portion of the eyeball.

Corticosteroid: Steroid hormones secreted by the adrenal glands.

Cretinism: Severe mental retardation of an infant caused by iodine deficiency during pregnancy.

Cystitis: Inflammation of the urinary bladder.

Dehydration: Loss of water from food or the body.

Delaney Clause: A clause in the Food Additive Amendment to the Food, Drug, and Cosmetic Act that states no substance can be added to foods that is known to cause cancer at any dose.

Dermis: A deeper layer of skin (beneath the epidermis) that contains nerves, blood vessels, and glands.

Dementia: Insanity or memory loss.

Dental Pulp: The soft tissue under the calcified enamel and dentin.

Dentin: The calcified tissue below the enamel of teeth that forms the greatest portion of the tooth structure.

Detoxify: To transform a toxic substance in the body into a form more easily excreted.

Diabetes: An hereditary metabolic disease characterized by inadequate supply of the hormone insulin or insensitivity of the cells to insulin's action that results in an inability to maintain normal blood sugar levels.

Diastolic Blood Pressure: The blood pressure in the heart and arteries when the heart relaxes between contractions.

Diuretic: An agent that increases the flow of urine and reduces the amount of water in the body.

Dopamine: A neurotransmitter and intermediate compound in the manufacture of adrenalin.

Dowager's Hump: The hunched appearance common in people with osteoporosis. The posture is further altered by collapse of the chest and protrusion of the abdomen.

Down's Syndrome: A syndrome of congenital defects that includes mental retardation and characteristic physical deformities.

Eclampsia: A disorder that sometimes develops in the later portion of pregnancy and is characterized by high blood pressure, protein in the urine, edema, salt retention, convulsions, and sometimes coma. Also called toxemia, pre-eclampsia, or pregnancy-induced hypertension.

Edema: The abnormal accumulation of water in the tissues.

Electrocardiogram (EKG): A graphic depiction on an electrocardiograph of the electrical impulses corresponding to the heartbeat.

Electrolyte: A substance or salt that dissolves into positive or negative charged particles and conducts an electrical charge. Sodium, potassium, and chloride are examples of electrolytes.

Electrolyte Balance: The distribution of electrolytes (salts) among the body fluids.

Emulsification: To disperse one liquid into a second liquid, such as oil into water.

Emulsifier: A compound that holds an oily substance in suspension in a watery fluid, such as lecithin used in commercial oil and vinegar salad dressings or bile in the digestive tract.

Enamel: The hard, calcified outer layer of the teeth.

Endocrine Glands: Ductless glands that secrete hormones, which in turn have profound effects on the regulation of body processes.

Endorphins: A group of neurotransmitter-like substances that produce a calming effect on the brain much like morphine.

Energy: The ability to do work.

Energy Nutrient: A nutrient that provides energy the body can use. Carbohydrate, protein, and fat.

Enkephalins: A group of neurotransmitter-like substances that have a calming effect on the brain.

Enriched: The addition to processed foods of a few nutrients to bring the level back to the original vitamin or mineral content. Not all nutrients usually are added back in the enrichment process.

Enzyme: Protein-like substances in the body that initiate and accelerate chemical reactions.

Epidermis: The outermost layer of skin.

Epinephrine: Adrenalin. A hormone secreted by the adrenal glands that aids in the release of stored sugar in the liver, contraction of muscles, and increased blood supply to the muscles; all in response to stress.

Epithelial: The internal and external surfaces of the body, including the skin, lining of the blood vessels, and outer surface of the eye.

Epithelial Tissue: The cells of most of the body surfaces, including the skin, eyes, and linings of the lungs, intestinal tract, and urinogenital tract. Examples of endocrine glands include, ovaries, testes, thyroid, and pancreas.

Esophagus: The passageway or tube from the throat to the stomach.

Essential Fatty Acid: A fat that cannot be manufactured by the body, i.e., linoleic acid found in safflower oil.

Essential Nutrient: A substance required by the body in minute amounts for growth, maintenance, and repair and that must be supplied in the diet.

Extracellular: Outside the cells. Extracellular fluid includes the blood, lymph, and fluid between the cells (interstitial fluid).

Extrinsic: From outside the body.

Extrinsic Factor: The name given to vitamin B12.

Fatigue: Feelings of physical or mental weariness, tiredness, or exhaustion.

Fatty Acid: A fat-soluble molecule that consists of a long chain of carbon atoms with hydrogens attached. Three fatty acids combined to a glycerol molecule comprise a triglyceride. Eicosapentaenoic acid (EPA) and linoleic acid are fatty acids.

Ferrous: Iron.

Fiber: The indigestible residue of food, composed of the carbohydrates cellulose, pectin, and hemicellulose, and the noncarbohydrate lignin.

Fibrocystic Breast Disease (FBD): An umbrella term for breast disorders characterized by tender, painful breasts that contain lumps or cysts.

Flatulence: Distension of the stomach or intestine with air or gas.

Folacin: Folic acid.

Follicle: A small cavity that secretes a substance.

Food and Drug Administration (FDA): An agency of the United States government responsible for monitoring the safety and effectiveness of food, drugs, and cosmetics sold in the United States.

Food Guide Pyramid: Outline of recommended amounts and types of foods a diet should include, prepared by the US Department of Agriculture and the US Department of Health and Human Services.

Food Intolerance: Inability to digest a food as a result of individual chemical idiosyncrasies, food contamination, psychological factors, or digestive enzyme deficiencies. Lactose intolerance is a food intolerance resulting from inadequate amounts of the digestive enzyme lactase.

Fortified: The addition of vitamins or minerals to a processed food to levels higher than naturally found. Milk is fortified with vitamin D.

Free Radical: A highly reactive compound derived from air pollution, radiation, cigarette smoke, or the incomplete breakdown of proteins and fats that is associated with tissue damage, disease, and premature aging.

Fructose: A simple sugar or carbohydrate sometimes known as fruit sugar.

Galactose: A simple sugar or carbohydrate. Part of the sugar lactose.

Gangrene: Inadequate blood supply to a tissue that results in the death of that tissue.

Gastritis: Inflammation of the stomach.

Gastrointestinal Tract: The stomach and intestinal tract.

Genetics: The branch of biology that studies heredity and biological variation.

Glaucoma: An eye disease characterized by increasing pressure within the eye and degeneration of the optic nerve.

Glucose: Sugar; blood sugar; the building block of starch.

Glucose Tolerance Factor (GTF): A compound containing chromium that aids the hormone insulin in regulating blood sugar levels.

Glutathione Peroxidase: An antioxidant enzyme.

Glycogen: The storage form of glucose in the body. Glycogen is formed and stored in the liver and muscles and is converted to glucose when energy is needed.

Goiter: Enlargement of the thyroid gland caused by iodine deficiency.

Goitrogen: A substance in food and in some medications that promotes goiter.

Gram: A unit of weight. Twenty-eight grams equal one ounce.

Growth Hormone: A hormone produced in the brain that promotes growth and aids in the regulation of carbohydrates, fat, and protein.

Hard Water: Water with a high calcium and magnesium concentration.

Hematocrit: The volume percent of red blood cells in blood.

Heme Iron: Iron associated with hemoglobin in red blood cells. This form of iron is found in meat, chicken, and fish and is well absorbed.

Hemochromatosis: A condition characterized by abnormal iron deposition in liver and other tissues.

Hemosiderosis: A disorder of iron metabolism where excessive iron is deposited into the liver and other tissues resulting in altered functioning of these tissues.

Hemoglobin: The oxygen-carrying protein in red blood cells. Each molecule of hemoglobin contains four atoms of iron.

Hemolytic: Separation of hemoglobin from the red blood cell as in hemolytic anemia caused by a vitamin E deficiency.

Hemorrhage: Seepage of blood from the blood vessels into the surrounding tissues.

Hepatitis: Inflammation of the liver.

HDL-Cholesterol: Cholesterol packaged in high-density lipoproteins. HDL is comprised of fats and protein and serves as a transport for fats in the blood. A high level of HDL is associated with a reduced risk for developing cardiovascular disease.

Homeostasis: The maintenance of a balanced state in the body regulated by automatic adjustment of physiological processes and feedback mechanisms.

Homocysteine: A by-product of the amino acid methionine.

Homocysteinuria: An inherited disorder characterized by excessive amounts of homocysteine in the urine, mental retardation, and blood clot formation.

Hormone: A substance produced by an organ called an endocrine gland that is released into the blood and transported to another organ or tissue, where it performs a specific action. Examples of hormones include adrenalin and estrogen.

Human Immunodeficiency Virus (HIV): The virus that causes AIDS. See Acquired Immunodeficiency Syndrome.

Human Papillomavirus: The virus that causes genital warts.

Humoral: Immunity and resistance to infection and disease maintained by antibodies produced by B lymphocytes and other cells in the bloodstream.

Huntington's Disease: An inherited disorder of the nervous system characterized by mental retardation and emotional disturbances in adulthood.

Hyperglycemia: High blood sugar levels.

Hyperoxaluria: Excessive accumulation of oxalates in the urine, associated with kidney stone formation.

Hypertension: High blood pressure.

Hypoglycemia: Low blood sugar levels.

Immune System: A complex system of substances and organs that protect the body against disease and infection.

Immunity: The body's resistance to disease provided by a complex system of specialized cells, tissues, organs, and chemicals, such as antibodies and interferon.

Immunosuppressant: Substance that impairs immune system function.

Inborn Errors of Metabolism: Inherited or congenital disorders in how the body metabolizes a substance. For example, phenylketonuria (PKU) is a disorder where the body does not metabolize the amino acid phenylalanine and its toxic metabolites accumulate in the body.

Indoles: A group of compounds in cruciferous vegetables (vegetables in the cabbage family) associated with a reduced risk for developing cancer.

Insomnia: Inability to sleep, to stay asleep, or to fall asleep.

Insulin: A hormone produced by the pancreas that regulates blood sugar levels.

Interferon: A substance in the body formed in response to a virus, or other invading agent, that prevents the virus from multiplying. A component of the cell-mediated immune response.

Intermittent Claudication: Cramps and weakness in the legs induced by walking, relieved by rest, and associated with atherosclerosis.

International Unit (IU): An arbitrary unit of measurement that signifies biological activity used for the fat-soluble vitamins D and E.

Interstitial Fluid: The fluid in the spaces between the cells.

Intracellular: Inside the cell.

Intrinsic: Inside the body.

Intrinsic Factor: A factor manufactured in the stomach that attaches to vitamin B12 and facilitates its absorption in the intestine.

Jaundice: The appearance of bile in the blood, indicating liver disease.

Keratin: A tough form of protein found in skin, hair, nails, and feathers.

Keratinization: The formation of a toughened tissue from overproduction of keratin. A symptom of vitamin A deficiency.

Ketoacidosis: A condition where the body becomes too acidic with accompanying increases in ketones in the blood. Also called ketosis.

Ketogenic Diet: A diet where a large portion of the calories comes from fat, which are converted to ketones in the body. Sometimes used in the treatment of epilepsy.

Ketones: Intermediate products of fat metabolism, acetone, or acetoacetic acid.

Kilocalorie: The amount of heat required to raise 1,000mg of water 1 degree Centigrade. Kilocalorie (kcalorie) and calorie are used interchangeably in nutrition.

Lactation: Breast-feeding.

Lactose: The sugar found in milk.

Lacto-Ovo Vegetarian Diet: A diet that omits meat, chicken, and fish and is derived from fruit, vegetables, whole grain breads and cereals, nuts, seeds, eggs, and dairy products.

Larynx: The organ of the voice located in the throat.

L-Carnitine: An amino acid that transports fats for energy production and might enhance exercise performance.

L-Dopa: A neurotransmitter and intermediate metabolite of adrenalin.

Lean Body Tissue: The muscles and internal organs.

Lecithin: A fatty substance that also contains a water-soluble component containing phosphorus. Lecithin is a constituent of cell membranes, is manufactured in the liver, and is found in food.

Legume: A plant of the bean or pea family having roots that can "fix" nitrogen, thus making these plants a good source of protein. Examples of legumes include dried beans and peas.

Lethargy: Tired, sluggish, lack of energy.

Leukotriene: A group of hormone-like substances involved in inflammation and produced from polyunsaturated fatty acids.

Linoleic Acid: An essential polyunsaturated fatty acid.

Lipid: Fat, including triglycerides, phospholipids, and cholesterol.

Lipoprotein: A compound comprised of fat and protein that carries fats, such as triglycerides and cholesterol, in the blood.

LDL-cholesterol: Low density lipoprotein. A molecule comprised of fats and protein that transports cholesterol in the blood. A high level of LDL is associated with an increased risk for developing cardiovascular disease.

Lymph: The fluid in the lymphatic vessels and lymph sacs. A colorless fluid derived from the blood that is filtered through special vessels and nodes to remove debris and cellular waste products. The filtered lymph is returned to the blood.

Lymphocyte: A specialized white blood cell that is a component of the immune system and aids in the protection of the body against disease and infection. There are B lymphocytes and T lymphocytes.

Lymphoma: Cancer of the lymph tissue.

Macrocytic: Large cell.

Macrophages: A large blood cell involved in the immune response and the body's resistance to infection and disease.

Macula Lutea: The point of clearest vision in the retina.

Macular Degeneration: Disease of the eyes characterized by deterioration of the macula lutea in the retina and a loss of central vision.

Major Mineral: An essential mineral found in the body in amounts greater that 0.0005 percent of body weight.

Mastalgia: Pain of the breasts.

Megadose: Large intake of a nutrient; more than 10 times the RDA for a vitamin or mineral.

Megaloblastic Anemia: Anemia characterized by large, misshapen red blood cells that results from a deficiency of folic acid or vitamin B12.

Melanin: Dark brown to black pigments produced by the eyes, skin, hair, and muscles.

Menstrual: Pertaining to menstruation or the monthly discharge of blood and tissue from the uterus occurring between puberty and menopause.

Menstruation: The monthly discharge of blood and tissue from the uterus.

Metabolism: The total of all body processes, whereby the body converts foods into tissues and breaks down and repairs tissues and converts complex substances into simple ones for energy.

Metabolite: Any product of metabolism.

Metastasis: The migration of a disease from the original site to a distant tissue by way of the bloodstream or lymph system.

Microgram (mcg): A metric unit of weight equivalent to 1/1000th of a milligram or one millionth of a gram.

Microorganism: Minute plants or animals, such as bacteria or viruses, that are visible only through a microscope.

Milligram (mg): A metric unit of weight equivalent to 1/1000th of a gram.

Mineral: An inorganic, fundamental substance found naturally in the soil with specific chemical and structural properties. Many minerals are essential nutrients for growth, maintenance, and repair of tissues.

Minimum Daily Requirements: An outdated system of nutrient requirements based on the minimum amount of nutrient necessary to prevent clinical signs of deficiency.

Molecule: Two or more atoms. The number and type of atoms varies with the compound. Examples of molecules include amino acids, calcium carbonate, the vitamins, carbohydrate, glucose, and fatty acids.

Monoamine Oxidase Inhibitors (MAOI): Antidepressant drug that prolongs the life of stimulating brain chemicals.

Monocytes: A specialized white blood cell important in the immune response.

Monosodium Glutamate (MSG): A food additive that causes a negative reaction in sensitive people.

Monounsaturated Fat: A type of fat that has one spot on the fatty acid for the addition of a hydrogen atom. An example of a monounsaturated fat is oleic acid in olive oil.

Mucus: A substance secreted by epithelial cells composed of carbohydrates called mucopolysaccharides.

Myelin: A sheath surrounding nerve cells that speeds the transmission of nerve impulses.

Myoglobin: An oxygen-storing compound within some cells, especially muscle cells.

Nasal: Pertaining to the nose.

Natural Killer Cell: A lymphocyte of the immune system that destroys cells invaded by bacteria and viruses.

Neural Tube Defect (NTD): A birth defect affecting the spinal cord or brain, including spina bifida and anencephaly.

Neuritis: Inflammation or infection of the nerves.

Neuromuscular: The junction where a nerve cell meets a muscle cell.

Neuropathy: Any non-inflammatory disease of the peripheral (hands and feet) nerves.

Neurotransmitter: A chemical that serves as a communication link between nerve cells or between a nerve cell and a muscle or organ. Serotonin and dopamine are examples of neurotransmitters.

Niacin Equivalent: The unit of measure of the niacin activity in food, computed by adding the amount of niacin preformed in the food plus the amount the body produces from ingested tryptophan.

Night Blindness: A symptom of vitamin A deficiency.

Nitrosamine: A carcinogenic substance found in foods and cigarette smoke and formed in the stomach from nitrites in foods.

Norepinephrine: A neurotransmitter that aids in the regulation of blood pressure and numerous body processes.

Nucleic Acid: A component of deoxyribonucleic acid (DNA) and ribonucleic acid (RNA), the genetic code found in every cell.

Nucleus: The center of each cell that contains the genetic code.

Nutrient: A substance in food that provides the body with energy, helps in the regulation of metabolism, or builds, maintains, or repairs tissues.

Nutrient Density: A relatively high proportion of nutrients for the calories provided.

Nutritious Food: A food that provides a high quantity of one or more essential nutrients, with a small quantity of calories. (See Nutrient Density.)

Obesity: Body fat weight more than 20 percent above ideal body weight.

Opiate: A substance that has a calming effect on the nervous system.

Oral: Pertaining to the mouth.

Orlistat: A compound that reduces the absorption of fat in the intestines.

Organic: A substance that contains carbon.

Ovary: A glandular organ in the female reproductive system that produces the ovum (egg) and secretes the female hormones estrogen and progesterone.

Over-The-Counter Medications (OTC): Nonprescription medications.

Oxalate: Compounds in some plants, such as spinach and chard, that bind to minerals in the intestine and reduce their absorption.

Ozone: A highly reactive modification of oxygen whereby the two atoms in oxygen ($O2$) are increased to three ($O3$).

Palpitation: A fluttering or throbbing of the heart associated with irregular heart beat.

Pancreas: The organ responsible for the production and secretion of numerous digestive enzymes and the hormone insulin.

Parathyroid Gland: A gland in the body that secretes a hormone called parathyroid hormone that regulates calcium metabolism.

Pellagra: A disease caused by a deficiency of niacin and characterized by dermatitis, mental disorders, diarrhea, and weakness.

Periodontal Disease: Diseases of the tissues (periodontium) that surround the teeth.

Pernicious Anemia: A type of macrocytic or megaloblastic anemia caused by a deficiency of vitamin B12 or intrinsic factor necessary for vitamin B12 absorption.

Peroxide: One of a number of highly reactive free radicals.

Petechial Hemorrhages: Minute spots of hemorrhage below the skin, associated with a vitamin C deficiency.

pH: A symbol used to express the hydrogen-ion concentration and therefore the acidity or alkalinity of a substance. A pH below 7 is associated with increasing acidity and a pH above 7 is associated with increasing alkalinity.

Pharmacologic Agent: A substance with drug-like activity.

Phenylethylamine (PEA): A substance in chocolate that might release endorphins in the brain, but also might cause migraine headaches in some people.

Phlegm: A thick fluid secreted by the mucous glands of the air passages. One of the four humors that caused disease described in ancient medicine.

Phospholipid: A fatty substance that has a fat-soluble end and a water-soluble end and that is an essential part of cell membranes.

Phytate: A compound in unleavened whole grains that binds to minerals in the intestine and inhibits their absorption.

Pica: The practice of eating nonfood items, such as dirt or clay.

Placebo: A medicine or pill that has no pharmacologic effect, but is given to please or humor the patient.

Placebo Effect: The healing effect that faith in medicine or supplementation, even inert medicine, often has.

Plaque: An accumulation of fat, calcium, and other substances in the lining of the artery.

Platelets: Blood cell fragments that aid in blood coagulation and wound healing under normal circumstances.

Polycythemia: The presence of excessive amounts of red blood cells in the blood.

Polydipsia: Excessive thirst persisting for long periods of time.

Polyphagia: Excessive hunger persisting for long periods of time.

Polyuria: Excessive urination.

Postmenopausal: After menopause.

Precursor: A substance used as a building block for another substance. Linoleic acid is a precursor for prostaglandins, tryptophan is the precursor for serotonin and niacin.

Premenopausal: Prior to the onset of menopause.

Premenstrual Syndrome (PMS): A combination of physical and emotional symptoms occurring the week or two prior to menstruation.

Primary Deficiency: A nutrient deficiency caused by inadequate dietary intake of a nutrient.

Prostaglandin: A group of hormone-like substances formed from polyunsaturated fatty acids that have a profound effect on the body, including contraction of smooth muscle and dilation or contraction of blood vessels in the regulation of blood pressure.

Protease: An enzyme that breaks down proteins to small fragments during digestion and absorption.

Prothrombin: A protein in blood necessary for normal blood clotting.

Provitamin: A substance in food that can be converted to a vitamin once it enters the body. Beta carotene is the provitamin for vitamin A.

Rapid Eye Movement (REM): Sleep stage with high brain activity.

Rectum: The lower portion of the large intestine extending to the anal canal.

Refined: The process whereby the coarse parts of plants are removed. For example, the refining of whole wheat into white wheat flour involves removing three of the four parts of the kernel: the chaff, the bran, and the germ, leaving only the endosperm or high-carbohydrate inner core.

Regional Ileitis: A chronic inflammation of the small intestine characterized by cramping, abdominal pain, diarrhea, fever, and loss of appetite.

Renal: Pertaining to the kidney.

Replication: To reproduce.

Requirement: The amount of a nutrient that will prevent clinical deficiency symptoms, in contrast to the Recommended Dietary Allowances (i.e., RDAs), which contain an extra allowance.

Respiratory Tract: Pertaining to the lungs and its passageways.

Retina: The layer of light-sensitive cells lining the back of the inside of the eye.

Retinal Pigment Epithelium (RPE): A layer of colored cells in the retina of the eye.

Retinitis Pigmentosa: A hereditary, degenerative disorder of the retina causing night blindness and loss of peripheral vision.

Retinoic Acid: A form of vitamin A.

Retinol: Vitamin A.

Retinol Equivalents (RE): A unit of measurement for vitamin A; one RE is equivalent to 1 mcg or 3.33IU of vitamin A as retinol.

Retinopathy: A disease of the retina of the eye.

Riboflavin: Vitamin B2.

Rickets: Abnormal bone development caused by a deficiency of vitamin D.

Salt: A compound composed of a positive and a negative electrical charge. For example sodium (has a positive charge) and chloride (has a negative charge) comprise table salt.

Saturated Fat: A type of fat that is solid at room temperature and is found in foods from animal sources, hydrogenated vegetable oils, and coconut or palm oil. A diet high in saturated fats is linked to the development of cardiovascular disease.

Sciatica: Pain associated with inflammation of the sciatic nerve often resulting from a damaged spinal disc and characterized by tingling, numbness, and tenderness along the nerve.

Scurvy: A diseased caused by a deficiency of vitamin C and characterized by bleeding gums, loosened teeth, small hemorrhages below the skin, and weakness.

Sebaceous Glands: Glands in the skin that secrete a greasy lubricating substance called sebum.

Sebum: An oily secretion from the sebaceous glands of the skin.

Secondary Deficiency: A nutrient deficiency caused by something other than diet, such as a disease condition that reduces absorption or excessive intake of another nutrient.

Serotonin: A neurotransmitter produced in the brain that regulates mood, sleep, food intake, and pain.

Serum: The fluid portion of blood that is left after the clotting factors have been removed. Serum is a straw colored fluid with red blood cells.

Sinusitis: Inflammation of the sinus.

Skeletal: Relating to the bones.

Soft Water: Water with low calcium and magnesium concentrations.

Spina Bifida: A type of neural tube defect characterized by an exposed spinal cord.

Spleen: The largest lymphatic tissue in the body which is responsible for red blood formation.

Sprue: An intestinal disorder characterized by malabsorption of foods and nutrients.

Steatorrhea: Excessive amount of fat in the stool.

Sterol: A general term for compounds that resemble cholesterol, such as the sex hormones, bile acids, vitamin D, and the adrenal corticosteroid hormones.

Strict Vegetarian Diet: A diet that contains only foods of plant origin, such as whole grain breads and cereals, cooked dried beans and peas, fruits, vegetables, and nuts and seeds. Also called a vegan diet.

Subclinical Deficiency: A nutrient deficiency that does not produce overt physical symptoms.

Sublingual: Beneath the tongue.

Sudden Infant Death Syndrome (SIDS): The unexpected death of an apparently healthy infant that might be caused by respiratory problems.

Superoxide Dismutase (SOD): An antioxidant enzyme.

Superoxides: A group of highly reactive compounds called free radicals.

Synthesize: The process of combining two or more substances into a new compound in the body.

Systolic Blood Pressure: The maximum pressure in the heart and arteries when the heart contracts.

T Lymphocyte (T Cell): A specialized white blood cell of the immune system that attacks bacteria, viruses, and infected cells.

T Helper Cell: A type of T lymphocyte that assists other cells of the immune system.

Tannin: Tannic acid. A yellowish, astringent compound in tea.

Tetany: Intermittent, painful spasms of the muscles.

Therapeutics: The art of healing.

Thiamin: Vitamin B1.

Thromboxane: A prostaglandin that causes constriction of blood vessel walls and encourages platelets to clump at the site of a damaged artery.

Thymus Gland: A gland located in the front, upper portion of the chest.

Thyroid Gland: A major endocrine gland in the body located in the front of the throat and responsible for regulation of metabolism and other endocrine glands and their hormones.

Thyroxin: The hormone of the thyroid gland.

Tocopherol: Vitamin E.

Toxemia: A disorder that sometimes develops in the later portion of pregnancy characterized by high blood pressure, protein in the urine, edema, salt retention, convulsions, or sometimes coma.

Toxicity: The ability of a substance to cause harmful effects.

Trace Mineral: An essential mineral found in the body in amounts less than 0.0005 percent of body weight.

Tricyclics: Antidepressant medication that prolongs the release of stimulating chemicals in the brain.

Triglyceride: One of the three classes of fats. Triglycerides are composed of three fatty acids (tri) and one glycerol (glyceride) molecule. They are either saturated or unsaturated.

Tryptophan: An amino acid essential for life and converted in the body to niacin.

Type A: Personality that is time driven, impatient, and aggressive.

Type B: Personality that is patient, not competitive, and lives life at a slow pace.

Tyramine: A metabolite of the amino acid tyrosine that is found in foods, such as cheese and red wine.

Ubiquinone: A fat-soluble substance involved in the production of energy from carbohydrates. Also called co-enzyme Q.

Ulcer: Damage to epithelial tissues, such as the skin or lining of the stomach or small intestine, characterized by pain and inflammation.

Unsaturated Fat: A type of fat that is liquid at room temperature and is primarily found in foods of plant origin, such as vegetable oils, nuts, and seeds.

Urea: The main nitrogen-containing excretion product of metabolism, generated primarily by the breakdown of amino acids.

Ureters: The tubes that transport fluids from the kidney to the urinary bladder.

Urethra: The canal through which the urine is excreted from the body.

Urinary: Pertaining to urine.

Urticaria: An allergic skin disorder characterized by itching and reddened patches.

USRDA: The RDA figures used on labels. In most cases, the highest RDA suggested in the RDA tables for any age or gender group is used for the USRDA.

Vegan: A strict vegetarian who consumes no foods of animal origin.

Vein: A blood vessel that carries blood, carbon dioxide, and other waste products from the tissues to the heart and lungs.

Virus: Any of a large group of minute particles that are capable of infecting plants, animals, and humans.

Vitamin: An essential nutrient which must be obtained from the diet and is required by the body in minute amounts.

VLDL-cholesterol: Cholesterol carried in the blood by a type of lipoprotein that is made in the liver and is converted to LDL-cholesterol.

Wernicke-Korsakoff Syndrome: A disorder associated with excessive alcohol consumption and characterized by loss of coordination and memory.

Whole Grain: An unrefined grain that retains its edible outside layers (the bran) and the highly nutritious inner germ.

Xerophthalmia: A disease that impairs vision and is caused by a deficiency of vitamin A. This disorder is characterized by a thickening and inflammation of the outer surface of the eye.

Yeast Infection: Vaginal infection caused by an overgrowth of the fungus Candida albicans and characterized by redness, and a thick, white discharge. See Candidiasis.

Index

Acne, 158–59
Acquired immunodeficiency syndrome (AIDS), 160–63
  dietary recommendations, 162–63
  nutrition and, 160–62
  zinc and, 161–62
Acrodermatitis enteropathica, 160
Acute glomerulonephritis, 251
Additives
  carcinogenic, 191
  food allergies, 166–67
  headaches and, 239
  nitrites, 182
Adriamycin, 51
Adult-onset diabetes, 15
Aerobic exercise, 246
Aflatoxin, 190
Aging
  degenerative diseases and, 16
  vitamin C and, 76
  vitamin E and, 34, 39
AIDS. See Acquired immunodeficiency syndrome
Alcohol/alcohol abuse, 9
  cancer and, 182
  effect on vitamin and mineral sta-
    tus, 287–89
  liver disorders and, 257
  nutrient deficiencies and, 13, 15,
    286
    vitamin A, 21
    vitamin B1, 44
    vitamin B2, 47
    vitamin B6 and, 58
    vitamin C and, 78
Alkalosis, 105
Allergies 76, 163–68
  eczema and, 214–15

nutrition and, 166–68
Alliance for Aging Research, 25, 38
Alpha tocopherol, 38
Aluminum, 142–43, 168–69
Alzheimer's disease, 168–70
  aluminum and, 143, 168–69
  choline and, 82, 169–70
  dementia and, 170
  dietary recommendations, 170
  nutrition and, 168–70
  vitamin B1, 169
  vitamin B12 and, 62–63, 169
Amino acids
  essential, 8, 9
  headaches and, 239
  herpes infections and, 241
  insomnia and, 248
  methionine, 143
  tryptophan, 10, 51, 52, 55, 249
  tyramine, 239
  vitamin B6 and, 56
  vitamin B12 and, 62
Amygdalin. See Laetrile
Anaphylactic shock, 47
Anatomical nutrient deficiency stage,
  14
Anemia, 171–74
  copper and, 100, 173
  dietary recommendations, 173–74
  folic acid and, 171
  hemolytic, 36
  in infants, 36
  iron deficiency, 15, 116, 172
  lead and, 144
  macrocytic, 66
  nutrition and, 171–73
  pernicious, 61, 63
  selenium deficiency and, 172–73

435

About the Author

Elizabeth Somer, M.A., R.D. is a registered dietitian and author of several books, including *Nutrition for a Healthy Pregnancy, Food & Mood, Nutrition For Women: The Complete Guide,* and is co-author of *The Nutrition Desk Reference.* For the past 14 years she has served as Editor and Editor in Chief of *Nutrition Report* and *Nutrition Alert!,* newsletters that abstract the current nutrition research from more than 6,000 journals. She currently is Contributing Editor to *Shape Magazine* and has written more than 75 articles in numerous magazines, including *Shape, Redbook, McCall's, Self, Fit Pregnancy, First for Women, Cosmopolitan, Better Homes and Gardens, Living Fit, Food & Wine,* and *Women's Sports and Fitness.* Ms. Somer is a regular guest on AM Northwest (KATU, Channel 2 in Portland, OR) and frequently conducts local and national radio talk shows, television interviews, public presentations, workshops, and seminars on current nutrition research, from women's issues and the food-mood link to the prevention of heart disease and cancer.